Healthy Heart Sourcebook for Women

Heart Diseases & Disorders Sourcebook, 2nd Edition

Household Safety Sourcebook

Immune System Disorders Sourcebook

Infant & Toddler Health Sourcebook

Infectious Diseases Sourcebook

Injury & Trauma Sourcebook

Kidney & Urinary Tract Diseases & Disorders Sourcebook

Learning Disabilities Sourcebook, 2nd Edition

Leukemia Sourcebook

Liver Disorders Sourcebook

Lung Disorders Sourcebook

Medical Tests Sourcebook, 2nd Edition

Men's Health Concerns Sourcebook, 2nd Edition

Mental Health Disorders Sourcebook, 2nd Edition

Mental Retardation Sourcebook

Movement Disorders Sourcebook

Obesity Sourcebook

Osteoporosis Sourcebook

Pain Sourcebook, 2nd Edition

Pediatric Cancer Sourcebook

Physical & Mental Issues in Aging Sourcebook

Podiatry Sourcebook

Pregnancy & Birth Sourcebook, 2nd Edition

Prostate Cancer

Public Health Sourcebook

Reconstructive & Cosmetic Surgery Sourcebook

Rehabilitation Sourcebook

Respiratory Diseases & Disorders Sourcebook

Sexually Transmitted Diseases Sourcebook, 2nd Edition

Skin Disorders Sourcebook

Sleep Disorders Sourcebook

Sports Injuries Sourcebook, 2nd Edition

Stress-Related Disorders Sourcebook

Stroke Sourcebook

Substance Abuse Sourcebook

Surgery Sourcebook

Transplantation Sourcebook

Traveler's Health Sourcebook

Vegetarian Sourcebook

Women's Health Concerns Sourcebook, 2nd Edition

Workplace Health & Safety Sourcebook

Worldwide Health Sourcebook

Teen Health Series

Cancer Information for Teens

Diet Information for Teens

Drug Information for Teens

Fitness Information for Teens

Mental Health Information for Teens

Sexual Health Information for Teens

Skin Health Information for Teens

Sports Injuries Information for Teens

Arthritis
SOURCEBOOK

Second Edition

Health Reference Series

Second Edition

Arthritis
SOURCEBOOK

*Basic Consumer Health Information
about Osteoarthritis, Rheumatoid Arthritis,
Other Rheumatic Disorders, Infectious
Forms of Arthritis, and Diseases with
Symptoms Linked to Arthritis, Featuring
Facts about Diagnosis, Pain Management,
and Surgical Therapies*

*Along with Coping Strategies, Research
Updates, a Glossary, and Resources for
Additional Help and Information*

Edited by
Amy L. Sutton

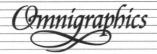

615 Griswold Street • Detroit, MI 48226

Bibliographic Note

Because this page cannot legibly accommodate all the copyright notices, the Bibliographic Note portion of the Preface constitutes an extension of the copyright notice.

Edited by Amy L. Sutton

Health Reference Series

Karen Bellenir, *Managing Editor*
David A. Cooke, M.D., *Medical Consultant*
Elizabeth Barbour, *Permissions Associate*
Dawn Matthews, *Verification Assistant*
Laura Pleva Nielsen, *Index Editor*
EdIndex, Services for Publishers, *Indexers*

* * *

Omnigraphics, Inc.

Matthew P. Barbour, *Senior Vice President*
Kay Gill, *Vice President—Directories*
Kevin Hayes, *Operations Manager*
Leif Gruenberg, *Development Manager*
David P. Bianco, *Marketing Director*

* * *

Peter E. Ruffner, *Publisher*

Frederick G. Ruffner, Jr., *Chairman*

Copyright © 2004 Omnigraphics, Inc.

ISBN 0-7808-0667-0

Library of Congress Cataloging-in-Publication Data

Arthritis sourcebook : basic consumer health information about osteoarthritis, rheumatoid arthritis, other rheumatic disorders, infectious forms of arthritis, and diseases with symptoms linked to arthritis, featuring facts about diagnosis, pain management, and surgical therapies; along with coping strategies, research updates, a glossary, and resources for additional help and information / edited by Amy L. Sutton.
    p. cm. -- (Health reference series)
  Includes index.
  ISBN 0-7808-0667-0 (hard cover : alk. paper)
  1. Arthritis--Popular works. I. Sutton, Amy L. II. Series.
  RC933.A665257 2005
  616.7'22--dc22

                                                              2004010229

Electronic or mechanical reproduction, including photography, recording, or any other information storage and retrieval system for the purpose of resale is strictly prohibited without permission in writing from the publisher.

The information in this publication was compiled from the sources cited and from other sources considered reliable. While every possible effort has been made to ensure reliability, the publisher will not assume liability for damages caused by inaccuracies in the data, and makes no warranty, express or implied, on the accuracy of the information contained herein.

This book is printed on acid-free paper meeting the ANSI Z39.48 Standard. The infinity symbol that appears above indicates that the paper in this book meets that standard.

Printed in the United States

Table of Contents

Visit www.healthreferenceseries.com to view *A Contents Guide to the Health Reference Series*, a listing of more than 10,000 topics and the volumes in which they are covered.

Part II: Forms of Arthritis and Other Rheumatic Disorders

Part III: Disorders with Symptoms Linked to Arthritis

Part IV: Management of Arthritis and Arthritis-Related Pain

Part VI: Additional Help and Information

Preface

About This Book

From 1985 to 2002, the number of Americans with arthritis doubled from 35 million to 70 million. The growing population of aging Americans has pushed arthritis to the forefront as a major public health problem, and today, the Arthritis Foundation estimates that one in three Americans experiences the joint inflammation that characterizes arthritis. In the United States, arthritis is the leading cause of workplace disability, costing the American economy more than $125 billion each year. Although arthritis limits everyday activities for many seniors, it is a disease that also affects children, teens, and young adults.

Despite the prevalence of arthritis, many people hold misconceptions. Arthritis is not just aches and pains associated with aging—instead, it is a condition that can affect individual joints and organs throughout the entire body. Although there is no cure for arthritis, new drugs and treatments, exercise programs, surgical techniques, and self-care strategies have made it possible to reduce the disability and pain associated with many forms of the disorder.

This *Sourcebook* provides basic consumer health information about arthritis and associated conditions that affect the joints, connective tissues, and muscles. Readers will learn essential information about the various forms of arthritis and arthritis pain in specific joints, as well as disorders with symptoms linked to arthritis. In addition, information about the management of arthritis and arthritis-related pain with medications, therapies, and surgery is included. It also offers arthritis patients practical tips for maintaining mobility and independence. A glossary of arthritis-related terms, directories of resources, and suggestions for additional reading help guide people seeking more information.

How to Use This Book

This book is divided into parts and chapters. Parts focus on broad areas of interest. Chapters are devoted to single topics within a part.

Part I: Understanding Arthritis identifies causes, prevalence, symptoms, and risk factors for arthritis and rheumatic diseases. This introductory part also offers information about arthritis research and identifies the characteristics of arthritis pain in specific joints, including the shoulder, elbow, hand, wrist, hip, knee, and foot.

Part II: Forms of Arthritis and Other Rheumatic Disorders describes common forms of arthritis, including osteoarthritis, adult and juvenile rheumatoid arthritis, and less prevalent rheumatic disorders like infectious arthritis, Reiter syndrome, ankylosing spondylitis, polymyalgia rheumatica and giant cell arteritis, and Still disease.

Part III: Disorders with Symptoms Linked to Arthritis identifies health problems that can cause arthritis symptoms, such as bursitis and tendinitis, fibromyalgia, gout and pseudogout, Lyme disease, psoriasis, scleroderma, and systemic lupus erythematosus.

Part IV: Management of Arthritis and Arthritis-Related Pain addresses health-related quality-of-life issues for people with arthritis. It explains medical tests that aid in arthritis diagnosis and discusses noninvasive arthritis pain management techniques, including medications, physical and occupational therapy, and alternative and complementary therapies such as acupuncture and homeopathic remedies. Surgeries for arthritis, including hip replacement, knee replacement, arthroscopy, osteotomy and unicondylar bone replacement, and total joint replacement, are also described.

Part V: Coping with Arthritis includes chapters on how patients with arthritis can seek symptom relief through strategies such as exercise, yoga, and dietary changes. It discusses stress management for arthritis patients and the impact of arthritis on occupational performance, pregnancy, sexuality, and daily tasks. Tips about maintaining independence and mobility are also provided.

Part VI: *Additional Help and Information* offers a glossary of important terms and directories of government agencies and private organizations that provide help and information to arthritis patients. Information about organizations that provide assistance to people disabled by arthritis or taking arthritis medications is also included along with a suggested list of books, magazines, and journal articles for further reading.

Bibliographic Note

This volume contains documents and excerpts from publications issued by the following U.S. government agencies: Agency for Healthcare Research and Quality (AHRQ); Centers for Disease Control and Prevention (CDC); National Center for Complementary and Alternative Medicine (NCCAM); National Institute of Arthritis and Musculoskeletal and Skin Diseases (NIAMS); National Institute of Neurological Disorders and Stroke (NINDS); National Institutes of Health Osteoporosis and Related Bone Diseases–National Resource Center; National Women's Health Information Center (NWHIC); and the U.S. Food and Drug Administration (FDA).

In addition, this volume contains copyrighted documents from the following organizations and individuals: About.com; A.D.A.M., Inc., American Academy of Orthopaedic Surgeons (AAOS); American Association for Clinical Chemistry; American College of Rheumatology (ACR); American Pain Foundation; American Podiatric Medical Association; Arthritis Foundation (AF); Arthritis Research Campaign; Cleveland Clinic Foundation; Colorado State University Cooperative Extension; Cornell University's Program on Employment and Disability; Carol Eustice; Hughston Sports Medicine Foundation; McKesson Health Solutions, LLC; The Myositis Association; National Pain Foundation; National Psoriasis Foundation; National Sleep Foundation; Rheumatology Division of the Hospital for Special Surgery; Spondylitis Association of America; University of Iowa's Virtual Hospital; and *Yoga Journal*.

Full citation information is provided on the first page of each chapter. Every effort has been made to secure all necessary rights to reprint the copyrighted material. If any omissions have been made, please contact Omnigraphics to make corrections for future editions.

Acknowledgements

Thanks go to the many organizations, agencies, and individuals who have contributed materials for this *Sourcebook* and to medical consultant Dr. David Cooke, verification assistant Dawn Matthews, and document engineer Bruce Bellenir. Special thanks go to managing editor Karen Bellenir and permissions specialist Liz Barbour for their help and support.

About the Health Reference Series

The *Health Reference Series* is designed to provide basic medical information for patients, families, caregivers, and the general public. Each volume takes a particular topic and provides comprehensive coverage. This is especially important for people who may be dealing with a newly diagnosed disease or a chronic disorder in themselves or in a family member. People looking for preventive guidance, information about disease warning signs, medical statistics, and risk factors for health problems will also find answers to their questions in the *Health Reference Series*. The *Series*, however, is not intended to serve as a tool for diagnosing illness, in prescribing treatments, or as a substitute for the physician/patient relationship. All people concerned about medical symptoms or the possibility of disease are encouraged to seek professional care from an appropriate health care provider.

Locating Information within the Health Reference Series

The *Health Reference Series* contains a wealth of information about a wide variety of medical topics. Ensuring easy access to all the fact sheets, research reports, in-depth discussions, and other material contained within the individual books of the series remains one of our highest priorities. As the *Series* continues to grow in size and scope, however, locating the precise information needed by a reader may become more challenging.

A *Contents Guide to the Health Reference Series* was developed to direct readers to the specific volumes that address their concerns. It presents an extensive list of diseases, treatments, and other topics of general interest compiled from the Tables of Contents and major index headings. To access *A Contents Guide to the Health Reference Series*, visit www.healthreferenceseries.com.

Medical Consultant

Medical consultation services are provided to the *Health Reference Series* editors by David A. Cooke, M.D. Dr. Cooke is a graduate of

Brandeis University, and he received his M.D. degree from the University of Michigan. He completed residency training at the University of Wisconsin Hospital and Clinics. He is board-certified in Internal Medicine. Dr. Cooke currently works as part of the University of Michigan Health System and practices in Brighton, MI. In his free time, he enjoys writing, science fiction, and spending time with his family.

Our Advisory Board

We would like to thank the following board members for providing guidance to the development of this series:

Dr. Lynda Baker,
Associate Professor of Library and Information Science,
Wayne State University, Detroit, MI

Nancy Bulgarelli,
William Beaumont Hospital Library, Royal Oak, MI

Karen Imarisio,
Bloomfield Township Public Library, Bloomfield Township, MI

Karen Morgan,
Mardigian Library, University of Michigan-Dearborn,
Dearborn, MI

Rosemary Orlando,
St. Clair Shores Public Library, St. Clair Shores, MI

Health Reference Series *Update Policy*

The inaugural book in the *Health Reference Series* was the first edition of *Cancer Sourcebook* published in 1989. Since then, the *Series* has been enthusiastically received by librarians and in the medical community. In order to maintain the standard of providing high-quality health information for the layperson the editorial staff at Omnigraphics felt it was necessary to implement a policy of updating volumes when warranted.

Medical researchers have been making tremendous strides, and it is the purpose of the *Health Reference Series* to stay current with the most recent advances. Each decision to update a volume will be made on an individual basis. Some of the considerations will include how much new information is available and the feedback we receive from people who use the books. If there is a topic you would like to see added to the update list, or an area of medical concern you feel has not been adequately addressed, please write to:

Editor
Health Reference Series
Omnigraphics, Inc.
615 Griswold Street
Detroit, MI 48226
E-mail: editorial@omnigraphics.com

Part One

Understanding Arthritis

Chapter 1

Do I Have Arthritis?

What Is Arthritis?

Many people start to feel pain and stiffness in their bodies over time. Sometimes their hands or knees or hips get sore and are hard to move. These people may have arthritis.

Arthritis is an illness that can cause pain and swelling in your joints. Over time, the joint can become severely damaged. Joints are places where two bones meet, such as your elbow or knee. Some kinds of arthritis can cause problems in other organs, such as your eyes, or in your chest. It can affect your skin, too.

These problems may be caused by inflammation, a swelling that can include pain or redness. They are telling you that something is wrong.

Some people may worry that arthritis means they won't be able to work or take care of their children and their family. Others think that you just have to accept things like arthritis.

It's true that arthritis can be painful. But there are things you can do to feel better. This information tells you some facts about arthritis and gives you some ideas about what to do, so you can keep doing the things you want to do.

There are several kinds of arthritis. The two most common ones are rheumatoid arthritis and osteoarthritis.

National Institute of Arthritis and Musculoskeletal and Skin Diseases (NIAMS), July 2001. Available online at http://www.niams.nih.gov; accessed December 2003.

Osteoarthritis is the most common form of arthritis. This is the form that usually comes with age and most often affects the fingers, knees, and hips. Sometimes osteoarthritis follows an injury to a joint. For example, a young person might hurt his knee badly playing soccer. Then, years after the knee has apparently healed, he might get arthritis in his knee joint.

Rheumatoid arthritis happens when the body's own defense system doesn't work properly. It affects joints, bones, and organs—often the hands and feet. You may feel sick or tired, and you may have a fever.

Other conditions can also cause arthritis. Some include:

- Gout, in which crystals build up in the joints. It usually affects the big toe.

- Lupus, in which the body's defense system can harm the joints, the heart, the skin, the kidneys, and other organs.

- Viral hepatitis, in which an infection of the liver can cause arthritis.

Do I Have Arthritis?

Pain is the way your body tells you that something is wrong. Most kinds of arthritis cause pain in your joints. You might have trouble moving around. Some kinds of arthritis can affect different parts of your body. So, along with the arthritis, you may:

- Have a fever.
- Lose weight.
- Have trouble breathing.
- Get a rash or itch.
- These symptoms may also be signs of other illnesses.

What Can I Do?

Go see a doctor. Many people use herbs or medicines that you can buy without a prescription for pain. You should tell your doctor if you do. Only a doctor can tell if you have arthritis or a related condition and what to do about it. It's important not to wait.

You'll need to tell the doctor how you feel and where you hurt. The doctor will examine you and may take x-rays (pictures) of your bones or joints. The x-rays don't hurt and aren't dangerous. You may also have to give a little blood for tests that will help the doctor decide if you have arthritis and what kind you have.

How Will the Doctor Help?

After the doctor knows what kind of arthritis you have, he or she will talk with you about the best way to treat it. The doctor may give you a prescription for medicine that will help with the pain, stiffness, and inflammation. Health insurance or public assistance may help you pay for the medicine, doctor visits, tests, and x-rays.

How Should I Use Arthritis Medicine?

Before you leave the doctor's office, make sure you ask about the best way to take the medicine the doctor prescribes. For example, you may need to take some medicines with milk, or you may need to eat something just before or after taking them, to make sure they don't upset your stomach.

You should also ask how often to take the medicine or to put cream on the spots that bother you. Creams might make your skin and joints feel better. Sometimes, though, they can make your skin burn or break out in a rash. If this happens, call the doctor.

What If I Still Hurt?

Sometimes you might still have pain after using your medicine. Here are some things to try:

- Take a warm shower.
- Do some gentle stretching exercises.
- Use an ice pack on the sore area.
- Rest the sore joint.

If you still hurt after using your medicine correctly and doing one or more of these things, call your doctor. Another kind of medicine might work better for you. Some people can also benefit from surgery, such as joint replacement.

You Can Feel Better

Arthritis can damage your joints, organs, and skin. There are things you can do to keep the damage from getting worse. They might also make you feel better.

- Try to keep your weight down. Too much weight can make your knees and hips hurt.

- Exercise. Moving all of your joints will help you. The doctor or nurse can show you how to move more easily. Going for a walk every day will help, too.

- Take your medicines when and how you are supposed to. They can help reduce pain and stiffness.

- Try taking a warm shower in the morning.

- See your doctor regularly.

- Seek information that can help you.

Chapter 2

Arthritis Overview

What Is Arthritis?

We can all feel a bit stiff in the morning. From time to time, we may even feel achy or sore. But with arthritis, a person can feel stiff, achy, or sore all the time. Arthritis means joint inflammation and refers to a group of diseases that cause pain, swelling, stiffness, and loss of motion in the joints (places in the body where bones meet like elbows, knees, and hips). Arthritis is often used as a more general term to refer to the more than 100 rheumatic diseases that may affect the joints but can also cause pain, swelling, and stiffness in other supporting structures of the body such as muscles, tendons, ligaments, bones, and internal organs. Throughout this chapter the terms arthritis and rheumatic diseases are sometimes used interchangeably.

The amount of discomfort caused by this disease varies from person to person. Some people can have pain so severe, they have to limit their daily activities. Other people have mild to moderate pain that doesn't limit them much or at all. Sometimes there are periods of time without any pain or discomfort.

Arthritis is a chronic, or lifelong, disease that has no cure. The good news is that many advances have been made in arthritis research. There are medicines and other treatments for the disease. Getting enough rest and exercise, controlling weight, and keeping a good diet

"Arthritis," from the National Woman's Health Information Center (NWHIC), August 2002. Available online at http://www.4woman.gov; accessed December 2003.

can also help ease symptoms. Other treatments include the use of pain relief methods and assistive devices, such as splints or braces. When arthritis is severe, surgery may be needed.

Are There Different Types of Arthritis?

There are over 100 different types of rheumatic diseases. The most common rheumatic diseases are:

Osteoarthritis. Also called degenerative joint disease, this is the most common type of arthritis, which occurs most often in older people. This disease affects cartilage, the tissue that cushions and protects the ends of bones in a joint. With osteoarthritis, the cartilage starts to wear away over time. In extreme cases, the cartilage can completely wear away, leaving nothing to protect the bones in a joint, causing bone-on-bone contact. Bones may also bulge, or stick out at the end of a joint, called a bone spur.

Osteoarthritis causes joint pain and can limit a person's normal range of motion (the ability to freely move and bend a joint). When severe, the joint may lose all movement, causing a person to become disabled. Disability most often happens when the disease affects the spine, knees, and hips.

Rheumatoid arthritis. This is an autoimmune disease in which the body's immune system (the body's way of fighting infection) attacks healthy joints, tissues, and organs. Occurring most often in women of childbearing age (15–44), this disease inflames the lining (or synovium) of joints. It can cause pain, stiffness, swelling, and loss of function in joints. When severe, rheumatoid arthritis can deform, or change, a joint. For example, the joints in a person's finger can become deformed, causing the finger to bend or curve.

Rheumatoid arthritis affects mostly joints of the hands and feet and tends to be symmetrical. This means the disease affects the same joints on both sides of the body (like both hands or both feet) at the same time and with the same symptoms. No other form of arthritis is symmetrical. About two to three times as many women as men have this disease.

Fibromyalgia. This chronic disorder causes pain throughout the tissues that support and move the bones and joints. Pain, stiffness, and localized tender points occur in the muscles and tendons, particularly those of the neck, spine, shoulders, and hips. Fatigue and sleep disturbances may also occur.

Gout. When a person has gout, they have higher than normal levels of uric acid in the blood. The body makes uric acid from many of the foods we eat. Too much uric acid causes deposits, called uric acid crystals, to form in the fluid and lining of the joints. The result is an extremely painful attack of arthritis. The most common joint gout affects is the big toe. This disease is more common in men than in women.

Infectious arthritis. Arthritis can be caused by an infection, either bacterial or viral, such as Lyme disease. When this disease is caused by bacteria, early treatment with antibiotics can ease symptoms and cure the disease.

Reactive arthritis. This is arthritis that develops after a person has an infection in the urinary tract, bowel, or other organs. People who have this disease often have eye problems, skin rashes, and mouth sores.

Psoriatic arthritis. Some people who have psoriasis, a common skin problem that causes scaling and rashes, also have arthritis. This disease often affects the joints at the ends of the fingers and can cause changes in the fingernails and toenails. Sometimes the spine can also be affected.

Systemic lupus erythematosus. Also called lupus or SLE, this is an autoimmune disease. When a person has an autoimmune disease, the immune system attacks itself, killing healthy cells and tissue, rather than doing its job to protect the body from disease and infection. Lupus can inflame and damage a person's joints, skin, kidneys, lungs, blood vessels, heart, and brain. African American women are three times more likely to get lupus than Caucasian women. It is also more common in Hispanic, Asian, and American Indian women.

Ankylosing spondylitis. This disease most often affects the spine, causing pain and stiffness. It can also cause arthritis in the hips, shoulders, and knees. It affects mostly men in their late teenage and early adult years.

Juvenile rheumatoid arthritis. The most common type of arthritis in children, this disease causes pain, stiffness, swelling, and loss of function in the joints. A young person can also have rashes and fevers with this disease.

Polymyalgia rheumatica. Because this disease involves tendons, muscles, ligaments, and tissues around the joint, symptoms often include pain, aching, and morning stiffness in the shoulders, hips, neck, and lower back. It is sometimes the first sign of giant cell arteritis, a disease of the arteries characterized by inflammation, weakness, weight loss, and fever.

Polymyositis. Causing inflammation and weakness in the muscles, this disease can affect the whole body and cause disability.

Psoriatic arthritis. This form of arthritis occurs in some persons with psoriasis, a scaling skin disorder, affecting the joints at the ends of the fingers and toes. It can also cause changes in the fingernails and toenails. Back pain may occur if the spine is involved.

Bursitis. This condition involves inflammation of the bursae, small, fluid-filled sacs that help reduce friction between bones and other moving structures in the joints. The inflammation may result from arthritis in the joint or injury or infection of the bursae. Bursitis produces pain and tenderness and may limit the movement of nearby joints.

Tendinitis. Also called tendonitis, this condition refers to inflammation of tendons (tough cords of tissue that connect muscle to bone) caused by overuse, injury, or a rheumatic condition. Tendinitis produces pain and tenderness and may restrict movement of nearby joints.

What Causes Arthritis?

For many types of arthritic diseases, no cause is known. Researchers are looking at possible causes for many of these diseases. With osteoarthritis, extreme stress on a joint may play a role in how this disease develops. Stress can be caused by weak cartilage (which runs in families) or from repeated injury to the joint. Biological makeup and family history may play a role in gout, rheumatoid arthritis, lupus, ankylosing spondylitis, and some other arthritic diseases.

Researchers are also looking at why some people develop these diseases and others do not. Being overweight and aging appear to increase a person's chances of getting osteoarthritis. And women are more likely than men to get lupus and rheumatoid arthritis.

What Does Arthritis Do to a Person's Joints?

Osteoarthritis and rheumatoid arthritis—the two most common types of rheumatic diseases—affect a person's joints, causing discomfort and pain. The range of motion in a joint can lessen, making it harder for a person to perform daily activities. Sometimes the joint can lose all function (not be able to move).

What Are the Symptoms of Arthritis?

Different types of arthritis have different symptoms. In general, people who have arthritis feel pain and stiffness in the joints. Some other common symptoms of arthritis are:

- Swelling in one or more joints
- Stiffness around the joints that lasts for a least one hour in the early morning
- Joint pain or tenderness that is constant or comes and goes
- Feeling like it's hard to use or move a joint
- Warmth or redness in a joint

Sometimes a person can lose weight, feel weak, and have fevers or joint pain for no reason. See a health care provider if you have any one of these symptoms for longer than two weeks.

How Is Arthritis Diagnosed?

Diagnosing rheumatic diseases can be difficult because some symptoms are common to many different diseases. Your health care provider will first do a complete physical exam, looking for any swelling, redness, warmth, deformity, ease of movement, and tenderness in your joints. Your heart, lungs, eyes, ears, throat and other parts of your body may be examined as well. This is because some types of arthritis can affect your organs. Lab tests may also be ordered and samples of blood, urine, or synovial fluid may be taken. Your doctor may have you also see a rheumatologist, a doctor who specializes in arthritis.

What Are the Treatments for Arthritis?

Treatments for arthritis help to reduce pain and swelling in the joints, keep the joints moving, and keep the disease from getting worse. When you have arthritis, it is important to develop a good relationship with your health care provider. Together, you can develop a treatment plan that will work best for you.
Treatments include:

- Over-the-counter medicines like analgesics (aspirin), other nonsteroidal anti-inflammatory drugs, or NSAIDs (Advil, Motrin, Nuprin), and acetaminophen (Tylenol).

11

- Prescription drugs to relieve pain, such as celecoxib (Celebrex) and rofecoxib (Vioxx).

- Over-the-counter creams and sprays for pain relief.

- Corticosteroids (prednisone, cortisone, Solu-Medrol, hydrocortisone) to decrease inflammation and suppress the immune system (used for rheumatoid arthritis) taken by mouth, injection, or applied as creams to the skin.

- Applying heat or ice to reduce pain and inflammation.

- Daily exercise (without overdoing it) to keep the joints moving and strengthen the muscles around the joints. Rest is also needed for joints affected by arthritis. You will need to find the right type of exercise and the right amount of rest. Your doctor can send you to a physical therapist to help you with an exercise and rest program. Walking and swimming in a heated pool can help arthritis. Stretching and gentle yoga can also help maintain flexibility.

- Controlling or losing weight to reduce stress on joints.

- Hydrotherapy, or exercising (swimming, water aerobics) or relaxing in warm water (baths, hot tubs) to help relax tense muscles and relieve pain.

- Mobilization therapy, including traction (gentle, steady pulling), massage, and manipulation (using the hands to restore normal movement to stiff joints) to help control pain and increase joint motion and flexibility.

- Relaxation therapy, or learning ways to release muscle tension by yourself, such as progressive relaxation where you tighten muscle groups one by one, relaxing tension throughout your body.

- Assistive devices for treating arthritis pain include splints and braces, which are used to support weakened joints or allow them to rest. Some of these devices prevent the joint from moving; others allow some movement.

- Surgery to repair or replace damaged joints. Knees and hips, for example, can be replaced. A new, artificial knee or hip is put in your body to take the place of the damaged joint (in severe cases).

- Nutritional supplements are often reported as helpful in treating rheumatic diseases. These include products such as

S-adenosylmethionine (SAM-e) for osteoarthritis and fibro-myalgia, dehydroepiandrosterone (DHEA) for lupus, and glucosamine and chondroitin sulfate for osteoarthritis. Reports on the safety and effectiveness of these products should be viewed with caution since very few claims have been carefully evaluated.

Be aware that there are many products you can buy that make lots of promises to cure arthritis, but don't. Some of these products, such as snake venom, are even harmful. Although not harmful, other products like copper bracelets don't cure the disease or ease symptoms.

What Research Is Being Done on Arthritis?

Scientists are looking at new ways to treat rheumatoid arthritis. They are experimenting with new drugs and biologic agents that selectively block certain immune system activities associated with inflammation. Newly developed drugs include etanercept (Enbrel) and infliximab (Remicade).

Some genetic and behavioral studies are focusing on factors that may lead to osteoarthritis. Researchers recently found that daughters of women who have knee osteoarthritis have a significant increase in cartilage breakdown, making them more susceptible to disease. This finding has important implications for identifying people who are susceptible to osteoarthritis. Other studies of risk factors for osteoarthritis have identified excessive weight and lack of exercise as contributing factors to knee and hip disability.

Chapter 3

Questions and Answers about Arthritis and Rheumatic Diseases

What Are Rheumatic Diseases and What Is Arthritis?

Rheumatic diseases are characterized by inflammation (signs are redness and/or heat, swelling, and pain) and loss of function of one or more connecting or supporting structures of the body. They especially affect joints, tendons, ligaments, bones, and muscles. Common symptoms are pain, swelling, and stiffness. Some rheumatic diseases can also involve internal organs. There are more than 100 rheumatic diseases.

Many people use the word arthritis to refer to all rheumatic diseases. However, the word literally means joint inflammation. The many different kinds of arthritis comprise just a portion of the rheumatic diseases. Some rheumatic diseases are described as connective tissue diseases because they affect the supporting framework of the body and its internal organs. Others are known as autoimmune diseases because they occur when the immune system, which normally protects the body from infection and disease, harms the body's own healthy tissues. Throughout this chapter the terms arthritis and rheumatic diseases are sometimes used interchangeably.

Examples of Rheumatic Diseases

- **Osteoarthritis**—This is the most common type of arthritis, affecting an estimated 21 million adults in the United States.

Excerpted from the publication by the National Institute of Arthritis and Musculoskeletal and Skin Diseases (NIAMS), February 2002. Available online at http://www.niams.nih.gov; accessed December 2003.

Osteoarthritis primarily affects cartilage, which is the tissue that cushions the ends of bones within the joint. In osteoarthritis, the cartilage begins to fray and may entirely wear away. Osteoarthritis can cause joint pain and stiffness. Disability results most often when the disease affects the spine and the weight-bearing joints (the knees and hips).

- **Rheumatoid arthritis**—This inflammatory disease of the synovium, or lining of the joint, results in pain, stiffness, swelling, joint damage, and loss of function of the joints. Inflammation most often affects joints of the hands and feet and tends to be symmetrical (occurring equally on both sides of the body). This symmetry helps distinguish rheumatoid arthritis from other forms of the disease. About 1 percent of the U.S. population (about 2.1 million people) has rheumatoid arthritis.

- **Juvenile rheumatoid arthritis**—This is the most common form of arthritis in childhood, causing pain, stiffness, swelling, and loss of function of the joints. The arthritis may be associated with rashes or fevers, and may affect various parts of the body.

- **Fibromyalgia**—Fibromyalgia is a chronic disorder that causes pain throughout the tissues that support and move the bones and joints. Pain, stiffness, and localized tender points occur in the muscles and tendons, particularly those of the neck, spine, shoulders, and hips. Patients may also experience fatigue and sleep disturbances.

- **Systemic lupus erythematosus**—Systemic lupus erythematosus (also known as lupus or SLE) is an autoimmune disease in which the immune system harms the body's own healthy cells and tissues. This can result in inflammation of and damage to the joints, skin, kidneys, heart, lungs, blood vessels, and brain.

- **Scleroderma**—Also known as systemic sclerosis, scleroderma means literally hard skin. The disease affects the skin, blood vessels, and joints. It may also affect internal organs, such as the lungs and kidneys. In scleroderma, there is an abnormal and excessive production of collagen (a fiber-like protein) in the skin or internal organs.

- **Spondyloarthropathies**—This group of rheumatic diseases principally affects the spine. One common form—ankylosing spondylitis—not only affects the spine, but may also affect the hips, shoulders, and knees as the tendons and ligaments around the bones and joints become inflamed, resulting in pain and stiffness. Ankylosing spondylitis tends to affect people in late adolescence or early adulthood. Reactive arthritis, sometimes called Reiter syndrome, is another spondyloarthropathy. It develops after an infection involving the lower urinary tract, bowel, or other organ and is commonly associated with eye problems, skin rashes, and mouth sores.

- **Gout**—This type of arthritis results from deposits of needle-like crystals of uric acid in the joints. The crystals cause inflammation, swelling, and pain in the affected joint, which is often the big toe.

- **Infectious arthritis**—This is a general term used to describe forms of arthritis that are caused by infectious agents, such as bacteria or viruses. Parvovirus arthritis and gonococcal arthritis are examples of infectious arthritis. Arthritis symptoms may also occur in Lyme disease, which is caused by a bacterial infection following the bite of certain ticks. In those cases of arthritis caused by bacteria, early diagnosis and treatment with antibiotics are crucial to get rid of the infection and minimize damage to the joints.

- **Polymyalgia rheumatica**—Because this disease involves tendons, muscles, ligaments, and tissues around the joint, symptoms often include pain, aching, and morning stiffness in the shoulders, hips, neck, and lower back. It is sometimes the first sign of giant cell arteritis, a disease of the arteries characterized by inflammation, weakness, weight loss, and fever.

- **Polymyositis**—This is a rheumatic disease that causes inflammation and weakness in the muscles. The disease may affect the whole body and cause disability.

- **Psoriatic arthritis**—This form of arthritis occurs in some patients with psoriasis, a scaling skin disorder. Psoriatic arthritis often affects the joints at the ends of the fingers and toes and is accompanied by changes in the fingernails and toenails. Back pain may occur if the spine is involved.

- **Bursitis**—This condition involves inflammation of the bursae, small, fluid-filled sacs that help reduce friction between bones and other moving structures in the joints. The inflammation may result from arthritis in the joint or injury or infection of

17

the bursae. Bursitis produces pain and tenderness and may limit the movement of nearby joints.

- **Tendinitis (Tendonitis)**—This condition refers to inflammation of tendons (tough cords of tissue that connect muscle to bone) caused by overuse, injury, or a rheumatic condition. Tendinitis produces pain and tenderness and may restrict movement of nearby joints.

What Causes Rheumatic Disease?

Scientists are studying risk factors that increase the likelihood of developing a rheumatic disease. Some of these factors have been identified. For example, in osteoarthritis, inherited cartilage weakness or excessive stress on the joint from repeated injury may play a role. In lupus, rheumatoid arthritis, and scleroderma, the combination of genetic factors that determine susceptibility and environmental triggers are believed to be important. Family history also plays a role in some diseases such as gout and ankylosing spondylitis.

Gender is another factor in some rheumatic diseases. Lupus, rheumatoid arthritis, scleroderma, and fibromyalgia are more common among women. This indicates that hormones or other male-female differences may play a role in the development of these conditions.

Who Is Affected by Arthritis and Rheumatic Conditions?

An estimated 43 million people in the United States have arthritis or other rheumatic conditions. By the year 2020, this number is expected to reach 60 million. Rheumatic diseases are the leading cause of disability among adults age 65 and older.

Rheumatic diseases affect people of all races and ages. Some rheumatic conditions are more common among certain populations. For example:

- Rheumatoid arthritis occurs two to three times more often in women than in men.
- Scleroderma is more common in women than in men.
- Nine out of 10 people who have lupus are women.
- Nine out of 10 people who have fibromyalgia are women.
- Gout is more common in men than in women.

- Lupus is three times more common in African American women than in Caucasian women.

- Ankylosing spondylitis is more common in men than in women.

What Are the Symptoms of Arthritis?

Different types of arthritis have different symptoms. In general, people who have arthritis feel pain and stiffness in the joints. Early diagnosis and treatment help decrease further joint damage and help control symptoms of arthritis and many other rheumatic diseases.

Common Symptoms of Arthritis

- Swelling in one or more joints
- Stiffness around the joints that lasts for at least 1 hour in the early morning
- Constant or recurring pain or tenderness in a joint
- Difficulty using or moving a joint normally
- Warmth and redness in a joint

What Are the Treatments?

Treatments for rheumatic diseases include rest and relaxation, exercise, proper diet, medication, and instruction about the proper use of joints and ways to conserve energy. Other treatments include the use of pain relief methods and assistive devices, such as splints or braces. In severe cases, surgery may be necessary. The doctor and the patient work together to develop a treatment plan that helps the patient maintain or improve his or her lifestyle. Treatment plans usually combine several types of treatment and vary depending on the rheumatic condition and the patient.

Rest, Exercise, and Diet

People who have a rheumatic disease should develop a comfortable balance between rest and activity. One sign of many rheumatic conditions is fatigue. Patients must pay attention to signals from their bodies. For example, when experiencing pain or fatigue, it is important to take a break and rest. Too much rest, however, may cause muscles and joints to become stiff.

People with a rheumatic disease such as arthritis can participate in a variety of sports and exercise programs. Physical exercise can reduce joint pain and stiffness and increase flexibility, muscle strength, and endurance. It also helps with weight reduction and contributes to an improved sense of well-being. Before starting any exercise program, people with arthritis should talk with their doctor. Exercises that doctors often recommend include:

- Range-of-motion exercises (e.g., stretching, dance) to help maintain normal joint movement, maintain or increase flexibility, and relieve stiffness.

- Strengthening exercises (e.g., weight lifting) to maintain or increase muscle strength. Strong muscles help support and protect joints affected by arthritis.

- Aerobic or endurance exercises (e.g., walking, bicycle riding) to improve cardiovascular fitness, help control weight, and improve overall well-being. Studies show that aerobic exercise can also reduce inflammation in some joints.

Another important part of a treatment program is a well-balanced diet. Along with exercise, a well-balanced diet helps people manage their body weight and stay healthy. Weight control is important to people who have arthritis because extra weight puts extra pressure on some joints and can aggravate many types of arthritis. Diet is especially important for people who have gout. People with gout should avoid alcohol and foods that are high in purines, such as organ meats (liver, kidney), sardines, anchovies, and gravy.

Medications

A variety of medications are used to treat rheumatic diseases. The type of medication depends on the rheumatic disease and on the individual patient. The medications used to treat most rheumatic diseases do not provide a cure, but rather limit the symptoms of the disease. Infectious arthritis and gout are exceptions if medications are used properly.

Another example is Lyme disease, caused by the bite of certain ticks, where symptoms of arthritis may be prevented or may disappear if the infection is caught early and treated with antibiotics.

Medications commonly used to treat rheumatic diseases provide relief from pain and inflammation. In some cases, the medication may slow the course of the disease and prevent further damage to joints or other parts of the body.

The doctor may delay using medications until a definite diagnosis is made because medications can hide important symptoms (such as fever and swelling) and thereby interfere with diagnosis. Patients taking any medication, either prescription or over-the-counter, should always follow the doctor's instructions. The doctor should be notified immediately if the medicine is making the symptoms worse or causing other problems, such as an upset stomach, nausea, or headache. The doctor may be able to change the dosage or medicine to reduce these side effects.

Analgesics (pain relievers) such as acetaminophen (Tylenol) and nonsteroidal anti-inflammatory drugs (NSAIDs) such as ibuprofen are used to reduce the pain caused by many rheumatic conditions. NSAIDs have the added benefit of decreasing the inflammation associated with arthritis.

A common side effect of NSAIDs is stomach irritation, which can often be reduced by changing the dosage or medication. New NSAIDs, including celecoxib (Celebrex) and rofecoxib (Vioxx), were introduced to reduce gastrointestinal side effects and offer additional options for treatment. However, even new medications are occasionally associated with reactions ranging from mild to severe, and their long-term effects are still being studied. The dosage will vary depending on the particular illness and the overall health of the patient. The doctor and patient must work together to determine which analgesic to use and the appropriate amount. If analgesics do not ease the pain, the doctor may use other medications. [Brand names included in this chapter are provided as examples only, and their inclusion does not mean that these products are endorsed by the National Institutes of Health or any other Government agency. Also, if a particular brand name is not mentioned, this does not mean or imply that the product is unsatisfactory.]

Depending on the type of arthritis, a person may be asked to take a disease-modifying antirheumatic drug (DMARD). This category includes several unrelated medications that are intended to slow or prevent damage to the joint and thereby prevent disability and discomfort. DMARDs include methotrexate, sulfasalazine, and leflunomide (Arava).

Biological response modifiers are new drugs used for the treatment of rheumatoid arthritis. They can help reduce inflammation and structural damage of the joints by blocking the reaction of a substance called tumor necrosis factor, a protein involved in immune system response. These drugs include etanercept (Enbrel), infliximab (Remicade), and anakinra (Kineret).

21

Corticosteroids, such as prednisone, cortisone, Solu-Medrol, and hydrocortisone, are used to treat many rheumatic conditions because they decrease inflammation and suppress the immune system. The dosage of these medications will vary depending on the diagnosis and the patient. Again, the patient and doctor must work together to determine the right amount of medication.

Corticosteroids can be given by mouth, in creams applied to the skin, or by injection. Short-term side effects of corticosteroids include swelling, increased appetite, weight gain, and emotional ups and downs.

These side effects generally stop when the drug is stopped. It can be dangerous to stop taking corticosteroids suddenly, so it is very important that the doctor and patient work together when changing the corticosteroid dose. Side effects that may occur after long-term use of corticosteroids include stretch marks, excessive hair growth, osteoporosis, high blood pressure, damage to the arteries, high blood sugar, infections, and cataracts.

Hyaluronic acid products like Hyalgan and Synvisc mimic a naturally occurring body substance that lubricates the knee joint. They are usually injected directly into the joint to help provide temporary relief of pain and flexible joint movement.

Devices Used in Treatment

Transcutaneous electrical nerve stimulation (TENS) has been found effective in modifying pain perception. TENS blocks pain messages to the brain with a small device that directs mild electric pulses to nerve endings that lie beneath the painful area of the skin.

A blood-filtering device called the Prosorba Column is used in some health care facilities for filtering out harmful antibodies in people with severe rheumatoid arthritis.

Heat and Cold Therapies

Heat and cold can both be used to reduce the pain and inflammation of arthritis. The patient and doctor can determine which one works best.

Heat therapy increases blood flow, tolerance for pain, and flexibility. Heat therapy can involve treatment with paraffin wax, microwaves, ultrasound, or moist heat. Physical therapists are needed for some of these therapies, such as microwave or ultrasound therapy, but patients can apply moist heat themselves. Some ways to apply moist heat include placing warm towels or hot packs on the inflamed joint or taking a warm bath or shower.

Cold therapy numbs the nerves around the joint (which reduces pain) and may relieve inflammation and muscle spasms. Cold therapy can involve cold packs, ice massage, soaking in cold water, or over-the-counter sprays and ointments that cool the skin and joints.

Capsaicin cream is a preparation put on the skin to relieve joint or muscle pain when only one or two joints are involved.

Hydrotherapy, Mobilization Therapy, and Relaxation Therapy

Hydrotherapy involves exercising or relaxing in warm water. The water takes some weight off painful joints, making it easier to exercise. It helps relax tense muscles and relieve pain.

Mobilization therapies include traction (gentle, steady pulling), massage, and manipulation. (Someone other than the patient moves stiff joints through their normal range of motion.) When done by a trained professional, these methods can help control pain, increase joint motion, and improve muscle and tendon flexibility.

Relaxation therapy helps reduce pain by teaching people various ways to release muscle tension throughout the body. In one method of relaxation therapy, known as progressive relaxation, the patient tightens a muscle group and then slowly releases the tension. Doctors and physical therapists can teach patients a variety of relaxation techniques.

Assistive Devices

The most common assistive devices for treating arthritis pain are splints and braces, which are used to support weakened joints or allow them to rest. Some of these devices prevent the joint from moving; others allow some movement. A splint or brace should be used only when recommended by a doctor or therapist, who will show the patient the correct way to put the device on, ensure that it fits properly, and explain when and for how long it should be worn. The incorrect use of a splint or brace can cause joint damage, stiffness, and pain.

A person with arthritis can use other kinds of devices to ease the pain. For example, the use of a cane when walking can reduce some of the weight placed on a knee or hip affected by arthritis. A shoe insert (orthotic) can ease the pain of walking caused by arthritis of the foot or knee. Other devices can help with activities such as opening jars, closing zippers, and holding pencils.

Surgery

Surgery may be required to repair damage to a joint after injury or to restore function or relieve pain in a joint damaged by arthritis. The doctor may recommend arthroscopic surgery, bone fusion (surgery in which bones in the joint are fused or joined together), or arthroplasty (also known as total joint replacement, in which the damaged joint is removed and replaced with an artificial one).

Nutritional Supplements

Nutritional supplements are often reported as helpful in treating rheumatic diseases. These include products such as S-adenosylmethionine (SAM-e) for osteoarthritis and fibromyalgia, dehydroepiandrosterone (DHEA) for lupus, and glucosamine and chondroitin sulfate for osteoarthritis. Reports on the safety and effectiveness of these products should be viewed with caution since very few claims have been carefully evaluated.

Myths about Treating Arthritis

At this time, the only type of arthritis that can be cured is that caused by infections. Although symptoms of other types of arthritis can be effectively managed with rest, exercise, and medication, there are no cures. Some people claim to have been cured by treatment with herbs, oils, chemicals, special diets, radiation, or other products. However, there is no scientific evidence that such treatments cure arthritis.

Moreover, some may lead to serious side effects. Patients should talk to their doctor before using any therapy that has not been prescribed or recommended by the health care team caring for the patient.

Work with Your Doctor to Limit Your Pain

The role you play in planning your treatment is very important. It is vital for you to have a good relationship with your doctor in order to work together. You should not be afraid to ask questions about your condition or treatment. You must understand the treatment plan and tell the doctor whether it is helping you. Research has shown that patients who are well informed and participate actively in their own care experience less pain and make fewer visits to the doctor.

What Can Be Done to Help?

Studies show that an estimated 18 percent of Americans who have arthritis or other rheumatic conditions believe that their condition limits their activities. People with arthritis may find that they can no longer participate in some of their favorite activities, which can affect their overall well-being. Even when arthritis impairs only one joint, a person may have to change many daily activities to protect that joint from further damage and reduce pain. When arthritis affects the entire body, as it does in people with rheumatoid arthritis or fibromyalgia, many daily activities have to be changed to deal with pain, fatigue, and other symptoms.

Changes in the home may help a person with chronic arthritis continue to live safely, productively, and with less pain. People with arthritis may become weak, lose their balance, or fall. In the bathroom, installing grab bars in the tub or shower and by the toilet, placing a secure seat in the tub, and raising the height of the toilet seat can help. Special kitchen utensils can accommodate hands affected by arthritis to make meal preparation easier. An occupational therapist can help people who have rheumatic conditions identify and make adjustments in their homes to create a safer, more comfortable, and more efficient environment.

Friends and family members can help a patient with a rheumatic condition by learning about that condition and understanding how it affects the patient's life. Friends and family can provide emotional and physical assistance. Their support, as well as support from other people who have the same disease, can make it easier to cope.

What Research Is Being Done on Arthritis?

The National Institute of Arthritis and Musculoskeletal and Skin Diseases (NIAMS), a part of the National Institutes of Health (NIH), leads the federal medical research effort in arthritis and rheumatic diseases. The NIAMS sponsors research and research training on the NIH campus in Bethesda, Maryland, and at universities and medical centers throughout the United States. Research activities include both basic (laboratory) and clinical (involving patients) research studies to better understand what causes these conditions and how best to treat and prevent them.

The NIAMS currently supports three types of research centers that study arthritis, rheumatic diseases, and other musculoskeletal conditions: Multidisciplinary Clinical Research Centers (MCRCs), Specialized Centers of Research (SCORs), and Core Centers. A list of these centers and their locations can be obtained from the Institute.

The MCRCs are programs that focus on clinical research designed to assess and improve outcomes for patients affected by arthritis and other rheumatic diseases, musculoskeletal disorders (including bone and muscle diseases), and skin diseases. Each center studies one or more of the diseases within the NIAMS mission and provides resources for developing clinical projects using more than one approach.

Each SCOR focuses on a single disease. Currently, rheumatoid arthritis, systemic lupus erythematosus, osteoarthritis, osteoporosis, and scleroderma are being studied. Combining laboratory and clinical studies under one roof speeds up research on the causes of these diseases and hastens transfer of advances from the laboratory to the bedside to improve patient care.

Core Centers promote interdisciplinary collaborative efforts among scientists doing high-quality research related to a common theme. By providing funding for facilities, pilot and feasibility studies, and program enrichment activities at the Core Center, the Institute reinforces investigations already underway in NIAMS program areas. Current centers include Rheumatic Diseases Research Core Centers, Skin Disease Research Core Centers, and Core Centers for Musculoskeletal Disorders.

Research registries provide a means for collecting clinical, demographic, and laboratory information from patients and, sometimes, their relatives. These registries facilitate studies that could ultimately lead to improved diagnosis, treatment, and prevention. NIAMS currently supports research registries for rheumatoid arthritis, antiphospholipid syndrome (an autoimmune disorder), ankylosing spondylitis, lupus and neonatal lupus, scleroderma, juvenile rheumatoid arthritis, and juvenile dermatomyositis.

Some current NIAMS research efforts in rheumatic diseases are outlined below.

Biomarkers

Recent scientific breakthroughs in basic research have provided new information about what happens to the body's cells and other structures as rheumatic diseases progress. Biomarkers (laboratory and imaging signposts that detect disease) help researchers determine the likelihood that a person will develop a specific disease and its possible severity and outcome. Biomarkers have the potential to lead to novel and more effective ways to predict and monitor disease activity and responses to treatment. The NIAMS supports research on biomarkers for rheumatic and skin diseases, including a new initiative on osteoarthritis. Additional studies on specific rheumatic diseases follow.

Rheumatoid Arthritis

Researchers are trying to identify the cause of rheumatoid arthritis in order to develop better and more specific treatments. They are examining the role that the endocrine (hormonal), nervous, and immune systems play, and the ways in which these systems interact with environmental and genetic factors in the development of rheumatoid arthritis. Some scientists are trying to determine whether an infectious agent triggers rheumatoid arthritis. Others are studying the role of certain enzymes (specialized proteins in the body that spark biochemical reactions) in breaking down cartilage. Researchers are also trying to identify the genetic factors that place some people at higher risk than others for developing rheumatoid arthritis.

Moreover, scientists are looking at new ways to treat rheumatoid arthritis. They are experimenting with new drugs and biologic agents that selectively block certain immune system activities associated with inflammation. Newly developed drugs include etanercept (Enbrel) and infliximab (Remicade). Followup studies show promise for their effectiveness in slowing disease progression. Studies for additional new drugs continue. Other investigators have shown that minocycline and doxycycline, two antibiotic medications in the tetracycline family, have a modest benefit for people with rheumatoid arthritis. Research continues in this area.

Novel studies using imaging technologies are underway as well. These techniques help identify targets for new drugs by allowing researchers to see changes in cells during the disease process.

Osteoarthritis

The NIAMS has embarked on several innovative approaches to understand the causes and identify effective treatment and prevention methods for osteoarthritis. Through a public/ private partnership, researchers are identifying biomarkers for osteoarthritis to help develop and test new drugs. Imaging studies designed to better identify joint disorders and assess their progression are taking place as well.

The National Center for Complementary and Alternative Medicine and the NIAMS at the National Institutes of Health are currently funding a study on the usefulness of the dietary supplements glucosamine and chondroitin sulfate for osteoarthritis. Previous studies suggest these substances may be effective for reducing pain in knee osteoarthritis. Researchers are also investigating whether they prevent the loss of cartilage.

Some genetic and behavioral studies are focusing on factors that may lead to osteoarthritis. Researchers recently found that daughters of women who have knee osteoarthritis have a significant increase in cartilage breakdown, thus making them more susceptible to disease. This finding has important implications for identifying people who are susceptible to osteoarthritis. Other studies of risk factors for osteoarthritis have identified excessive weight and lack of exercise as contributing factors to knee and hip disability.

Researchers are working to understand what role certain enzymes play in the breakdown of joint cartilage in osteoarthritis and are testing drugs that block the action of these enzymes.

Studies of injuries in young adults show that those who have had a previous joint injury are more likely to develop osteoarthritis. These studies underscore the need for increased education about joint injury prevention and use of proper sports equipment.

Systemic Lupus Erythematosus

Researchers are looking at how genetic, environmental, and hormonal factors influence the development of systemic lupus erythematosus. They are trying to find out why lupus is more common in certain populations, and they have made progress in identifying the genes that may be responsible for lupus. Researchers also continue to study the cellular and molecular basis of autoimmune disorders such as lupus. Promising areas of research on treatment include biologic agents; newer, more selective drugs that suppress the immune system; and bone transplants to correct immune abnormalities. Contrary to the widely held belief that estrogens can make the disease worse, clinical studies are revealing that it may be safe to use estrogens for hormone replacement therapy and birth control in women with lupus.

Scleroderma

Current studies on scleroderma are focusing on overproduction of collagen, blood vessel injury, and abnormal immune system activity.

Researchers hope to discover how these three elements interact to cause and promote scleroderma. In one study, researchers found evidence of fetal cells within the blood and skin lesions of women who had been pregnant years before developing scleroderma. The study suggests that fetal cells may play a role in scleroderma by fostering the maturation of immune cells that promote the overproduction of collagen. Scientists are continuing to study the implications of this finding.

Treatment studies are underway as well. One study in particular is looking at the effectiveness of oral collagen in treating scleroderma.

Fibromyalgia

Scientists are looking at the basic causes of chronic pain and the health status of young women affected by fibromyalgia. The effectiveness of behavior therapy, acupuncture, and some alternative medical approaches for dealing with pain and loss of sleep are being tested. Researchers are also studying whether certain genes contribute to this disease.

Spondyloarthropathies

Researchers are working to understand the genetic and environmental causes of spondyloarthropathies, which include ankylosing spondylitis, psoriatic arthritis, inflammatory bowel disease, and reactive arthritis (Reiter syndrome), as well as related conditions of the eye. They are also looking at new imaging methods that will help with early and accurate diagnosis, guide treatment, and detect responses to treatment. Research on new treatments is also underway.

Where Can People Find More Information about Arthritis and Rheumatic Diseases?

National Institute of Arthritis and Musculoskeletal and Skin Diseases
1 AMS Circle
Bethesda, MD 20892-3675
Toll-Free: (877) 22-NIAMS (226-4267)
Phone: (301) 495-4484
TTY: (301) 565-2966
Fax: (301) 718-6366
Website: http://www.niams.nih.gov
E-mail: niamsinfo@mail.nih.gov

American Academy of Orthopaedic Surgeons (AAOS)
6300 North River Road
Rosemont, IL 60018-4262
Toll-Free: (800) 824-BONE (2663)
Phone: (847) 823-7186
Fax: (847) 823-8125
Website: http://www.aaos.org
E-mail: custserv@aaos.org

American College of Rheumatology
1800 Century Place, Suite 250
Atlanta, GA 30345-4300
Phone: (404) 633-3777
Fax: (404) 633-1870
Website: http://www.rheumatology.org

Arthritis Foundation
1330 West Peachtree Street
Atlanta, GA 30309
Toll-Free: (800) 283-7800
Phone: (404) 872-7100
Website: http://www.arthritis.org

Chapter 4

The Pain of Arthritis

Chapter Contents

Section 4.1

Questions and Answers about Arthritis Pain

National Institute of Arthritis and Musculoskeletal and Skin Diseases
(NIAMS), February 2001. Available online at http://www.niams.nih.gov;
accessed December 2003.

What Is Arthritis?

The word arthritis literally means joint inflammation, but it is often used to refer to a group of more than 100 rheumatic diseases that can cause pain, stiffness, and swelling in the joints. These diseases may affect not only the joints but also other parts of the body, including important supporting structures such as muscles, bones, tendons, and ligaments, as well as some internal organs. This information focuses on pain caused by two of the most common forms of arthritis—osteoarthritis and rheumatoid arthritis.

What Is Pain?

Pain is the body's warning system, alerting you that something is wrong. The International Association for the Study of Pain defines it as an unpleasant experience associated with actual or potential tissue damage to a person's body. Specialized nervous system cells (neurons) that transmit pain signals are found throughout the skin and other body tissues. These cells respond to things such as injury or tissue damage. For example, when a harmful agent such as a sharp knife comes in contact with your skin, chemical signals travel from neurons in the skin through nerves in the spinal cord to your brain, where they are interpreted as pain.

Most forms of arthritis are associated with pain that can be divided into two general categories: acute and chronic. Acute pain is temporary. It can last a few seconds or longer but wanes as healing occurs. Some examples of things that cause acute pain include burns, cuts, and fractures. Chronic pain, such as that seen in people with osteoarthritis and rheumatoid arthritis, ranges from mild to severe and can last weeks, months, and years to a lifetime.

How Many Americans Have Arthritis Pain?

Chronic pain is a major health problem in the United States and is one of the most weakening effects of arthritis. More than 40 million Americans are affected by some form of arthritis, and many have chronic pain that limits daily activity. Osteoarthritis is by far the most common form of arthritis, affecting over 20 million Americans, whereas rheumatoid arthritis, which affects about 2.1 million Americans, is the most disabling form of the disease.

What Causes Arthritis Pain? Why Is It So Variable?

The pain of arthritis may come from different sources. These may include inflammation of the synovial membrane (tissue that lines the joints), the tendons, or the ligaments; muscle strain; and fatigue. A combination of these factors contributes to the intensity of the pain.

The pain of arthritis varies greatly from person to person, for reasons that doctors do not yet understand completely. Factors that contribute to the pain include swelling within the joint, the amount of heat or redness present, or damage that has occurred within the joint. In addition, activities affect pain differently so that some patients note pain in their joints after first getting out of bed in the morning, whereas others develop pain after prolonged use of the joint. Each individual has a different threshold and tolerance for pain, often affected by both physical and emotional factors. These can include depression, anxiety, and even hypersensitivity at the affected sites due to inflammation and tissue injury. This increased sensitivity appears to affect the amount of pain perceived by the individual. Social support networks can make an important contribution to pain management.

How Do Doctors Measure Arthritis Pain?

Pain is a private, unique experience that cannot be seen. The most common way to measure pain is for the doctor to ask you, the patient, about your difficulties. For example, the doctor may ask you to describe the level of pain you feel on a scale of 1 to 10. You may use words like aching, burning, stinging, or throbbing. These words will give the doctor a clearer picture of the pain you are experiencing.

Because doctors rely on your description of pain to help guide treatment, you may want to keep a pain diary to record your pain sensations. You can begin a week or two before your visit to the doctor. On a daily basis, you can describe the situations that cause or alter the intensity of your pain, the sensations and severity of your pain, and your reactions to the pain. For example: "On Monday night, sharp pains in my knees produced by housework interfered with my sleep; on Tuesday morning, because of the pain, I had a hard time getting out bed. However, I coped with the pain by taking my medication and applying ice to my knees." The diary will give the doctor some insight into your pain and may play a critical role in the management of your disease.

What Will Happen When You First Visit a Doctor for Your Arthritis Pain?

The doctor will usually do the following:

- Take your medical history and ask questions such as: How long have you been experiencing pain? How intense is the pain? How often does it occur? What causes it to get worse? What causes it to get better?

- Review the medications you are using.

- Conduct a physical examination to determine causes of pain and how this pain is affecting your ability to function.

- Take blood and/or urine samples and request necessary laboratory work.

- Ask you to get x rays taken or undergo other imaging procedures such as a CAT scan (computerized axial tomography) or MRI (magnetic resonance imaging) to see how much joint damage has been done.

Once the doctor has done these things and reviewed the results of any tests or procedures, he or she will discuss the findings with you and design a comprehensive management approach for the pain caused by your osteoarthritis or rheumatoid arthritis.

Who Can Treat Arthritis Pain?

A number of different specialists may be involved in the care of a patient with arthritis—often a team approach is used. The team may include doctors who treat people with arthritis (rheumatologists), surgeons (orthopaedists), and physical and occupational therapists. Their goal is to treat all aspects of arthritis pain and help you learn to manage your pain. The physician, other health care professionals, and you, the patient, all play an active role in the management of arthritis pain.

How Is Arthritis Pain Treated?

There is no single treatment that applies to everyone with arthritis, but rather the doctor will develop a management plan designed to minimize your specific pain and improve the function of your joints. A number of treatments can provide short-term pain relief.

Short-Term Relief

- **Medications**—Because people with osteoarthritis have very little inflammation, pain relievers such as acetaminophen (Tylenol) [Brand names included in this chapter are provided as examples only and their inclusion does not mean that these products are endorsed by the National Institutes of Health or any other Government agency. Also, if a particular brand name is not mentioned, this does not mean or imply that the product is unsatisfactory.] may be effective. Patients with rheumatoid arthritis generally have pain caused by inflammation and often benefit from aspirin or other nonsteroidal anti-inflammatory drugs (NSAIDs) such as ibuprofen (Motrin or Advil).

- **Heat and cold**—The decision to use either heat or cold for arthritis pain depends on the type of arthritis and should be discussed with your doctor or physical therapist. Moist heat, such as a warm bath or shower, or dry heat, such as a heating pad, placed on the painful area of the joint for about 15 minutes may relieve the pain. An ice pack (or a bag of frozen vegetables) wrapped in a towel and placed on the sore area for about 15 minutes may help to reduce swelling and stop the pain. If you have poor circulation, do not use cold packs.

- **Joint protection**—Using a splint or a brace to allow joints to rest and protect them from injury can be helpful. Your physician or physical therapist can make recommendations.

- **Transcutaneous electrical nerve stimulation (TENS)**—A small TENS device that directs mild electric pulses to nerve endings that lie beneath the skin in the painful area may relieve some arthritis pain. TENS seems to work by blocking pain messages to the brain and by modifying pain perception.

35

- **Massage**—In this pain-relief approach, a massage therapist will lightly stroke and/or knead the painful muscle. This may increase blood flow and bring warmth to a stressed area. However, arthritis-stressed joints are very sensitive, so the therapist must be familiar with the problems of the disease.

Osteoarthritis and rheumatoid arthritis are chronic diseases that may last a lifetime. Learning how to manage your pain over the long term is an important factor in controlling the disease and maintaining a good quality of life. Some sources of long-term pain relief follow.

Long-Term Relief

- **Biological response modifiers**—These new drugs used for the treatment of rheumatoid arthritis reduce inflammation in the joints by blocking the reaction of a substance called tumor necrosis factor, an immune system protein involved in immune system response. These drugs include Enbrel and Remicade.

- **Nonsteroidal anti-inflammatory drugs (NSAIDs)**—These are a class of drugs including aspirin and ibuprofen that are used to reduce pain and inflammation and may be used for both short-term and long-term relief in people with osteoarthritis and rheumatoid arthritis. NSAIDs also include Celebrex and Vioxx, so-called COX-2 inhibitors that block an enzyme known to cause an inflammatory response.

- **Disease-modifying antirheumatic drugs (DMARDs)**— These are drugs used to treat people with rheumatoid arthritis who have not responded to NSAIDs. Some of these include the new drug Arava and methotrexate, hydroxychloroquine, penicillamine, and gold injections. These drugs are thought to influence and correct abnormalities of the immune system responsible for a disease like rheumatoid arthritis. Treatment with these medications requires careful monitoring by the physician to avoid side effects.

- **Corticosteroids**—These are hormones that are very effective in treating arthritis but cause many side effects. Corticosteroids can be taken by mouth or given by injection. Prednisone is the corticosteroid most often given by mouth to reduce the inflammation of rheumatoid arthritis. In both rheumatoid arthritis and osteoarthritis, the doctor also may inject a corticosteroid into the affected joint to stop pain. Because frequent injections may cause damage to the cartilage, they should be done only once or twice a year.

- **Other products**—Hyaluronic acid products like Hyalgan and Synvisc mimic a naturally occurring body substance that lubricates the knee joint and permits flexible joint movement without pain. A blood-filtering device called the Prosorba Column is used in some health care facilities for filtering out harmful antibodies in people with severe rheumatoid arthritis.

- **Weight reduction**—Excess pounds put extra stress on weight-bearing joints such as the knees or hips. Studies have shown that overweight women who lost an average of 11 pounds substantially reduced the development of osteoarthritis in their knees. In addition, if osteoarthritis has already affected one knee, weight reduction will reduce the chance of it occurring in the other knee.

- **Exercise**—Swimming, walking, low-impact aerobic exercise, and range-of-motion exercises may reduce joint pain and stiffness. In addition, stretching exercises are helpful. A physical therapist can help plan an exercise program that will give you the most benefit.

- **Surgery**—In select patients with arthritis, surgery may be necessary. The surgeon may perform an operation to remove the synovium (synovectomy), realign the joint (osteotomy), or in advanced cases replace the damaged joint with an artificial one (arthroplasty). Total joint replacement has provided not only dramatic relief from pain but also improvement in motion for many people with arthritis.

What Alternative Therapies May Relieve Arthritis Pain?

Many people seek other ways of treating their disease, such as special diets or supplements. Although these methods may not be harmful in and of themselves, no research to date shows that they help. Some people have tried acupuncture, in which thin needles are inserted at specific points in the body. Others have tried glucosamine and chondroitin sulfate, two natural substances found in and around cartilage cells, for osteoarthritis of the knee.

Some alternative or complementary approaches may help you to cope with or reduce some of the stress of living with a chronic illness.

It is important to inform your doctor if you are using alternative thera-pies. If the doctor feels the approach has value and will not harm you, it can be incorporated into your treatment plan. However, it is impor-tant not to neglect your regular health care or treatment of serious symptoms.

How Can You Cope with Arthritis Pain?

The long-term goal of pain management is to help you cope with a chronic, often disabling disease. You may be caught in a cycle of pain, depression, and stress. To break out of this cycle, you need to be an active participant with the doctor and other health care professionals in managing your pain. This may include physical therapy, cognitive-behavioral therapy, occupational therapy, biofeedback, relaxation tech-niques (for example, deep breathing and meditation), and family counseling therapy.

Things you can do to manage arthritis pain:

- Eat a healthy diet.

- Get 8 to 10 hours of sleep at night.

- Keep a daily diary of pain and mood changes to share with your physician.

- Choose a caring physician.

- Join a support group.

- Stay informed about new research on managing arthritis pain.

What Research Is Being Conducted on Arthritis Pain?

The NIAMS, part of the National Institutes of Health, is sponsor-ing research that will increase understanding of the specific ways to diagnose, treat, and possibly prevent arthritis pain. As part of its com-mitment to pain research, the Institute joined with many other NIH institutes and offices in 1998 in a special announcement to encour-age more studies on pain.

At the Specialized Center of Research in Osteoarthritis at Rush-Presbyterian-St. Luke's Medical Center in Chicago, Illinois, research-ers are studying the human knee and analyzing how injury in one joint may affect other joints. In addition, they are analyzing the effect of pain and analgesics on gait (walking) and comparing pain and gait before and after surgical treatment for knee osteoarthritis.

At the University of Maryland Pain Center in Baltimore, NIAMS researchers are evaluating the use of acupuncture on patients with osteoarthritis of the knee. Preliminary findings suggest that traditional Chinese acupuncture is both safe and effective as an additional therapy for osteoarthritis, and it significantly reduces pain and improves physical function.

At Duke University in Durham, North Carolina, NIAMS researchers have developed cognitive-behavioral therapy (CBT) involving both patients and their spouses. The goal of CBT for arthritis pain is to help patients cope more effectively with the long-term demands of a chronic and potentially disabling disease. Researchers are studying whether aerobic fitness, coping abilities, and spousal responses to pain behaviors diminish the patient's pain and disability.

NIAMS-supported research on arthritis pain also includes projects in the Institute's Multipurpose Arthritis and Musculoskeletal Diseases Centers. At the University of California at San Francisco, researchers are studying stress factors, including pain, that are associated with rheumatoid arthritis. Findings from this study will be used to develop patient education programs that will improve a person's ability to deal with rheumatoid arthritis and enhance quality of life. At the Indiana University School of Medicine in Indianapolis, health care professionals are looking at the causes of pain and joint disability in patients with osteoarthritis. The goal of the project is to improve doctor-patient communication about pain management and increase patient satisfaction.

The list of pain studies continues. A NIAMS-funded project at Stanford University in California is evaluating the effects of a patient education program that uses a book and videotape to control chronic pain. At Indiana University in Indianapolis, Institute-supported scientists are determining whether strength training can diminish the risk of severe pain from knee osteoarthritis. And a multicenter study funded by the National Center for Complementary and Alternative Medicine and NIAMS, and coordinated by the University of Utah School of Medicine, is investigating the effects of the dietary supplements glucosamine and chondroitin sulfate for knee osteoarthritis.

Section 4.2

Keeping a Pain Diary

This information is reprinted with permission from the American Pain Foundation © 2002 American Pain Foundation. For additional information, call 1-888-615-PAIN (7246), or visit www.painfoundation.org.

You are the only one who knows how much pain you are feeling. When your doctor asks you about the pain, you probably won't remember how hard some days were. You may not remember how bad the pain was. The diary is to help you describe what is happening to you while it is happening. It will be very helpful to your doctor to know when the pain was bad, what made you feel better, and what didn't make you feel better.

Don't worry about how much to write. You don't even have to write sentences. Just write the words that describe how you are feeling. Don't worry if you miss a day. Do it when you can. If thinking about your pain every day is too hard, put the diary away for a few days and go back to it when you are ready. This is your diary. Write when you can for as many days as you can and then stop.

Keep a small notebook or tape recorder with you all day and, during the course of the day, write down what you are feeling. The following questions might help you. Write the date and time every time you write in the diary. If writing is too painful, ask a family member or friend to do it for you or record the diary on a tape recorder.

1. Where does it hurt? List every place that hurts. Does the pain move? Does the pain feel different in different places?

2. How does the pain feel? The following words might be helpful: burning, stabbing, sharp, aching, throbbing, tingling, dull, pounding, or pressing.

3. Did you have pain when you woke up or did it start later?

4. Does the pain change during the day?

5. What, if anything, makes the pain better or worse?

6. What medicines are you taking? Do they help—never, sometimes, always? List all of the medicines your doctor gave you and all of the medicines you bought for yourself at the store.

7. Have you stopped taking any medicines because they made you constipated, sleepy or sick, or for other reasons?

8. Do you do anything to help make the pain go away other than taking medicine such as getting a massage or meditating?

9. Do you have trouble sleeping because of the pain?

10. Does the pain keep you from spending time with family or friends?

11. Do you skip meals because of the pain?

12. How has the pain changed your life?

Section 4.3

An Overview of Arthritis Pain Research

"Pain Research: An Overview," National Institute of Arthritis and Musculoskeletal and Skin Diseases (NIAMS), May 2003. Available online at http://www.niams.nih.gov; accessed March 2004.

About Pain

Throbbing, burning, aching, stinging—the terms patients use to describe pain are often different because pain is personal and subjective and influenced by age, gender, race/ethnicity, and psychosocial factors. The International Association for the Study of Pain defines it as an unpleasant experience associated with actual or potential tissue damage to a person's body.

There are two basic forms of physical pain: acute and chronic. Acute pain, for the most part, results from disease, inflammation, or injury to tissues. It is immediate and usually of a short duration. Acute pain is a normal response to injury and may be accompanied by anxiety or emotional distress. The cause of acute pain can usually be diagnosed and treated.

Chronic pain is continuous pain that persists for more than 3 months, and beyond the time of normal healing. It ranges from mild to severe and can last weeks, months, or years to a lifetime. The cause of chronic pain is not always evident, although it can be brought on by chronic conditions such as arthritis and fibromyalgia. Chronic pain can often interfere with a patient's quality of life, sleep, and productivity.

A Symptom of Many Diseases

Pain often accompanies diseases of the bones, muscles, joints, and skin, which affect millions of Americans. Most of these diseases are chronic and may cause lifelong pain. In certain cases, such as with some rheumatic diseases, the sources of pain may include inflammation of the synovial membrane (tissue that lines the joints), the tendons, or the ligaments; muscle strain; and muscle fatigue. A combination of these factors contributes to the intensity of the pain. Muscle inflammation characterizes other painful disorders such as polymyositis (characterized by inflamed and tender muscles throughout the body, particularly those of the shoulder and hip) and dermatomyositis (characterized by patchy red rashes around the knuckles, eyes, and other parts of the body, along with chronic inflammation of the muscles).

In other cases, such as with myofascial pain syndromes, the cause of the pain is unknown. Myofascial pain syndromes affect sensitive areas known as trigger points, located within the body's muscles. It is important to consult with a physician to help determine the cause and treatment for your pain.

Talking to Your Doctor about Pain

Pain is managed by the patient and his or her health care providers. In order to help assess the cause and treatment for your pain, a doctor will usually do the following:

- Take your medical history.

- Review any medications you are using.

- Conduct a physical examination to determine the causes of pain and how this pain is affecting your ability to function.

- Take blood and/or urine samples and request necessary laboratory work.

- Ask you to have x-rays taken or undergo other imaging procedures such as a CAT (computerized axial tomography) scan or MRI (magnetic resonance imaging).

There is no medical test that can convey the level of pain you are feeling. Only you can describe your pain. In order to provide an accurate description of your pain, it may be helpful to share the answers to the following questions with your doctor:

- How long have you had pain?
- Where is the pain located?
- Does the pain come and go or is it continuous?
- What makes the pain better or worse?
- Has the pain changed since your last visit with your doctor?
- What medications or treatments have you tried for the pain?

After you have been evaluated by your doctor, he or she will discuss the findings with you and design a comprehensive management plan for your pain. There are currently many treatment options available for pain, and scientists believe that research can help lead to more and better treatments for pain in the future.

Research on Pain

Pain research is conducted and funded by the Department of Health and Human Services' National Institutes of Health (NIH) by many of its institutes and centers, including the National Institute of Arthritis and Musculoskeletal and Skin Diseases (NIAMS). Although some of this research on pain is not linked to any disease specifically, certain aspects of pain research are applicable to many diseases.

The research on pain supported by NIAMS covers a broad spectrum from basic research to clinical studies to behavioral interventions. This research is needed to:

- determine the most effective drug and nondrug therapies and interventions, including complementary and alternative treatments
- remove barriers to effective treatment
- identify assessment tools for patients unable to describe their pain

• identify effective pain management strategies for individuals with disabilities and in underserved populations

NIAMS currently supports research on pain conducted by scientists in laboratories on the NIH campus, and through grants and contracts to researchers in universities, research institutions, and medical centers across the United States. This research includes basic and behavioral investigations, such as pain processing mechanisms in the brain and central nervous system; stress response systems and pain; gender and hormonal influences on pain; and coping methods for pain.

Grant and contract applications submitted to NIH go through a two-step peer review process. Applications from researchers are first reviewed by panels of outside experts for their scientific merit. Applications are then reviewed by the Institute's Advisory Council, which assesses the relevance and priority of proposed projects, and makes recommendations on funding particular meritorious applications. This process is used throughout NIH for applications in all diseases and areas of science.

Why Is Basic Research Important to Understanding Pain?

Basic research is work undertaken primarily to acquire new knowledge of the biological, behavioral, and social mechanisms that underlie health and disease. This type of research, which is often conducted using animal models, provides the broad base of knowledge necessary to advance the diagnosis, treatment, and prevention of many diseases. NIAMS supports a wide and diverse body of basic research, since it is hard to know where scientific advances will come from. Progress in one research area provides data for other areas. Similarly, progress in areas supported by other NIH institutes provides valuable information for diseases within the NIAMS mission. That is why it is essential to support basic studies across the research spectrum and to encourage sharing of knowledge from experts in many disciplines.

Why Is Behavioral Research Important to Understanding Pain?

Pain has a profound effect on the quality of human life. Pain can cause disruptions in sleep, eating, mobility, and overall ability to function. Progress is being made in understanding the physiological

44

mechanisms involved in pain. However, understanding individuals' pain experience presents unique scientific challenges. The levels of pain different people experience and their reactions to it vary widely, perhaps due to psychological state, age, gender, social environment, and cultural background, as well as genetic or physiological differences. Thus, the pain experience needs to be examined at all levels of basic and clinical research, including behavioral research, with the goal of developing interventions to manage or prevent pain.

Behavioral and social sciences research include a wide array of disciplines. The field uses such techniques as:

- surveys and questionnaires
- randomized clinical trials
- direct observation
- descriptive methods
- economic analyses
- laboratory and field experiments
- standardized tests
- evaluation

Highlights of Current and Planned Initiatives

NIH Pain Research Consortium. The NIH Pain Research Consortium encourages information sharing and collaborative research efforts across NIH in the field of pain research. Directors of participating NIH Institutes meet to exchange information, propose topics for workshops and conferences, and support program announcements in the field of pain research. These meetings help to provide coordination of pain research across all NIH components, and ensure that results of NIH-sponsored pain research are widely communicated.

Sex and Gender Factors Affecting Women's Health—Specialized Centers of Research (SCORS). In conjunction with the NIH Office of Research on Women's Health and other NIH institutes, NIAMS is co-funding research on the role of sex- and gender-related health effects. As part of this initiative, a multidisciplinary SCOR is devoted to studying the mechanisms of chronic pain, with special focus on sex-related factors that influence pain and painful clinical conditions that show a high prevalence in women. This center will help apply basic knowledge to the study of persistent pain in humans, and ultimately to developing new ways to diagnose and treat these conditions in the general population.

The Management of Chronic Pain—Program Announcement. NIAMS is co-sponsoring an announcement for grants to study management of chronic pain across the lifespan. It has been estimated that 4 out of every 10 people with moderate to severe pain do not get enough relief for chronic pain. The announcement's goal is to encourage research to find effective interventions, effective drug and nondrug treatments, assessment tools, and management strategies for pain.

Information Resources

National Institute of Arthritis and Musculoskeletal and Skin Diseases
National Institutes of Health
1 AMS Circle
Bethesda, MD 20892-3675
Toll-Free: (877) 226-4267
Phone: (301) 495-4484
Fax: (301) 718-6366
Website: http://www.niams.nih.gov

The National Institute of Arthritis and Musculoskeletal and Skin Diseases provides information about rheumatic, bone, muscle, and skin diseases. It distributes patient and professional education materials and refers people to other sources of information. Additional information and updates can also be found on the NIAMS website.

National Institute of Dental and Craniofacial Research
National Institutes of Health
45 Center Drive, MSC 6400
Building 45, Room 4AS-25
Bethesda, MD 20892-6400
Phone: (301) 496-4261
http://www.nidcr.nih.gov

The National Institute of Dental and Craniofacial Research (NIDCR) provides information about craniofacial-oral-dental diseases and disorders. It distributes patient and professional education materials and refers people to other sources of information. Additional information and updates can also be found on the NIDCR website.

National Institute of Neurological Disorders and Stroke
National Institutes of Health
Office of Communications and Public Liaison
P.O. Box 5801
Bethesda, MD 20824
Toll-Free: (800) 352-9424
Phone: (301) 496-5751
Fax: (301) 402-2186
Website: http://www.ninds.nih.gov

The National Institute of Neurological Disorders and Stroke (NINDS) provides information about neurological disorders. It distributes patient and professional education materials and refers people to other sources of information. Additional information and updates can also be found on the NINDS website.

American Chronic Pain Association
P.O. Box 850
Rocklin, CA 95677
Phone: (916) 632-0922
Website: http://www.theacpa.org

This association provides information on positive ways to deal with chronic pain and can provide guidelines on selecting a pain management center.

American Pain Society
4700 West Lake Avenue
Glenview, IL 60025-1485
Phone: (847) 375-4715
Website: http://www.ampainsoc.org

This society provides general information to the public and maintains a directory of resources, including referrals to pain centers.

National Chronic Pain Outreach Association, Inc.
7979 Old Georgetown Road, Suite 100
Bethesda, MD 20814-2429
Phone: (301) 652-4948
Fax: (301) 907-0745
Website: http://neurosurgery.mgh.harvard.edu/ncpainoa.htm

This association operates an information clearinghouse offering publications and cassette tapes for people with pain. It also publishes a newsletter that includes information on pain management techniques, coping strategies, book reviews, and support groups.

National Foundation for the Treatment of Pain
1330 Skyline Drive, Suite #21
Monterey, CA 93940
Phone: (831) 655-8812
Fax: (831) 655-2823
Website: http://www.paincare.org

This organization provides support for patients who are suffering from pain, their families and friends, and the physicians who treat them. They also offer a patient forum, advocacy programs, information, support resources, and direct medical intervention.

Chapter 5

Arthritis Pain in Specific Joints

Chapter Contents

Section 5.1

Arthritis and Chronic Joint Symptoms More Common Than Previously Thought

Centers for Disease Control and Prevention, October 24, 2002. Available online at http://www.cdc.gov; accessed November 2003.

The first state-by-state survey of arthritis and chronic joint symptoms shows that 1 in 3 U.S. adults are affected, the Centers for Disease Control and Prevention (CDC) reported today.

The new data put the number of adults with arthritis and chronic joint symptoms at 70 million (33.0 percent), a substantial increase over the previous estimate that 43 million had arthritis. Researchers said the earlier estimate was probably too low and that arthritis-related questions on the new survey more accurately capture undiagnosed persons with chronic joint symptoms—pain, aching, stiffness, or swelling in or around their joints.

"Arthritis is the number one cause of disability, and the new data confirm that arthritis and chronic joint symptoms are one of our most common public health problems," said CDC Director Dr. Julie L. Gerberding. "CDC is committed to continuing to support the states in finding ways to reduce the arthritis-associated pain and limitations that affect so many Americans."

As part of the CDC's 2001 Behavioral Risk Factor Surveillance System telephone survey, more than 212,000 U.S. adults aged 18 years and older were asked if their doctor had ever told them they had arthritis or if they had chronic joint symptoms during the past 12 months.

The percentages of people reporting arthritis and chronic joint symptoms varied widely among the states: Hawaii had the lowest rate (17.8 percent) and West Virginia had the highest (42.6 percent).

More women than men (37.3 percent and 28.4 percent, respectively) reported having arthritis and chronic joint symptoms, and whites (35.3 percent) and blacks (31.5 percent) were more likely to report them than Hispanics (23.3 percent) and other races or ethnic groups. (27.8). The 33 percent of adults with arthritis and chronic joint

50

symptoms comprised 10.6 percent reporting doctor-diagnosed arthritis, 10.0 percent reporting chronic joint symptoms, and 12.4 percent reporting both.

These data will be invaluable to states in planning health services and arthritis intervention programs, said Dr. Charles Helmick of CDC's arthritis program and coauthor of the study. "Efforts to promote early diagnosis and appropriate clinical and self management are needed to reduce the impact of arthritis."

CDC currently provides funds to 36 health departments to improve the quality of life of people with arthritis through state-based programs and to more broadly disseminate self-management techniques, including appropriate physical activity programs. All 50 states conduct surveillance for arthritis and chronic joint symptoms in odd numbered years.

"These numbers show us that now, more than ever, arthritis is a fact of life," said Dr. John H. Klippel, medical director of the Arthritis Foundation. "The Arthritis Foundation, in partnership with the CDC, is committed to identifying the millions of Americans with arthritis and chronic joint symptoms so that we can help them take control of this chronic condition. Americans must take their joint health seriously, and see a health care provider at the earliest warning signs of arthritis, so that they can continue to enjoy active lives and avoid any future limitations."

Arthritis encompasses more than 100 diseases and conditions that affect joints and other connective tissue.

Section 5.2

Arthritis of the Shoulder

Although most people think of the shoulder as a single joint, there are really two joints in the area of the shoulder. One is located where the collarbone (clavicle) meets the tip of the shoulder bone (acromion). This is called the acromioclavicular or AC joint. The junction of the upper arm bone (humerus) with the shoulder blade (scapula) is called the glenohumeral joint. Both joints may be affected by arthritis.

To provide you with effective treatment, your physician will need to determine which joint is affected and what type of arthritis you have. Three major types of arthritis generally affect the shoulder.

- Osteoarthritis, or wear-and-tear arthritis, is a degenerative condition that destroys the smooth outer covering (articular cartilage) of bone. It usually affects people over 50 years of age and is more common in the AC joint than in the glenohumeral shoulder joint.

- Rheumatoid arthritis is a systemic inflammatory condition of the joint lining. It can affect people of any age and usually affects multiple joints on both sides of the body.

- Posttraumatic arthritis is a form of osteoarthritis that develops after an injury such as a fracture or dislocation of the shoulder. Arthritis can also develop after a rotator cuff tear.

Signs and Symptoms

The most common symptom of arthritis of the shoulder is pain, which is aggravated by activity and progressively worsens. If the glenohumeral shoulder joint is affected, the pain is centered in the back of the shoulder and may intensify with changes in the weather. The pain of arthritis in the AC joint is focused on the front of the shoulder.

Someone with rheumatoid arthritis may have pain in all of these areas if both shoulder joints are affected.

Limited motion is another symptom. It may become more difficult to lift your arm to comb your hair or reach up to a shelf. You may hear a clicking or snapping sound (crepitus) as you move your shoulder.

As the disease progresses, any movement of the shoulder causes pain, night pain is common and sleeping may be difficult.

Diagnosis

A physical examination and x-rays are needed to properly diag nose arthritis of the shoulder. During the physical examination, your physician will look for:

- Weakness (atrophy) in the muscles

- Tenderness to touch

- Extent of passive (assisted) and active (self-directed) range of motion

- Any signs of injury to the muscles, tendons, and ligaments surrounding the joint as well as signs of previous injuries

- Involvement of other joints (an indication of rheumatoid arthritis)

- Crepitus with movement

- Pain when pressure is placed on the joint x-rays of an arthritic shoulder show a narrowing of the joint space, changes in the bone, and the formation of bone spurs (osteophytes). If an injection of a local anesthetic into the joint temporarily relieves the pain, the diagnosis is confirmed.

Treatment

As with other arthritic conditions, initial treatment of arthritis of the shoulder is conservative:

- Rest or change activities to avoid provoking pain; you may need to modify the way you move your arm to do things.

- Take nonsteroidal anti-inflammatory medications such as aspirin or ibuprofen to reduce inflammation.

- Ice the shoulder for 20 to 30 minutes two or three times a day to reduce inflammation and ease pain.

- If you have rheumatoid arthritis, your doctor may prescribe a disease-modifying drug such as methotrexate or recommend a series of corticosteroid injections.

- Dietary supplements such as glucosamine and chondroitin sulfate may be helpful.

If conservative treatment does not reduce pain, there are surgical options. As with all surgeries, there are some risks and possible complications. Your orthopaedic surgeon will do all that is possible to minimize these risks.

Arthritis of the glenohumeral joint can be treated by replacing the entire shoulder joint with a prosthesis (total shoulder arthroplasty) or by replacing the head of the upper arm bone (hemiarthroplasty). The most common surgical procedure used to treat arthritis of the AC joint is a resection arthroplasty. In this procedure, a small piece of bone from the end of the collarbone is removed, leaving a space that later fills with scar tissue. Surgical treatment of arthritis of the shoulder is generally very effective in reducing pain and restoring motion.

Section 5.3

Arthritis of the Flbow

How many times a day do you bend your elbow? Every time you eat or drink, sit at a desk to type or write, point the remote at the TV to change the channel—hundreds of times a day, you bend your elbow without even thinking about it. Now imagine if every time you bent your elbow, you felt the pain of arthritis.

For many Americans, this scenario is all too true. Arthritis of the elbow can cause pain not only when they bend their elbow, but when they straighten it, such as to carry a briefcase. The most common cause of arthritis of the elbow is rheumatoid arthritis (RA). Osteoarthritis (OA or wear-and-tear arthritis) and trauma can also cause arthritis in the elbow joint.

- RA is a disease of the joint linings, or synovia. As the joint lining swells, the joint space narrows. The disease gradually destroys the bones and soft tissues. Usually, RA affects both elbows, as well other joints such as the hand, wrist, and shoulder.

- OA affects the cushioning cartilage on the ends of the bones that enables them to move smoothly in the joint. As the cartilage is destroyed, the bones begin to rub against each other. Loose fragments within the joint may accelerate degeneration.

- Trauma or injury to the elbow can also damage the articular cartilage. This eventually leads to the development of posttraumatic arthritis. Usually, this form of arthritis is confined to the injured joint.

Signs and Symptoms

- Pain. In the early stages of RA, pain may be primarily on the outer (lateral) side of the joint. Pain generally worsens as you turn (rotate) your forearm. The pain of OA may intensify as you extend your arm. Pain that continues during the night or when you are at rest indicates a more advanced stage of OA.

- Swelling, particularly with RA.

- An inability to perform daily activities because the elbow is unstable and gives way.

- Inability to straighten (extend) or bend (flex) the elbow.

- Catching or locking of the elbow, particularly with OA.

- Stiffness, particularly with posttraumatic arthritis.

- Involvement of both elbows or pain at the wrists and/or shoulders as well as the elbows indicates RA.

Diagnosis and Tests

During the physical examination, your physician will look for signs of tenderness and swelling. He or she will also assess your range of motion. The physician may try to recreate the pain by moving the joint. X-rays will show the joint narrowing as well as the presence of any loose bodies. If your pain is due to posttraumatic arthritis, the x-rays may show a malunion or nonunion of bones.

Nonsurgical Treatments

The initial treatment is nonsurgical and depends on the type of arthritis. Your physician will discuss the options with you and develop an individualized program of medical and physical activities. Among the therapies that can be used are:

- Activity modification. OA may be linked to repetitive overuse of the joint, so modifying job or sports activities can be helpful. Intermittent periods of rest can relieve stress on the elbow.

- Medical management. Acetaminophen or ibuprofen can provide short-term pain relief. More potent agents can be prescribed to treat RA. These include antimalarial agents, gold salts, immunosuppressive drugs, and corticosteroids. An injection of a corticosteroid into the joint can often help.

- Physical therapies. Heat or cold applications and gentle exercises may be prescribed. A splint worn at night or one that permits movement as it protects the elbow from stresses may also be helpful. Other assistive devices, such as handle extensions, can be used to maintain daily activities.

Surgical Options

If your arthritis does not respond to the above treatments, you and your physician may discuss surgical options. Because several nerves are near the elbow, a skilled orthopaedic surgeon should be consulted. Surgery usually results in improved pain control and increased range of motion.

The exact procedure will depend on the type of arthritis you have, the stage of the disease, and your own age, expectations, and activity requirements. Some of the options include:

- Arthroscopy. Using pencil-sized instruments and two or three small incisions, the surgeon can remove bone spurs, loose fragments, or a portion of the diseased synovium. This procedure can be used with both RA and OA.

- Synovectomy. The surgeon removes the diseased synovium. Sometimes, a portion of bone is also removed to provide a greater range of motion. This procedure is often used in the early stages of RA.

- Osteotomy. The surgeon removes part of the bone to relieve pressure on the joint. This procedure is often used to treat OA.

- Arthroplasty. The surgeon creates an artificial joint using either an internal prosthesis or an external fixation device. A total joint replacement is usually reserved for patients over 60 years old or patients with RA in advanced stages.

Section 5.4

Arthritis of the Hand

Arthritis can affect any joint in the body, but it is most visible when it strikes the hands and fingers. Each hand has 27 bones plus the two bones of the forearm that help define the wrist. Joints are created whenever two or more bones come together, so there is plenty of potential for arthritic problems in the hand.

Arthritis of the hand can be both painful and disabling. The most common forms of arthritis in the hand are osteoarthritis and rheumatoid arthritis.

Osteoarthritis of the Hand

Osteoarthritis is a degenerative joint disease in which the cushioning cartilage that covers the bone surfaces at joints begins to wear out. It may be caused by simple wear and tear on joints, or it may develop after an injury to a joint. In the hand, osteoarthritis most often develops in three sites:

- at the base of the thumb, where the thumb and wrist come together (the trapeziometacarpal joint)

- at the middle joint of a finger (the proximal interphalangeal or PIP joint)

- at the finger tip (the distal interphalangeal or DIP joint)

Rheumatoid Arthritis of the Hand

Rheumatoid arthritis affects the cells that line and normally lubricate the joints (synovial tissue). It is a systemic condition, which means that it affects multiple joints, usually on both sides of the body. The joint lining (synovium) becomes inflamed and swollen. The swollen tissue may stretch the surrounding ligaments, which are connective tissues that hold bones together, resulting in deformity and instability. The inflammation may also spread to the tendons, which are the connective tissues that link muscles and bones. This can result in tears (ruptures) in the tendons. Rheumatoid arthritis of the hand is most common in the wrist and finger knuckles (the metacarpophalangeal or MP joints).

Signs and Symptoms

Stiffness, swelling, loss of motion, and pain are symptoms common to both osteoarthritis and rheumatoid arthritis in the hand. With osteoarthritis, bony nodules may develop at the middle joints of one or more fingers (Bouchard nodes) and at the fingertip (Heberden nodes). The joints become enlarged and the fingers crooked. In rheumatoid arthritis, some joints may be more swollen than others. There is often a sausage-shaped (fusiform) swelling of the finger. Other symptoms of rheumatoid arthritis of the hand include:

- a soft, lumpy mass over the back of the hand
- a creaking sound (crepitus) during movement
- a shift in the position of the fingers as they drift away from the direction of the thumb
- inflammation of the finger tendons, resulting in a permanent bending (boutonnière) deformity
- a swan-neck deformity caused by hyperextension (swayback) at the middle joint of the finger associated with a bent fingertip

Diagnosis and Treatment

Your doctor will examine you and ask whether you have similar symptoms in other joints. X-rays will show certain characteristics of arthritis, such as a narrowing of the joint space, the formation of cysts or bony outgrowths (osteophytes or nodes), and the development of hard (sclerotic) areas of bone. If your doctor suspects rheumatoid arthritis, he or she may request blood or other lab tests to confirm the diagnosis.

Treatment is designed to relieve pain and restore function. Treatment decisions are based on the type of arthritis you have, its progression, and its impact on your life. Anti-inflammatory medications such as aspirin or ibuprofen may help reduce swelling and relieve pain; prescription medications or steroid (cortisone) injections may be recommended. Your physician may refer you to a physical or occupational therapist because changing the way you do things with your hands may help relieve pain and pressure.

Osteoarthritis Treatments

If you have osteoarthritis, your physician may recommend a period of rest. You may also be advised to wear finger or wrist splints at night and for selected activities. Surgery is usually not advised unless these treatments fail. Several surgical options are available:

- Surgery may be used to drain or remove the cysts associated with the nodes and to remove excess bone growth.

- Joint fusion (stiffening the problem joint) may be used to correct deformities that interfere with functioning or that are cosmetically unacceptable.

- A joint replacement may be advised.

Rheumatoid Arthritis Treatments

If you have rheumatoid arthritis in your hands, medications can help decrease inflammation, relieve pain and retard the progress of the disease. Rest, controlled exercise, and wearing finger or wrist splints may also be part of your treatment program. Several disease-modifying treatments are now available. These include cortisone injections, antimalarial drugs, methotrexate, cyclosporine, gold, and some other drugs that help suppress the body's immune system to reduce the inflammation. Adaptive devices may help you cope with the activities of daily living.

Rheumatoid arthritis often affects the connective tissues (tendons) as well as the joints. The tendons that become inflamed may rupture. If this happens, you may be unable to bend or straighten your fingers or to grip properly. In certain cases, specific preventive surgery may be recommended. Preventive surgery options include removing nodules, releasing pressure on tendons by removing the inflamed tissue, and strengthening the tendons. If a tendon rupture occurs, an orthopaedic hand surgeon may be able to repair it with a tendon transfer or graft. Unfortunately, there is no cure for rheumatoid arthritis. However, surgical procedures can often help correct deformities, relieve pain, and improve function. These options include joint replacements, joint fusion and, in some cases, removing damaged bone.

Section 5.5

Arthritis of the Wrist

Arthritis affects millions of people in the United States. Often, arthritis strikes at the weightbearing joints of the body, such as the knees and the shoulders. But a significant number of people suffer from arthritis in their wrists and hands that make it difficult for them to perform the activities of daily living.

Although there are hundreds of kinds of arthritis, most wrist pain is caused by just two types:

- Osteoarthritis (OA) is a progressive condition that destroys the smooth articular cartilage covering the ends of bones. The bare bones rub against each other, resulting in pain, stiffness, and weakness. OA can develop due to normal wear and tear on the wrist or as a result of a traumatic injury to the forearm, wrist, or ligaments.

- Rheumatoid arthritis (RA) is a systemic inflammatory disease that affects the joint linings and destroys bones, tissues, and joints. Rheumatoid arthritis often starts in smaller joints, like those found in the hand and wrist, and is symmetrical, meaning that it usually affects the same joint on both sides of the body.

Signs and Symptoms

- OA of the wrist joint manifests with swelling, pain, limited motion, and weakness. These symptoms are usually limited to the wrist joint itself.

- RA of the wrist joint usually manifests with swelling, tenderness, limited motion, and decreased grip strength. In addition, hand function may be impaired and there may be pain in the knuckle joints (metacarpophalangeal or MP joints).

61

- Joint swelling may also put pressure on the nerves that travel through the wrist. This can cause a lesion to develop (compression neuropathy) or lead to carpal tunnel syndrome.

Diagnosis and Treatment

Six bones make up the wrist joint: the two bones of the lower arm (the radius and the ulna) and four wrist bones (the carpals). Your physician will use a combination of physical examination, patient history, and tests to diagnose arthritis of the wrist. X-rays can help distinguish among various forms of arthritis. Some, but not all, forms of RA can be confirmed by a laboratory blood test.

In general, early treatment is nonsurgical and designed to help relieve pain and swelling. Several therapies can be used to treat arthritis, including:

- Modifying your activities.

- Immobilizing the wrist for a short time in a splint.

- Taking anti-inflammatory medications such as aspirin or ibuprofen.

- Following a prescribed exercise program.

- Getting a steroid injection into the joint.

Your physician may prescribe other therapies, depending on the type of arthritis you have. For example, additional therapies for patients with rheumatoid arthritis include antimalarial drugs, antimetabolites, gold, immunosuppressive drugs (both nonsteroidal and corticosteroids), and newer genetically engineered medications.

When such conservative methods are no longer effective or if hand function decreases, surgery is an option. The goal of surgery is to relieve pain; depending on the type of surgery, joint function may also be affected. Surgical options include removing the arthritic bones, joint fusion (making the joint solid and preventing any movement at the wrist), and joint replacement. You and your physician should discuss the options and select the one that is best for you.

Section 5.6

Back Pain Caused by Arthritis

"Low Back Pain Fact Sheet," National Institute of Neurological
Disorders and Stroke, July 2003. Available online at http://
www.ninds.nih.gov; accessed March 2004.

If you have lower back pain, you are not alone. Nearly everyone at
some point has back pain that interferes with work, routine daily activities, or recreation. Americans spend at least $50 billion each year
on low back pain, the most common cause of job-related disability and
a leading contributor to missed work. Back pain is the second most
common neurological ailment in the United States—only headache
is more common. Fortunately, most occurrences of low back pain go
away within a few days. Others take much longer to resolve or lead
to more serious conditions.

Acute or short-term low back pain generally lasts from a few days
to a few weeks. Most acute back pain is mechanical in nature—the
result of trauma to the lower back or a disorder such as arthritis. Pain
from trauma may be caused by a sports injury, work around the house
or in the garden, or a sudden jolt such as a car accident or other stress
on spinal bones and tissues. Symptoms may range from muscle ache
to shooting or stabbing pain, limited flexibility and/or range of motion, or an inability to stand straight. Occasionally, pain felt in one
part of the body may radiate from a disorder or injury elsewhere in
the body. Some acute pain syndromes can become more serious if left
untreated.

Chronic back pain is measured by duration—pain that persists for
more than 3 months is considered chronic. It is often progressive and
the cause can be difficult to determine.

What Structures Make up the Back?

The back is an intricate structure of bones, muscles, and other tissues that form the posterior part of the body's trunk, from the neck
to the pelvis. The centerpiece is the spinal column, which not only
supports the upper body's weight but houses and protects the spinal

cord—the delicate nervous system structure that carries signals that control the body's movements and convey its sensations. Stacked on top of one another are more than 30 bones—the vertebrae—that form the spinal column, also known as the spine. Each of these bones contains a roundish hole that, when stacked in register with all the others, creates a channel that surrounds the spinal cord. The spinal cord descends from the base of the brain and extends in the adult to just below the rib cage. Small nerves (roots) enter and emerge from the spinal cord through spaces between the vertebrae. Because the bones of the spinal column continue growing long after the spinal cord reaches its full length in early childhood, the nerve roots to the lower back and legs extend many inches down the spinal column before exiting. This large bundle of nerve roots was dubbed by early anatomists as the cauda equina, or horse's tail. The spaces between the vertebrae are maintained by round, spongy pads of cartilage called intervertebral disks that allow for flexibility in the lower back and act much like shock absorbers throughout the spinal column to cushion the bones as the body moves. Bands of tissue known as ligaments and tendons hold the vertebrae in place and attach the muscles to the spinal column.

Starting at the top, the spine has four regions:

- the seven cervical or neck vertebrae (labeled C1–C7),
- the 12 thoracic or upper back vertebrae (labeled T1–T12),
- the five lumbar vertebrae (labeled L1–L5), which we know as the lower back, and
- the sacrum and coccyx, a group of bones fused together at the base of the spine.

The lumbar region of the back, where most back pain is felt, supports the weight of the upper body.

What Causes Lower Back Pain?

As people age, bone strength and muscle elasticity and tone tend to decrease. The disks begin to lose fluid and flexibility, which decreases their ability to cushion the vertebrae.

Pain can occur when, for example, someone lifts something too heavy or overstretches, causing a sprain, strain, or spasm in one of the muscles or ligaments in the back. If the spine becomes overly strained or compressed, a disk may rupture or bulge outward. This rupture may put pressure on one of the more than 50 nerves rooted to the spinal cord that control body movements and transmit signals from the body to the brain. When these nerve roots become compressed or irritated, back pain results.

Low back pain may reflect nerve or muscle irritation or bone lesions. Most low back pain follows injury or trauma to the back, but pain may also be caused by degenerative conditions such as arthritis or disk disease, osteoporosis or other bone diseases, viral infections, irritation to joints and disks, or congenital abnormalities in the spine. Obesity, smoking, weight gain during pregnancy, stress, poor physical condition, posture inappropriate for the activity being performed, and poor sleeping position also may contribute to low back pain. Additionally, scar tissue created when the injured back heals itself does not have the strength or flexibility of normal tissue. Buildup of scar tissue from repeated injuries eventually weakens the back and can lead to more serious injury.

Occasionally, low back pain may indicate a more serious medical problem. Pain accompanied by fever or loss of bowel or bladder control, pain when coughing, and progressive weakness in the legs may indicate a pinched nerve or other serious condition. People with diabetes may have severe back pain or pain radiating down the leg related to neuropathy. People with these symptoms should contact a doctor immediately to help prevent permanent damage.

Who Is Most Likely to Develop Low Back Pain?

Nearly everyone has low back pain some time. Men and women are equally affected. It occurs most often between ages 30 and 50, due in part to the aging process but also as a result of sedentary lifestyles with too little (sometimes punctuated by too much) exercise. The risk of experiencing low back pain from disk disease or spinal degeneration increases with age.

What Conditions Are Associated with Low Back Pain?

Conditions that may cause low back pain and require treatment by a physician or other health specialist include:

Bulging disk (also called protruding, herniated, or ruptured disk). The intervertebral disks are under constant pressure. As disks degenerate and weaken, cartilage can bulge or be pushed into the space containing the spinal cord or a nerve root, causing pain. Studies have shown that most herniated disks occur in the lower, lumbar portion of the spinal column.

Cauda equina syndrome. A much more serious complication of a ruptured disk is cauda equina syndrome, which occurs when disk material is pushed into the spinal canal and compresses the bundle of lumbar and sacral nerve roots. Permanent neurological damage may result if this syndrome is left untreated.

Sciatica is a condition in which a herniated or ruptured disk presses on the sciatic nerve, the large nerve that extends down the spinal column to its exit point in the pelvis and carries nerve fibers to the leg. This compression causes shock-like or burning low back pain combined with pain through the buttocks and down one leg to below the knee, occasionally reaching the foot. In the most extreme cases, when the nerve is pinched between the disk and an adjacent bone, the symptoms involve not pain but numbness and some loss of motor control over the leg due to interruption of nerve signaling. The condition may also be caused by a tumor, cyst, metastatic disease, or degeneration of the sciatic nerve root.

Spinal degeneration from disk wear and tear can lead to a narrowing of the spinal canal. A person with spinal degeneration may experience stiffness in the back upon awakening or may feel pain after walking or standing for a long time.

Spinal stenosis related to congenital narrowing of the bony canal predisposes some people to pain related to disk disease.

Osteoporosis is a metabolic bone disease marked by progressive decrease in bone density and strength. Fracture of brittle, porous bones in the spine and hips results when the body fails to produce new bone and/or absorbs too much existing bone. Women are four times more likely than men to develop osteoporosis. Caucasian women of northern European heritage are at the highest risk of developing the condition.

Skeletal irregularities produce strain on the vertebrae and supporting muscles, tendons, ligaments, and tissues supported by spinal column. These irregularities include scoliosis, a curving of the spine to the side; kyphosis, in which the normal curve of the upper back is severely rounded; lordosis, an abnormally accentuated arch in the lower back; back extension, a bending backward of the spine; and back flexion, in which the spine bends forward.

Fibromyalgia is a chronic disorder characterized by widespread musculoskeletal pain, fatigue, and multiple tender points, particularly in the neck, spine, shoulders, and hips. Additional symptoms may include sleep disturbances, morning stiffness, and anxiety.

Spondylitis refers to chronic back pain and stiffness caused by a severe infection to or inflammation of the spinal joints. Other painful inflammations in the lower back include osteomyelitis (infection in the bones of the spine) and sacroiliitis (inflammation in the sacroiliac joints).

How Is Back Pain Treated?

Most low back pain can be treated without surgery. Treatment involves using analgesics, reducing inflammation, restoring proper function and strength to the back, and preventing recurrence of the injury. Most patients with back pain recover without residual functional loss. Patients should contact a doctor if there is not a noticeable reduction in pain and inflammation after 72 hours of self-care.

Quick Tips to a Healthier Back

Following any period of prolonged inactivity, begin a program of regular low-impact exercises. Speed walking, swimming, or stationary bike riding 30 minutes a day can increase muscle strength and flexibility. Yoga can also help stretch and strengthen muscles and improve posture. Ask your physician or orthopaedist for a list of low-impact exercises appropriate for your age and designed to strengthen lower back and abdominal muscles.

- Always stretch before exercise or other strenuous physical activity.

- Don't slouch when standing or sitting. When standing, keep your weight balanced on your feet. Your back supports weight most easily when curvature is reduced.

- At home or work, make sure your work surface is at a comfortable height for you.

- Sit in a chair with good lumbar support and proper position and height for the task. Keep your shoulders back. Switch sitting positions often and periodically walk around the office or gently stretch muscles to relieve tension. A pillow or rolled-up towel placed behind the small of your back can provide some lumbar support. If you must sit for a long period of time, rest your feet on a low stool or a stack of books.

- Wear comfortable, low-heeled shoes.

- Sleep on your side to reduce any curve in your spine. Always sleep on a firm surface.

- Ask for help when transferring an ill or injured family member from a reclining to a sitting position or when moving the patient from a chair to a bed.

- Don't try to lift objects too heavy for you. Lift with your knees, pull in your stomach muscles, and keep your head down and in line with your straight back. Keep the object close to your body. Do not twist when lifting.

- Maintain proper nutrition and diet to reduce and prevent excessive weight, especially weight around the waistline that taxes lower back muscles. A diet with sufficient daily intake of calcium, phosphorus, and vitamin D helps to promote new bone growth.

- If you smoke, quit. Smoking reduces blood flow to the lower spine and causes the spinal disks to degenerate.

Section 5.7

Arthritis of the Hip

Arthritis literally means inflammation of a joint. In some forms of arthritis, such as osteoarthritis, the inflammation arises because the smooth covering (articular cartilage) on the ends of bones wears away. In other forms of arthritis, such as rheumatoid arthritis, the joint lining becomes inflamed as part of a systemic disease. These diseases are considered the inflammatory arthritides.

The three most common types of inflammatory arthritis that affect the hip are:

- Rheumatoid arthritis (RA): RA is a systemic disease of the immune system that usually affects multiple joints on both sides of the body at the same time.

- Ankylosing spondylitis (AS): AS is a chronic inflammation of the spine and the sacroiliac joint (the point where the spine meets the pelvic bone) that can also cause inflammation in other joints.

- Systemic lupus erythematosus (SLE or lupus): SLE is an autoimmune disease in which the body harms its own healthy cells and tissues.

Signs and Symptoms

The classic sign of arthritis is joint pain. Inflammatory arthritis of the hip is characterized by a dull, aching pain in the groin, outer thigh, or buttocks. Pain is usually worse in the morning and lessens with activity; however, vigorous activity can result in increased pain and stiffness. The pain may limit your movements or make walking difficult.

Diagnostic Tests

During the physical examination, your physician may ask you to move your hip in various ways to see which motions are restricted or painful. Your physician will want to know if you walk with a limp, if one or both hips are painful, and if you experience pain in any other joints. X-rays and laboratory studies will be needed. The x-rays will show if there is any thinning or erosion in the bones, any loss of joint space, or any excess fluid in the joint. Laboratory studies will show whether a rheumatoid factor or other antibodies are present.

Treatment

Treatment depends on the diagnosis. If you have an infection in the hip joint, it must be eliminated, either through the use of medications or through surgical draining. Nonoperative treatments may provide some relief with relatively few side effects or complications:

- Anti-inflammatory medications, such as aspirin or ibuprofen, may help reduce the inflammation.

- Corticosteroids are potent anti-inflammatories, part of a drug category known as symptom-modifying antirheumatic drugs, or SMARDs. They can be taken by mouth, by injection, or in creams applied to the skin.

- Methotrexate and sulfasalazine may be prescribed to help retard the progression of the disease. These medications are part of a drug category called DMARDs, or disease-modifying antirheumatic drugs. For example, tumor necrosis factor is one of the substances that seem to cause inflammation in people with arthritis. Newer drugs that work against this factor seem to have a positive effect on arthritis in some patients as well.

- Physical therapy may help you increase the range of motion and strengthening exercises may help maintain muscle tone. Swimming is a preferred exercise for people with AS.

- Assistive devices, such as a cane, walker, long shoehorn, or reacher, may make it easier for you to do daily living activities.

If these treatments do not relieve the pain, surgery may be recommended. The type of surgery depends on several factors, including your age, the condition of the hip joint, the type of inflammatory arthritis you have, and the progression of the disease. Your orthopaedic surgeon will discuss the various options with you. Do not hesitate to ask why a specific procedure is being recommended and what outcome you can expect. Although complications are possible in any surgery, your orthopaedic surgeon will take steps to minimize the risks.

The most common surgical procedures performed for inflammatory arthritis of the hip include:

- Total hip replacement is often recommended for patients with RA or AS because it provides pain relief and improves motion.

- Bone grafts may help patients with SLE to build new bone cells to replace those affected by osteonecrosis. People with SLE have a higher incidence of this disease, which causes bone cells to die and weakens bone structure.

- Another option for patients with SLE and osteonecrosis is core decompression, which reduces bone marrow pressure and encourages blood flow.

- Synovectomy (removing part or all of the joint lining) may be effective if the disease is limited to the joint lining and has not affected the cartilage.

Section 5.8

Arthritis of the Knee

"Questions and Answers about Knee Problems," National Institute of Arthritis and Musculoskeletal and Skin Diseases (NIAMS), May 2001. Available online at http://www.niams.nih.gov; accessed January 2004.

What Do the Knees Do? How Do They Work?

The knees provide stable support for the body and allow the legs to bend and straighten. Both flexibility and stability are needed for standing and for motions like walking, running, crouching, jumping, and turning.

Several kinds of supporting and moving parts, including bones, cartilage, muscles, ligaments, and tendons, help the knees do their job. Any of these parts can be involved in pain or dysfunction.

What Causes Knee Problems?

There are two general kinds of knee problems: mechanical and inflammatory.

Mechanical Knee Problems

Some knee problems result from injury, such as a direct blow or sudden movements that strain the knee beyond its normal range of movement. Other problems, such as osteoarthritis in the knee, result from wear and tear on its parts.

Inflammatory Knee Problems

Inflammation that occurs in certain rheumatic diseases, such as rheumatoid arthritis and systemic lupus erythematosus, can damage the knee.

Joint Basics

The point at which two or more bones are connected is called a joint. In all joints, the bones are kept from grinding against each other by padding called cartilage. Bones are joined to bones by strong, elastic bands of tissue called ligaments. Tendons are tough cords of tissue that connect muscle to bone. Muscles work in opposing pairs to bend and straighten joints. While muscles are not technically part of a joint, they're important because strong muscles help support and protect joints.

What Are the Parts of the Knee?

Like any joint, the knee is composed of bones and cartilage, ligaments, tendons, and muscles.

Bones and Cartilage

The knee joint is the junction of three bones: the femur (thighbone or upper leg bone), the tibia (shinbone or larger bone of the lower leg), and the patella (kneecap). The patella is 2 to 3 inches wide and 3 to 4 inches long. It sits over the other bones at the front of the knee joint and slides when the leg moves. It protects the knee and gives leverage to muscles.

The ends of the three bones in the knee joint are covered with articular cartilage, a tough, elastic material that helps absorb shock and allows the knee joint to move smoothly. Separating the bones of the knee are pads of connective tissue. One pad is called a meniscus. The plural is menisci. The menisci are divided into two crescent-shaped discs positioned between the tibia and femur on the outer and inner sides of each knee. The two menisci in each knee act as shock absorbers, cushioning the lower part of the leg from the weight of the rest of the body as well as enhancing stability.

Muscles

There are two groups of muscles at the knee. The quadriceps muscle comprises four muscles on the front of the thigh that work to straighten the leg from a bent position. The hamstring muscles, which bend the leg at the knee, run along the back of the thigh from the hip to just below the knee. Keeping these muscles strong with exercises such as walking up stairs or riding a stationary bicycle helps support and protect the knee.

Tendons and Ligaments

The quadriceps tendon connects the quadriceps muscle to the patella and provides the power to extend the leg. Four ligaments connect the femur and tibia and give the joint strength and stability:

- The medial collateral ligament (MCL) provides stability to the inner (medial) part of the knee.

- The lateral collateral ligament (LCL) provides stability to the outer (lateral) part of the knee.

- The anterior cruciate ligament (ACL), in the center of the knee, limits rotation and the forward movement of the tibia.

- The posterior cruciate ligament (PCL), also in the center of the knee, limits backward movement of the tibia.

Other ligaments are part of the knee capsule, which is a protective, fiber-like structure that wraps around the knee joint. Inside the capsule, the joint is lined with a thin, soft tissue called synovium.

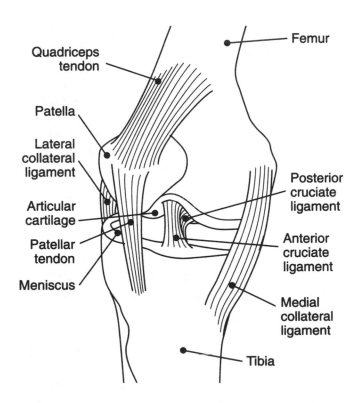

Figure 5.1. The Parts of the Knee

How Are Knee Problems Diagnosed?

Doctors use several methods to diagnose knee problems.

- Medical history—The patient tells the doctor details about symptoms and about any injury, condition, or general health problem that might be causing the pain.

- Physical examination—The doctor bends, straightens, rotates (turns), or presses on the knee to feel for injury and discover the limits of movement and the location of pain. The patient may be asked to stand, walk, or squat to help the doctor assess the knee's function.

- Diagnostic tests—The doctor uses one or more tests to determine the nature of a knee problem.

  - X-ray (radiography)—An x-ray beam is passed through the knee to produce a two-dimensional picture of the bones.

  - Computerized axial tomography (CAT) scan—X-rays lasting a fraction of a second are passed through the knee at different angles, detected by a scanner, and analyzed by a computer. This produces a series of clear cross-sectional images (slices) of the knee tissues on a computer screen. CAT scan images show soft tissues such as ligaments or muscles more clearly than conventional x-rays. The computer can combine individual images to give a three-dimensional view of the knee.

  - Bone scan (radionuclide scanning)—A very small amount of radioactive material is injected into the patient's bloodstream and detected by a scanner. This test detects blood flow to the bone and cell activity within the bone and can show abnormalities in these processes that may aid diagnosis.

  - Magnetic resonance imaging (MRI)—Energy from a powerful magnet (rather than x-rays) stimulates knee tissue to produce signals that are detected by a scanner and analyzed by a computer. This creates a series of cross-sectional images of a specific part of the knee. An MRI is particularly useful for detecting soft tissue damage or disease. Like a CAT scan, a computer is used to produce three-dimensional views of the knee during MRI.

75

- Arthroscopy—The doctor manipulates a small, lighted optic tube (arthroscope) that has been inserted into the joint through a small incision in the knee. Images of the inside of the knee joint are projected onto a television screen. While the arthroscope is inside the knee joint, removal of loose pieces of bone or cartilage or the repair of torn ligaments and menisci is also possible.

- Biopsy—The doctor removes tissue to examine under a microscope.

Arthritis

What Is Arthritis of the Knee?

Arthritis of the knee is most often osteoarthritis. In this disease, the cartilage in the joint gradually wears away. In rheumatoid arthritis, which can also affect the knees, the joint becomes inflamed and cartilage may be destroyed. Arthritis not only affects joints; it can also affect supporting structures such as muscles, tendons, and ligaments.

Osteoarthritis may be caused by excess stress on the joint from deformity, repeated injury, or excess weight. It most often affects middle-aged and older people. A young person who develops osteoarthritis may have an inherited form of the disease or may have experienced continuous irritation from an unrepaired torn meniscus or other injury. Rheumatoid arthritis often affects people at an earlier age than osteoarthritis.

Signs and Diagnosis

Someone who has arthritis of the knee may experience pain, swelling, and a decrease in knee motion. A common symptom is morning stiffness that lessens as the person moves around. Sometimes the joint locks or clicks when the knee is bent and straightened, but these signs may occur in other knee disorders as well. The doctor may confirm the diagnosis by performing a physical examination and examining x-rays, which typically show a loss of joint space. Blood tests may be helpful for diagnosing rheumatoid arthritis, but other tests may be needed too. Analyzing fluid from the knee joint may be helpful in diagnosing some kinds of arthritis. The doctor may use arthroscopy to directly see damage to cartilage, tendons, and ligaments and to confirm a diagnosis, but arthroscopy is usually done only if a repair procedure is to be performed.

Treatment

Most often osteoarthritis of the knee is treated with pain-reducing medicines, such as aspirin or acetaminophen (Tylenol); nonsteroidal anti-inflammatory drugs (NSAIDs), such as ibuprofen (Motrin, Nuprin, Advil); and exercises to restore joint movement and strengthen the knee. Losing excess weight can also help people with osteoarthritis.

Rheumatoid arthritis of the knee may require physical therapy and more powerful medications. In people with arthritis of the knee, a seriously damaged joint may need to be replaced with an artificial one. (A new procedure designed to stimulate the growth of cartilage by using a patient's own cartilage cells is being used experimentally to repair cartilage injuries at the end of the femur at the knee. It is not, however, a treatment for arthritis.)

Section 5.9

Arthritis of the Feet

Reprinted with permission from, "Your Podiatric Physician Talks about Arthritis," a brochure produced by the American Podiatric Medical Association, www.apma.org. © 2002 APMA. Reprinted by permission.

What Is Arthritis?

Arthritis, in general terms, is inflammation and swelling of the cartilage and lining of the joints, generally accompanied by an increase in the fluid in the joints. Arthritis has multiple causes; just as a sore throat may have its origin in a variety of diseases, so joint inflammation and arthritis are associated with many different illnesses.

Arthritis and the Feet

Arthritis is a frequent component of complex diseases that may involve more than 100 identifiable disorders. If the feet seem more susceptible to arthritis than other parts of the body, it is because each foot has 33 joints that can be afflicted, and there is no way to avoid the pain of the tremendous weight-bearing load on the feet.

Arthritis is a disabling and occasionally crippling disease; it afflicts almost 40 million Americans. In some forms, it appears to have hereditary tendencies. Although the prevalence of arthritis increases with age, all people from infancy to middle age are potential victims. People over 50 are the primary targets.

Arthritic feet can result in loss of mobility and independence, but that may be avoided with early diagnosis and proper medical care.

Some Causes

Besides heredity, arthritic symptoms may arise in a number of ways:

- Through injuries, notably in athletes and industrial workers, especially if the injuries have been ignored (which injuries of the feet tend to be).

- Through bacterial and viral infections that strike the joints. The same organisms that are present in pneumonia, gonorrhea, staphylococcal infections, and Lyme disease cause the inflammations.

- In conjunction with bowel disorders such as colitis and ileitis, frequently resulting in arthritic conditions in the joints of the ankles and toes. Such inflammatory bowel diseases seem distant from arthritis, but treating them can relieve arthritic pain.

- Using drugs, both prescription drugs and illegal street drugs, can induce arthritis.

- As part of a congenital autoimmune disease syndrome of undetermined origin. Recent research has suggested, for instance, that a defective gene may play a role in osteoarthritis.

Symptoms

Because arthritis can affect the structure and function of the feet it is important to see a doctor of podiatric medicine if any of the following symptoms occur in the feet:

- Swelling in one or more joints
- Recurring pain or tenderness in any joint
- Redness or heat in a joint

- Limitation in motion of joint
- Early morning stiffness
- Skin changes, including rashes and growths

Some Forms of Arthritis

Osteoarthritis is the most common form of arthritis. It is frequently called degenerative joint disease or wear-and-tear arthritis. Although it can be brought on suddenly by an injury, its onset is generally gradual; aging brings on a breakdown in cartilage, and pain gets progressively more severe, although it can be relieved with rest. Dull, throbbing nighttime pain is characteristic, and it may be accompanied by muscle weakness or deterioration. Walking may become erratic.

It is a particular problem for the feet when people are overweight, simply because there are so many joints in each foot. The additional weight contributes to the deterioration of cartilage and the development of bone spurs.

Rheumatoid arthritis (RA) is a major crippling disorder, and perhaps the most serious form of arthritis. It is a complex, chronic inflammatory system of diseases, often affecting more than a dozen smaller joints during the course of the disease, frequently in a symmetrical pattern—both ankles or the index fingers of both hands, for example. It is often accompanied by signs and symptoms—lengthy morning stiffness, fatigue, and weight loss—and it may affect various systems of the body, such as the eyes, lungs, heart, and nervous system. Women are three or four times more likely than men to suffer RA.

RA has a much more acute onset than osteoarthritis. It is characterized by alternating periods of remission, during which symptoms disappear, and exacerbation, marked by the return of inflammation, stiffness, and pain. Serious joint deformity and loss of motion frequently result from acute rheumatoid arthritis. However, the disease system has been known to be active for months, or years, then abate, sometimes permanently.

Gout (gouty arthritis) is a condition caused by a buildup of the salts of uric acid—a normal byproduct of the diet—in the joints. A single big toe joint is commonly the affected area, possibly because it is subject to so much pressure in walking; attacks of gouty arthritis are extremely painful, perhaps more so than any other form of arthritis. Men are much more likely to be afflicted than women, an indication that heredity may play a role in the disease. Although a rich diet that contains lots of red meat, rich sauces, shellfish, and brandy is popularly associated with gout, there are other protein compounds in foods such as lentils and beans that may play a role.

Diagnosis

Different forms of arthritis affect the body in different ways; many have distinct systemic effects that are not common to other forms. Early diagnosis is important to effective treatment of any form. Destruction of cartilage is not reversible, and if the inflammation of arthritic disease isn't treated, both cartilage and bone can be damaged, which makes the joints increasingly difficult to move. Most forms of arthritis cannot be cured, but can be controlled or brought into remission; perhaps only five percent of the most serious cases, usually of rheumatoid arthritis, result in such severe crippling so that walking aids or wheelchairs are required.

Treatment

The objectives in the treatment of arthritis are controlling inflammation, preserving joint function (or restoring it if it has been lost), and curing the disease if that is possible.

Because the foot is such a frequent target, the doctor of podiatric medicine is often the first physician to encounter some of the complaints—inflammation, pain, stiffness, excessive warmth, and injuries. Even bunions can be manifestations of arthritis.

Arthritis may be treated in many ways. Patient education is important. Physical therapy and exercise may be indicated, accompanied by medication. In such a complex disease system, it is no wonder that a wide variety of drugs have been used effectively to treat it; likewise, a given treatment may be very effective in one patient and almost no help at all to another. Aspirin is still the first-line drug of choice for most forms of arthritis, and the benchmark against which other therapies are measured.

The control of foot functions with shoe inserts called orthoses, or with braces or specially prescribed shoes, may be recommended. Surgical intervention is a last resort in arthritis, as it is with most disease conditions; the replacement of damaged joints with artificial joints is a possible surgical procedure.

Arthritis Tips

- Wear comfortable shoes that conform to the shape of your foot.

- Wear shoes with a wide and deep toe box.

- Always fit the larger foot and have your feet sized each time you purchase shoes.

- Avoid high-heeled shoes over two inches tall.

- Seek professional podiatric evaluation and assistance if your feet are uncomfortable or painful.

Your podiatric physician/surgeon has been trained specifically and extensively in the diagnosis and treatment of all manners of foot conditions. This training encompasses all of the intricately related systems and structures of the foot and lower leg including neurological, circulatory, skin, and the musculoskeletal system, which includes bones, joints, ligaments, tendons, muscles, and nerves.

Part Two

Forms of Arthritis and Other Rheumatic Disorders

Chapter 6

Osteoarthritis

Chapter Contents

Section 6.1

Understanding the Basics of Osteoarthritis

"Handout on Health: Osteoarthritis," National Institute of Arthritis and Musculoskeletal and Skin Diseases (NIAMS), July 2002. Available online at http://www.niams.nih.gov; accessed January 2004.

What Is Osteoarthritis?

Osteoarthritis is the most common type of arthritis, especially among older people. Sometimes it is called degenerative joint disease or osteoarthrosis.

Osteoarthritis is a joint disease that mostly affects the cartilage. Cartilage is the slippery tissue that covers the ends of bones in a joint. Healthy cartilage allows bones to glide over one another. It also absorbs energy from the shock of physical movement. In osteoarthritis, the surface layer of cartilage breaks down and wears away. This allows bones under the cartilage to rub together, causing pain, swelling, and loss of motion of the joint. Over time, the joint may lose its normal shape. Also, bone spurs—small growths called osteophytes—may grow on the edges of the joint. Bits of bone or cartilage can break off and float inside the joint space. This causes more pain and damage.

People with osteoarthritis usually have joint pain and limited movement. Unlike some other forms of arthritis, osteoarthritis affects only joints and not internal organs. For example, rheumatoid arthritis—the second most common form of arthritis—affects other parts of the body besides the joints. It begins at a younger age than osteoarthritis, causes swelling and redness in joints, and may make people feel sick, tired, and (uncommonly) feverish.

Who Has Osteoarthritis?

Osteoarthritis is one of the most frequent causes of physical disability among adults. More than 20 million people in the United States have the disease. By 2030, 20 percent of Americans—about 70 million people—will have passed their 65th birthday and will be at risk for osteoarthritis. Some younger people get osteoarthritis from joint injuries, but osteoarthritis most often occurs in older people. In fact, more than half of the population age 65 or older would show x-ray evidence of osteoarthritis in at least one joint. Both men and women have the disease. Before age 45, more men than women have osteoarthritis, whereas after age 45, it is more common in women.

How Does Osteoarthritis Affect People?

Osteoarthritis affects each person differently. In some people, it progresses quickly; in others, the symptoms are more serious. Scientists do not know yet what causes the disease, but they suspect a combination of factors, including being overweight, the aging process, joint injury, and stresses on the joints from certain jobs and sports activities.

Osteoarthritis hurts people in more than their joints: their finances and lifestyles also are affected.

Financial effects include:

- The cost of treatment
- Wages lost because of disability

Lifestyle effects include:

- Depression
- Anxiety
- Feelings of helplessness
- Limitations on daily activities
- Job limitations
- Trouble participating in everyday personal and family joys and responsibilities

Despite these challenges, most people with osteoarthritis can lead active and productive lives. They succeed by using osteoarthritis treatment strategies, such as the following:

- Pain relief medications
- Rest and exercise
- Patient education and support programs
- Learning self-care and having a good attitude

Osteoarthritis Basics: The Joint and Its Parts

Most joints—the place where two moving bones come together— are designed to allow smooth movement between the bones and to absorb shock from movements like walking or repetitive movements. The joint is made up of:

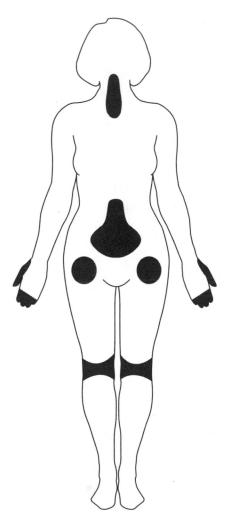

Figure 6.1. *Body Parts Most Often Affected by Osteoarthritis. Osteoarthritis most often occurs at the ends of the fingers, thumbs, neck, lower back, knees, and hips.*

- Cartilage: a hard but slippery coating on the end of each bone.

- Joint capsule: a tough membrane sac that holds all the bones and other joint parts together.

- Synovium: a thin membrane inside the joint capsule.

- Synovial fluid: a fluid that lubricates the joint and keeps the cartilage smooth and healthy.

- Ligaments, tendons, and muscles: tissues that keep the bones stable and allow the joint to bend and move. Ligaments are tough, cord-like tissues that connect one bone to another. Tendons are tough, fibrous cords that connect muscles to bones. Muscles are bundles of specialized cells that contract to produce movement when stimulated by nerves.

How Do You Know If You Have Osteoarthritis?

Usually, osteoarthritis comes on slowly. Early in the disease, joints may ache after physical work or exercise. Osteoarthritis can occur in any joint. Most often it occurs at the hands, knees, hips, or spine.

Hands: Osteoarthritis of the fingers is one type of osteoarthritis that seems to have some hereditary characteristics; that is, it runs in families. More women than men have it, and they develop it especially after menopause. In osteoarthritis, small, bony knobs appear on the end joints of the fingers. They are called Heberden nodes. Similar knobs, called Bouchard nodes, can appear on the middle joints of the fingers. Fingers can become enlarged and gnarled, and they may ache or be stiff and numb. The base of the thumb joint also is commonly affected by osteoarthritis. Osteoarthritis of the hands can be helped by medications, splints, or heat treatment.

Knees: The knees are the body's primary weight-bearing joints. For this reason, they are among the joints most commonly affected by osteoarthritis. They may be stiff, swollen, and painful, making it hard to walk, climb, and get in and out of chairs and bathtubs. If not treated, osteoarthritis in the knees can lead to disability. Medications, weight loss, exercise, and walking aids can reduce pain and disability. In severe cases, knee replacement surgery may be helpful.

Hips: Osteoarthritis in the hip can cause pain, stiffness, and severe disability. People may feel the pain in their hips, or in their groin,

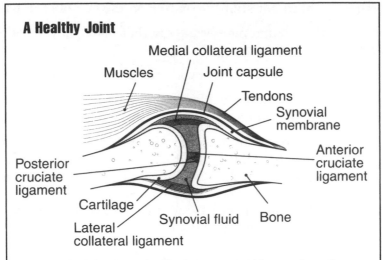

A Healthy Joint

In a healthy joint, the ends of bones are encased in smooth cartilage. Together, they are protected by a joint capsule lined with a synovial membrane that produces synovial fluid. The capsule and fluid protect the cartilage, muscles, and connective tissues.

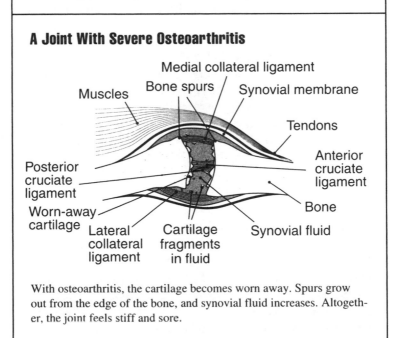

A Joint With Severe Osteoarthritis

With osteoarthritis, the cartilage becomes worn away. Spurs grow out from the edge of the bone, and synovial fluid increases. Altogether, the joint feels stiff and sore.

Figure 6.2. *Comparison of a Healthy Joint and a Joint Affected by Osteoarthritis*

inner thigh, buttocks, or knees. Walking aids, such as canes or walkers, can reduce stress on the hip. Osteoarthritis in the hip may limit moving and bending. This can make daily activities such as dressing and foot care a challenge. Walking aids, medication, and exercise can help relieve pain and improve motion. The doctor may recommend hip replacement if the pain is severe and not relieved by other methods.

Spine: Stiffness and pain in the neck or in the lower back can result from osteoarthritis of the spine. Weakness or numbness of the arms or legs also can result. Some people feel better when they sleep on a firm mattress or sit using back support pillows. Others find it helps to use heat treatments or to follow an exercise program that strengthens the back and abdominal muscles. In severe cases, the doctor may suggest surgery to reduce pain and help restore function.

How Do Doctors Diagnose Osteoarthritis?

No single test can diagnose osteoarthritis. Most doctors use a combination of the following methods to diagnose the disease and rule out other conditions:

Clinical history: The doctor begins by asking the patient to describe the symptoms, and when and how the condition started. Good doctor-patient communication is important. The doctor can give a better assessment if the patient gives a good description of pain, stiffness, and joint function, and how they have changed over time. It also is important for the doctor to know how the condition affects the patient's work and daily life. Finally, the doctor also needs to know about other medical conditions and whether the patient is taking any medicines.

Physical examination: The doctor will check the patient's general health, including checking reflexes and muscle strength. Joints bothering the patient will be examined. The doctor will also observe the patient's ability to walk, bend, and carry out activities of daily living.

X-rays: Doctors take x-rays to see how much joint damage has been done. X-rays of the affected joint can show such things as cartilage loss, bone damage, and bone spurs. But there often is a big difference between the severity of osteoarthritis as shown by the x-ray and the degree of pain and disability felt by the patient. Also, x-rays may not show early osteoarthritis damage, before much cartilage loss has taken place.

Other tests: The doctor may order blood tests to rule out other causes of symptoms. Another common test is called joint aspiration, which involves drawing fluid from the joint for examination.

It usually is not difficult to tell if a patient has osteoarthritis. It is more difficult to tell if the disease is causing the patient's symptoms. Osteoarthritis is so common—especially in older people—that symptoms seemingly caused by the disease actually may be due to other medical conditions. The doctor will try to find out what is causing the symptoms by ruling out other disorders and identifying conditions that may make the symptoms worse. The severity of symptoms in osteoarthritis is influenced greatly by the patient's attitude, anxiety, depression, and daily activity level.

How Is Osteoarthritis Treated?

Most successful treatment programs involve a combination of treatments tailored to the patient's needs, lifestyle, and health. Osteoarthritis treatment has four general goals:

- Improve joint care through rest and exercise.
- Maintain an acceptable body weight.
- Control pain with medicine and other measures.
- Achieve a healthy lifestyle.

Osteoarthritis treatment plans often include ways to manage pain and improve function. Such plans can involve exercise, rest and joint care, pain relief, weight control, medicines, surgery, and nontraditional treatment approaches.

Exercise

Research shows that exercise is one of the best treatments for osteoarthritis. Exercise can improve mood and outlook, decrease pain, increase flexibility, improve the heart and blood flow, maintain weight, and promote general physical fitness. Exercise is also inexpensive and, if done correctly, has few negative side effects. The amount and form of exercise will depend on which joints are involved, how stable the joints are, and whether a joint replacement has already been done.

You can use exercises to keep strong and limber, extend your range of movement, and reduce your weight. Some different types of exercise include the following:

- Strength exercises: These can be performed with exercise bands, inexpensive devices that add resistance.

- Aerobic activities: These keep your lungs and circulation systems in shape.

- Range of motion activities: These keep your joints limber.

- Agility exercises: These can help you maintain daily living skills.

- Neck and back strength exercises: These can help you keep your spine strong and limber.

Ask your doctor or physical therapist what exercises are best for you. Ask for guidelines on exercising when a joint is sore or if swelling is present. Also, check if you should (1) use pain-relieving drugs, such as analgesics or anti-inflammatories (also called NSAIDs), to make exercising easier, or (2) use ice afterward.

Rest and Joint Care

Treatment plans include regularly scheduled rest. Patients must learn to recognize the body's signals, and know when to stop or slow down, which prevents pain caused by overexertion. Some patients find that relaxation techniques, stress reduction, and biofeedback help. Some use canes and splints to protect joints and take pressure off them. Splints or braces provide extra support for weakened joints. They also keep the joint in proper position during sleep or activity. Splints should be used only for limited periods because joints and muscles need to be exercised to prevent stiffness and weakness. An occupational therapist or a doctor can help the patient get a properly fitting splint.

Nondrug Pain Relief

People with osteoarthritis may find nondrug ways to relieve pain. Warm towels, hot packs, or a warm bath or shower to apply moist heat to the joint can relieve pain and stiffness. In some cases, cold packs (a bag of ice or frozen vegetables wrapped in a towel) can relieve pain or numb the sore area. (Check with a doctor or physical therapist to find out if heat or cold is the best treatment.) Water therapy in a heated pool or whirlpool also may relieve pain and stiffness. For osteoarthritis in the knee, patients may wear insoles or cushioned shoes to redistribute weight and reduce joint stress.

Weight Control

Osteoarthritis patients who are overweight or obese need to lose weight. Weight loss can reduce stress on weight-bearing joints and limit further injury. A dietitian can help patients develop healthy eating habits. A healthy diet and regular exercise help reduce weight.

Medicines

Doctors prescribe medicines to eliminate or reduce pain and to improve functioning. Doctors consider a number of factors when choosing medicines for their patients with osteoarthritis. Two important factors are the intensity of the pain and the potential side effects of the medicine. Patients must use medicines carefully and tell their doctors about any changes that occur.

The following types of medicines are commonly used in treating osteoarthritis:

- Acetaminophen: Acetaminophen is a pain reliever (for example, Tylenol) that does not reduce swelling. Acetaminophen does not irritate the stomach and is less likely than nonsteroidal anti-inflammatory drugs (NSAIDs) to cause long-term side effects. Research has shown that acetaminophen relieves pain as effectively as NSAIDs for many patients with osteoarthritis. [Warning: People with liver disease, people who drink alcohol heavily, and those taking blood-thinning medicines or NSAIDs should use acetaminophen with caution.]

- NSAIDs (nonsteroidal anti-inflammatory drugs): Many NSAIDs are used to treat osteoarthritis. Patients can buy some over the counter (for example, aspirin, Advil, Motrin IB, Aleve, ketoprofen). Others require a prescription. All NSAIDs work similarly: they fight inflammation and relieve pain. However, each NSAID is a different chemical, and each has a slightly different effect on the body. Side effects: NSAIDs can cause stomach irritation or, less often, they can affect kidney function. The longer a person uses NSAIDs, the more likely he or she is to have side effects, ranging from mild to serious. Many other drugs cannot be taken when a patient is being treated with NSAIDs because NSAIDs alter the way the body uses or eliminates these other drugs. Check with your health care provider or pharmacist before you take NSAIDs in addition to another medication. Also, NSAIDs sometimes are associated with serious gastrointestinal problems, including ulcers, bleeding, and perforation of the stomach or intestine. People over age 65 and those with any history of ulcers or gastrointestinal bleeding should use NSAIDs with caution.

- COX-2 inhibitors: Several new NSAIDs—valdecoxib (Bextra), celecoxib (Celebrex), and rofecoxib (Vioxx)—from a class of drugs known as COX-2 inhibitors are now being used to treat osteoarthritis. These medicines reduce inflammation similarly to traditional NSAIDs, but they cause fewer gastrointestinal side effects. However, these medications occasionally are associated with harmful reactions ranging from mild to severe.

- Other medications: Doctors may prescribe several other medicines for osteoarthritis, including the following: topical pain-relieving creams, rubs, and sprays (for example, capsaicin cream), which are applied directly to the skin; mild narcotic painkillers, which—although very effective—may be addictive and are not commonly used; and corticosteroids, powerful anti-inflammatory hormones made naturally in the body or man-made for use as medicine. Corticosteroids may be injected into the affected joints to temporarily relieve pain. This is a short-term measure, generally not recommended for more than two or three treatments per year. Oral corticosteroids should not be used to treat osteoarthritis. Doctors may also prescribe hyaluronic acid, a medicine for joint injection, used to treat osteoarthritis of the knee. This substance is a normal component of the joint, involved in joint lubrication and nutrition.

Most medicines used to treat osteoarthritis have side effects, so it is important for people to learn about the medicines they take. Even nonprescription drugs should be checked. Several groups of patients are at high risk for side effects from NSAIDs, such as people with a history of peptic ulcers or digestive tract bleeding, people taking oral corticosteroids or anticoagulants (blood thinners), smokers, and people who consume alcohol. Some patients may be able to help reduce side effects by taking some medicines with food. Others should avoid stomach irritants such as alcohol, tobacco, and caffeine. Some patients try to protect their stomachs by taking other medicines that coat the stomach or block stomach acids. These measures help, but they are not always completely effective.

Surgery

For many people, surgery helps relieve the pain and disability of osteoarthritis. Surgery may be performed to:

- Remove loose pieces of bone and cartilage from the joint if they are causing mechanical symptoms of buckling or locking

- Resurface (smooth out) bones

- Reposition bones

- Replace joints

Surgeons may replace affected joints with artificial joints called prostheses. These joints can be made from metal alloys, high-density plastic, and ceramic material. They can be joined to bone surfaces by special cements. Artificial joints can last 10 to 15 years or longer. About 10 percent of artificial joints may need revision. Surgeons choose the design and components of prostheses according to their patient's weight, sex, age, activity level, and other medical conditions.

The decision to use surgery depends on several things. Both the surgeon and the patient consider the patient's level of disability, the intensity of pain, the interference with the patient's lifestyle, the patient's age, and occupation. Currently, more than 80 percent of osteoarthritis surgery cases involve replacing the hip or knee joint. After surgery and rehabilitation, the patient usually feels less pain and swelling, and can move more easily.

Nontraditional Approaches

Among the alternative therapies used to treat osteoarthritis are the following:

- Acupuncture: Some people have found pain relief using acupuncture (the use of fine needles inserted at specific points on the skin). Preliminary research shows that acupuncture may be a useful component in an osteoarthritis treatment plan for some patients.

- Folk remedies: Some patients seek alternative therapies for their pain and disability. Some of these alternative therapies have included wearing copper bracelets, drinking herbal teas, and taking mud baths. Although these practices are not harmful, some can be expensive. They also cause delays in seeking medical treatment. To date, no scientific research shows these approaches to be helpful in treating osteoarthritis.

- Nutritional supplements: Nutrients such as glucosamine and chondroitin sulfate have been reported to improve the symptoms of people with osteoarthritis, as have certain vitamins. Additional studies are being carried out to further evaluate these claims.

Self-Care for People with Arthritis

People with osteoarthritis can enjoy good health despite having the disease. How? By learning self-care skills and developing a good-health attitude. Self-care is central to successfully managing the pain and disability of osteoarthritis. People have a much better chance of having a rewarding lifestyle when they educate themselves about the disease and take part in their own care. Working actively with a team of health care providers enables people with the disease to minimize pain, share in decision making about treatment, and feel a sense of control over their lives. Research shows that people with osteoarthritis who take part in their own care report less pain and make fewer doctor visits. They also enjoy a better quality of life.

Self-Help and Education Programs

Three kinds of programs help people learn about osteoarthritis, learn self-care, and improve their good-health attitude. These programs include

- Patient education programs
- Arthritis self-management programs
- Arthritis support groups

These programs teach people about osteoarthritis, its treatments, exercise and relaxation, patient and health care provider communication, and problem solving. Research has shown that these programs have clear and long-lasting benefits.

Exercise

Regular physical activity plays a key role in self-care and wellness. Two types of exercise are important in osteoarthritis management.

The first type, therapeutic exercises, keeps joints working as well as possible. The other type, aerobic conditioning exercises, improves strength and fitness and controls weight. Patients should be realistic when they start exercising. They should learn how to exercise correctly because exercising incorrectly can cause problems.

Most people with osteoarthritis exercise best when their pain is least severe. Start with an adequate warmup and begin exercising slowly. Resting frequently ensures a good workout. It also reduces the risk of injury. A physical therapist can evaluate how a patient's muscles are working. This information helps the therapist develop a safe, personalized exercise program to increase strength and flexibility.

Many people enjoy sports or other activities in their exercise program. Good activities include swimming and aquatic exercise, walking, running, biking, cross-country skiing, and using exercise machines and exercise videotapes.

People with osteoarthritis should check with their doctor or physical therapist before starting an exercise program. Health care providers will suggest what exercises are best for you, how to warm up safely, and when to avoid exercising a joint affected by arthritis. Pain medications and applying ice after exercising may make exercising easier.

Body, Mind, Spirit

Making the most of good health requires careful attention to the body, mind, and spirit. People with osteoarthritis must plan and develop daily routines that maximize their quality of life and minimize disability. They also need to evaluate these routines periodically to make sure they are working well.

Good health also requires a positive attitude. People must decide to make the most of things when faced with the challenges of osteoarthritis. This attitude—a good-health mindset—doesn't just happen. It takes work, every day. And with the right attitude, you will achieve it.

Current Research

The leading role in osteoarthritis research is played by the National Institute of Arthritis and Musculoskeletal and Skin Diseases (NIAMS), within the National Institutes of Health (NIH). The NIAMS funds many researchers across the United States to study osteoarthritis. It has established a Specialized Center of Research devoted to osteoarthritis. Also, many researchers study arthritis at NIAMS Multipurpose Arthritis and Musculoskeletal Diseases Centers and Multidisciplinary Clinical Research Centers. These centers conduct

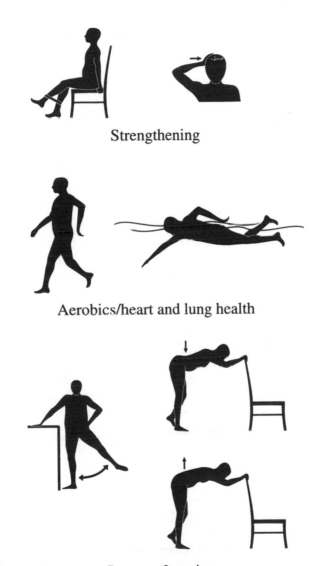

Strengthening

Aerobics/heart and lung health

Range of motion

Figure 6.3. *Exercises for osteoarthritis. People with osteoarthritis should do different kinds of exercise for different benefits to the body.*

basic, laboratory, and clinical research aimed at understanding the causes, treatment options, and prevention of arthritis and musculoskeletal diseases. Center researchers also study epidemiology, health services, and professional, patient, and public education. The NIAMS also supports multidisciplinary clinical research centers that expand clinical studies for diseases like osteoarthritis.

For years, scientists thought that osteoarthritis was simply a disease of wear and tear that occurred in joints as people got older. In the last decade, however, research has shown that there is more to the disorder than aging alone. The production, maintenance, and breakdown of cartilage, as well as bone changes in osteoarthritis, are now seen as a series or cascade of events. Many researchers are trying to discover where in that cascade of events things go wrong. By understanding what goes wrong, they hope to find new ways to prevent or treat osteoarthritis. Some key areas of research are described below.

Animal Models: Animals help researchers understand how diseases work and why they occur. Animal models help researchers learn many things about osteoarthritis, such as what happens to cartilage, how treatment strategies might work, and what might prevent the disease. Animal models also help scientists study osteoarthritis in very early stages before it causes detectable joint damage.

Diagnostic Tools: Some scientists want to find ways to detect osteoarthritis at earlier stages so that they can treat it earlier. They seek specific abnormalities in the blood, joint fluid, or urine of people with the disease. Other scientists use new technologies to analyze the differences between the cartilage from different joints. For example, many people have osteoarthritis in the knees or hips, but few have it in the ankles. Can ankle cartilage be different? Does it age differently? Answering these questions will help us understand the disease better.

Genetics Studies: Researchers suspect that inheritance plays a role in 25 to 30 percent of osteoarthritis cases. Researchers have found that genetics may play a role in approximately 40 to 65 percent of hand and knee osteoarthritis cases. They suspect inheritance might play a role in other types of osteoarthritis, as well. Scientists have identified a mutation (a gene defect) affecting collagen, an important part of cartilage, in patients with an inherited kind of osteoarthritis that starts at an early age. The mutation weakens collagen protein, which may break or tear more easily under stress. Scientists are looking for other gene mutations in osteoarthritis. Recently, researchers found that the daughters of women who have knee osteoarthritis have a significant increase in cartilage breakdown, thus making them more susceptible to disease. In the future, a test to determine who carries the genetic defect (or defects) could help people reduce their risk for osteoarthritis with lifestyle adjustments.

Tissue Engineering: This technology involves removing cells from a healthy part of the body and placing them in an area of diseased or damaged tissue in order to improve certain body functions. Currently, it is used to treat small traumatic injuries or defects in cartilage, and, if successful, could eventually help treat osteoarthritis. Researchers at the NIAMS are exploring three types of tissue engineering. The two most common methods being studied today include cartilage cell replacement and stem cell transplantation. The third method is gene therapy.

- *Cartilage cell replacement:* In this procedure, researchers remove cartilage cells from the patient's own joint and then clone or grow new cells using tissue culture and other laboratory techniques. They then inject the newly grown cells into the patient's joint. Patients with cartilage cell replacement have fewer symptoms of osteoarthritis. Actual cartilage repair is limited, however.

- *Stem cell transplantation:* Stem cells are primitive cells that can transform into other kinds of cells, such as muscle or bone cells. They usually are taken from bone marrow. In the future, researchers hope to insert stem cells into cartilage, where the cells will make new cartilage. If successful, this process could be used to repair damaged cartilage and avoid the need for surgical joint replacements with metal or plastics.

- *Gene therapy:* Scientists are working to genetically engineer cells that would inhibit the body chemicals, called enzymes, that may help break down cartilage and cause joint damage. In gene therapy, cells are removed from the body, genetically changed, and then injected back into the affected joint. They live in the joint and protect it from damaging enzymes.

Comprehensive Treatment Strategies: Effective treatment for osteoarthritis takes more than medicine or surgery. Getting help from a variety of care professionals often can improve patient treatment and self-care. Research shows that adding patient education and social support is a low-cost, effective way to decrease pain and reduce the amount of medicine used.

Exercise plays a key part in comprehensive treatment. Researchers are studying exercise in greater detail and finding out just how to use it in treating or preventing osteoarthritis. For example, several scientists have studied knee osteoarthritis and exercise. Their results included the following:

- Strengthening the thigh muscle (quadriceps) can relieve symptoms of knee osteoarthritis and prevent more damage.

- Walking can result in better functioning, and the more you walk, the farther you will be able to walk.

- People with knee osteoarthritis who were active in an exercise program feel less pain. They also function better.

Research has shown that losing extra weight can help people who already have osteoarthritis. Moreover, overweight or obese people who do not have osteoarthritis may reduce their risk of developing the disease by losing weight.

Using NSAIDs: Many people who have osteoarthritis have persistent pain despite taking simple pain relievers such as acetaminophen. Some of these patients take NSAIDs instead. Health care providers are concerned about long-term NSAID use because it can lead to an upset stomach, heartburn, nausea, and more dangerous side effects, such as ulcers.

Scientists are working to design and test new, safer NSAIDs. One example currently available is a class of selective NSAIDs called COX-2 inhibitors. Traditional NSAIDs prevent inflammation by blocking two related enzymes in the body called COX-1 and COX-2. The gastrointestinal side effects associated with traditional NSAIDs seems to be associated mainly with blocking the COX-1 enzyme, which helps protect the stomach lining. The new selective COX-2 inhibitors, however, primarily block the COX-2 enzyme, which helps control inflammation in the body. As a result, COX-2 inhibitors reduce pain and inflammation but are less likely than traditional NSAIDs to cause gastrointestinal ulcers and bleeding. However, research shows that some COX-2 inhibitors may not protect against heart disease as well as traditional NSAIDs, so check with your doctor if you have concerns.

Drugs to Prevent Joint Damage: No treatment actually prevents osteoarthritis or reverses or blocks the disease process once it begins. Present treatments just relieve the symptoms. Researchers are looking for drugs that would prevent, slow down, or reverse joint damage. One experimental antibiotic drug, doxycycline, may stop certain enzymes from damaging cartilage. The drug has shown some promise in clinical studies, but more studies are needed. Researchers also are studying growth factors and other natural chemical messengers. These potential medicines may be able to stimulate cartilage growth or repair.

Acupuncture: During an acupuncture treatment, a licensed acupuncture therapist inserts very fine needles into the skin at various points on the body. Scientists think the needles stimulate the release of natural, pain-relieving chemicals produced by the brain or the nervous system. Researchers are studying acupuncture treatment of patients who have knee osteoarthritis. Early findings suggest that traditional Chinese acupuncture is effective for some patients as an additional therapy for osteoarthritis, reducing pain and improving function.

Nutritional Supplements: Nutritional supplements are often reported as helpful in treating osteoarthritis. Such reports should be viewed with caution, however, since very few studies have carefully evaluated the role of nutritional supplements in osteoarthritis.

- *Glucosamine and chondroitin sulfate*: Both of these nutrients are found in small quantities in food and are components of normal cartilage. Scientific studies on these two nutritional supplements have not yet shown that they affect the disease. They may relieve symptoms and reduce joint damage in some patients, however. The National Center for Complementary and Alternative Medicine at the NIH is supporting a clinical trial to test whether glucosamine, chondroitin sulfate, or the two nutrients in combination reduce pain and improve function. Patients using this therapy should do so only under the supervision of their doctor, as part of an overall treatment program with exercise, relaxation, and pain relief.

- *Vitamins D, C, E, and beta carotene:* The progression of osteoarthritis may be slower in people who take higher levels of vitamin D, C, E, or beta carotene. More studies are needed to confirm these reports.

- *Hyaluronic acid:* Injecting this substance into the knee joint provides long-term pain relief for some people with osteoarthritis.

Hyaluronic acid is a natural component of cartilage and joint fluid. It lubricates and absorbs shock in the joint. The Food and Drug Administration (FDA) approved this therapy for patients with osteoarthritis of the knee who do not get relief from exercise, physical therapy, or simple analgesics. Researchers are presently studying the benefits of using hyaluronic acid to treat osteoarthritis.

- Estrogen: In studies of older women, scientists found a lower risk of osteoarthritis in women who had used oral estrogens for hormone replacement therapy. The researchers suspect having low levels of estrogen could increase the risk of developing osteoarthritis. Additional studies are needed to answer this question.

Hope for the Future

Research is opening up new avenues of treatment for people with osteoarthritis. A balanced, comprehensive approach is still the key to staying active and healthy with the disease. People with osteoarthritis should combine exercise, relaxation education, social support, and medicines in their treatment strategies. Meanwhile, as scientists unravel the complexities of the disease, new treatments and prevention methods should appear. They will improve the quality of life for people with osteoarthritis and their families.

Additional Resources

National Institute of Arthritis and Musculoskeletal and Skin Diseases
1 AMS Circle
Bethesda, MD 20892-3675
Toll-Free: (877) 22-NIAMS (226-4267)
Phone: (301) 495-4484
TTY: (301) 565-2966
Fax: (301) 718-6366
Website: http://www.niams.nih.gov
E-mail: niamsinfo@mail.nih.gov

American College of Rheumatology
1800 Century Place, Suite 250
Atlanta, GA 30345-4300
Phone: (404) 633-3777
Fax: (404) 633-1870
Website: http://www.rheumatology.org

American Academy of Orthopaedic Surgeons (AAOS)
6300 North River Road
Rosemont, IL 60018-4262
Toll-Free: (800) 824-BONE (2663)
Phone: (847) 823-7186
Fax: (847) 823-8125
Website: http://www.aaos.org
E-mail: custserv@aaos.org

Arthritis Foundation
1330 West Peachtree Street
Atlanta, GA 30309
Toll-Free: (800) 283-7800
Phone: (404) 872-7100
Website: http://www.arthritis.org

Section 6.2

Knee and Hip Injuries in Youth Increase Risk of Osteoarthritis Later

"Knee, Hip Injuries in Youth Increase Risk of Osteoarthritis Later," National Institute of Arthritis and Musculoskeletal and Skin Diseases (NIAMS), March, 6, 2001. Available online at http://www.niams.nih.gov; accessed December 2003.

Knee and hip injuries in adolescents and young adults have been linked to osteoarthritis (OA) in those joints later in life, according to an article in a recent [2001] issue of the *Annals of Internal Medicine*.

The Johns Hopkins Precursors Study, conducted over a 46-year period, was designed to identify the body's predictors of the aging process. The study, funded by the National Institute on Aging with investigator support by NIAMS [National Institute of Arthritis and Musculoskeletal and Skin Diseases], found that participants with a history of athletic or traumatic injury to the knee joint before age 22 had a higher rate of subsequent knee OA. In addition, knee and hip injuries during followup, in the participants' mid thirties, were also related to future knee and hip OA.

Dr. Allan Gelber of Johns Hopkins was the lead author on the paper. He and his colleagues recommend that physicians who treat young patients with athletic or traumatic injuries include stabilizing the joint with braces and temporarily reducing high-impact exercise to minimize further damage of the injured joint as part of the treatment regimen. In addition, they advise physicians to advocate use of proper sports equipment under safe conditions to prevent joint injuries from occurring and decrease the long-term risk of OA disease later in life.

OA or degenerative joint disease mostly affects the cartilage, which is the padding between two bones. It is the most common type of arthritis and a leading cause of disability, especially among older people. Over 20 million Americans have OA.

Chapter 7

Rheumatoid Arthritis (RA)

Features of Rheumatoid Arthritis

Rheumatoid arthritis is an inflammatory disease that causes pain, swelling, stiffness, and loss of function in the joints. It has several special features that make it different from other kinds of arthritis. For example, rheumatoid arthritis generally occurs in a symmetrical pattern. This means that if one knee or hand is involved, the other one is also. The disease often affects the wrist joints and the finger joints closest to the hand. It can also affect other parts of the body besides the joints. In addition, people with the disease may have fatigue, occasional fever, and a general sense of not feeling well (malaise).

Another feature of rheumatoid arthritis is that it varies a lot from person to person. For some people, it lasts only a few months or a year or two and goes away without causing any noticeable damage. Other people have mild or moderate disease, with periods of worsening symptoms, called flares, and periods in which they feel better, called remissions. Still others have severe disease that is active most of the time, lasts for many years, and leads to serious joint damage and disability.

Although rheumatoid arthritis can have serious effects on a person's life and well-being, current treatment strategies—including pain

"Handout on Health: Rheumatoid Arthritis," National Institute of Arthritis and Musculoskeletal and Skin Diseases (NIAMS), November 1999. Available online at http://www.niams.nih.gov; accessed November 2003. Reviewed and revised by David A. Cooke, M.D. on November 27, 2003.

relief and other medications, a balance between rest and exercise, and patient education and support programs—allow most people with the disease to lead active and productive lives. In recent years, research has led to a new understanding of rheumatoid arthritis and has increased the likelihood that, in time, researchers can find ways to greatly reduce the impact of this disease.

Features of rheumatoid arthritis include:

- Tender, warm, swollen joints.

- Symmetrical pattern. For example, if one knee is affected, the other one is also.

- Joint inflammation often affecting the wrist and finger joints closest to the hand; other affected joints can include those of the neck, shoulders, elbows, hips, knees, ankles, and feet.

- Fatigue, occasional fever, a general sense of not feeling well (malaise).

- Pain and stiffness lasting for more than 30 minutes in the morning or after a long rest.

- Symptoms that can last for many years.

- Symptoms in other parts of the body besides the joints.

- Variability of symptoms among people with the disease.

How Rheumatoid Arthritis Develops and Progresses

The Joints

A normal joint (the place where two bones meet) is surrounded by a joint capsule that protects and supports it. Cartilage covers and cushions the ends of the two bones. The joint capsule is lined with a type of tissue called synovium, which produces synovial fluid. This clear fluid lubricates and nourishes the cartilage and bones inside the joint capsule.

In rheumatoid arthritis, the immune system, for unknown reasons, attacks a person's own cells inside the joint capsule. White blood cells that are part of the normal immune system travel to the synovium and cause a reaction. This reaction, or inflammation, is called synovitis, and it results in the warmth, redness, swelling, and pain that are typical symptoms of rheumatoid arthritis. During the inflammation process, the cells of the synovium grow and divide abnormally, making the normally thin synovium thick and resulting in a joint that is swollen and puffy to the touch.

As rheumatoid arthritis progresses, these abnormal synovial cells begin to invade and destroy the cartilage and bone within the joint. The surrounding muscles, ligaments, and tendons that support and stabilize the joint become weak and unable to work normally. All of these effects lead to the pain and deformities often seen in rheumatoid arthritis. Doctors studying rheumatoid arthritis now believe that damage to bones begins during the first year or two that a person has the disease. This is one reason early diagnosis and treatment are so important in the management of rheumatoid arthritis.

A joint (the place where two bones meet) is surrounded by a capsule that protects and supports it. The joint capsule is lined with a type of tissue called synovium, which produces synovial fluid that lubricates and nourishes joint tissues. In rheumatoid arthritis, the synovium becomes inflamed, causing warmth, redness, swelling, and pain. As the disease progresses, abnormal synovial cells invade and erode, or destroy, cartilage and bone within the joint. Surrounding muscles, ligaments, and tendons become weakened. Rheumatoid arthritis can also cause more generalized bone loss that may lead to osteoporosis (fragile bones that are prone to fracture).

Other Parts of the Body

Some people also experience the effects of rheumatoid arthritis in places other than the joints. About one quarter develop rheumatoid nodules. These are bumps under the skin that often form close to the joints. Many people with rheumatoid arthritis develop anemia, or a decrease in the normal number of red blood cells. Other effects, which occur less often, include neck pain and dry eyes and mouth. Very rarely, people may have inflammation of the blood vessels, the lining of the lungs, or the sac enclosing the heart.

Occurrence and Impact of Rheumatoid Arthritis

Scientists estimate that about 2.1 million people, or 1 percent of the U.S. adult population, have rheumatoid arthritis. Interestingly, some recent studies have suggested that the overall number of new cases of rheumatoid arthritis may actually be going down. Scientists are now investigating why this may be happening.

Rheumatoid arthritis occurs in all races and ethnic groups. Although the disease often begins in middle age and occurs with increased frequency in older people, children and young adults also develop it. Like some other forms of arthritis, rheumatoid arthritis occurs much more frequently in women than in men. About two to three times as many women as men have the disease.

By all measures, the financial and social impact of all types of arthritis, including rheumatoid arthritis, is substantial, both for the

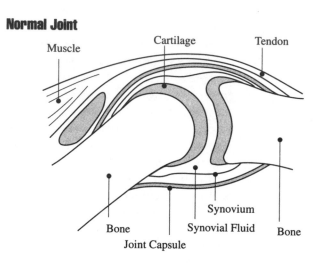

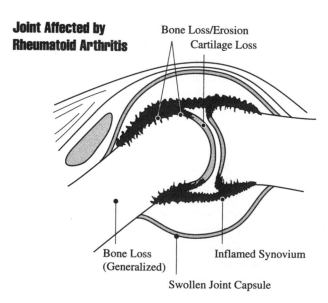

Figure 7.1. *Comparison of Normal Joint and Joint Affected by Rheumatoid Arthritis*

nation and for individuals. From an economic standpoint, the medical and surgical treatment for rheumatoid arthritis and the wages lost because of disability caused by the disease add up to millions of dollars. Daily joint pain is an inevitable consequence of the disease, and most patients also experience some degree of depression, anxiety, and feelings of helplessness. In some cases, rheumatoid arthritis can interfere with a person's ability to carry out normal daily activities, limit job opportunities, or disrupt the joys and responsibilities of family life. However, there are arthritis self-management programs that help people cope with the pain and other effects of the disease and help them lead independent and productive lives.

Searching for the Cause of Rheumatoid Arthritis

Rheumatoid arthritis is one of several autoimmune diseases ("auto" means self), so-called because a person's immune system attacks his or her own body tissues. Scientists still do not know exactly what causes this to happen, but research over the last few years has begun to unravel the factors involved.

Genetic (inherited) factors. Scientists have found that certain genes that play a role in the immune system are associated with a tendency to develop rheumatoid arthritis. At the same time, some people with rheumatoid arthritis do not have these particular genes, and other people have these genes but never develop the disease. This suggests that a person's genetic makeup is an important part of the story but not the whole answer. It is clear, however, that more than one gene is involved in determining whether a person develops rheumatoid arthritis and, if so, how severe the disease will become.

Environmental factors. Many scientists think that something must occur to trigger the disease process in people whose genetic makeup makes them susceptible to rheumatoid arthritis. An infectious agent such as a virus or bacterium appears likely, but the exact agent is not yet known. Note, however, that rheumatoid arthritis is not contagious: A person cannot catch it from someone else.

Other factors. Some scientists also think that a variety of hormonal factors may be involved. These hormones, or possibly deficiencies or changes in certain hormones, may promote the development of rheumatoid arthritis in a genetically susceptible person who has been exposed to a triggering agent from the environment.

Even though all the answers aren't known, one thing is certain: Rheumatoid arthritis develops as a result of an interaction of many factors. Much research is going on now to understand these factors and how they work together.

Diagnosing and Treating Rheumatoid Arthritis

Diagnosing and treating rheumatoid arthritis is a team effort between the patient and several types of health care professionals. A person can go to his or her family doctor or internist or to a rheumatologist. A rheumatologist is a doctor who specializes in arthritis and other diseases of the joints, bones, and muscles. As treatment progresses, other professionals often help. These may include nurses, physical or occupational therapists, orthopedic surgeons, psychologists, and social workers.

Studies have shown that people who are well informed and participate actively in their own care experience less pain and make fewer visits to the doctor than do other people with rheumatoid arthritis.

Patient education and arthritis self-management programs, as well as support groups, help people to become better informed and to participate in their own care. An example of a self-management program is the arthritis self-help course offered by the Arthritis Foundation and developed at one of the NIAMS-supported Multipurpose Arthritis and Musculoskeletal Diseases Centers. Self-management programs teach about rheumatoid arthritis and its treatments, exercise and relaxation approaches, patient/health care provider communication, and problem solving. Research on these programs has shown that they have the following clear and long-lasting benefits:

- They help people understand the disease.

- They help people reduce their pain while remaining active.

- They help people cope physically, emotionally, and mentally.

- They help people feel greater control over their disease and help build a sense of confidence in the ability to function and lead a full, active, and independent life.

Diagnosis

Rheumatoid arthritis can be difficult to diagnose in its early stages for several reasons. First, there is no single test for the disease. In addition, symptoms differ from person to person and can be more severe in some people than in others. Also, symptoms can be similar to those of other types of arthritis and joint conditions, and it may take some time for other conditions to be ruled out as possible diagnoses. Finally, the full range of symptoms develops over time, and only a few symptoms may be present in the early stages. As a result, doctors use a variety of tools to diagnose the disease and to rule out other conditions.

Medical history. This is the patient's description of symptoms and when and how they began. Good communication between patient and doctor is especially important here. For example, the patient's description of pain, stiffness, and joint function and how these change over time is critical to the doctor's initial assessment of the disease and his or her assessment of how the disease changes.

Physical examination. This includes the doctor's examination of the joints, skin, reflexes, and muscle strength.

Laboratory tests. One common test is for rheumatoid factor, an antibody that is eventually present in the blood of most rheumatoid arthritis patients. (An antibody is a special protein made by the immune system that normally helps fight foreign substances in the body.) Not all people with rheumatoid arthritis test positive for rheumatoid factor, however, especially early in the disease. And some others who do test positive never develop the disease. Other common tests include one that indicates the presence of inflammation in the body (the erythrocyte sedimentation rate), a white blood cell count, and a blood test for anemia.

X-rays. X-rays are used to determine the degree of joint destruction. They are not useful in the early stages of rheumatoid arthritis before bone damage is evident, but they can be used later to monitor the progression of the disease.

Treatment

Doctors use a variety of approaches to treat rheumatoid arthritis. These are used in different combinations and at different times during the course of the disease and are chosen according to the patient's individual situation. No matter what treatment the doctor and patient choose, however, the goals are the same: relieve pain, reduce inflammation, slow down or stop joint damage, and improve the person's sense of well-being and ability to function.

Treatment is another key area for communication between patient and doctor. Talking to the doctor can help ensure that exercise and pain management programs are provided as needed and that drugs are prescribed appropriately. Talking can also help in making decisions about surgery.

Lifestyle

This approach includes several activities that help improve a person's ability to function independently and maintain a positive outlook.

Rest and Exercise

Both rest and exercise help in important ways. People with rheumatoid arthritis need a good balance between the two, with more rest when the disease is active and more exercise when it is not. Rest helps to reduce active joint inflammation and pain and to fight fatigue. The length of time needed for rest will vary from person to person, but in general, shorter rest breaks every now and then are more helpful than long times spent in bed.

Exercise is important for maintaining healthy and strong muscles, preserving joint mobility, and maintaining flexibility. Exercise can also help people sleep well, reduce pain, maintain a positive attitude, and lose weight. Exercise programs should be planned and carried out to take into account the person's physical abilities, limitations, and changing needs.

Care of Joints

Some people find that using a splint for a short time around a painful joint reduces pain and swelling by supporting the joint and letting it rest. Splints are used mostly on wrists and hands, but also on ankles and feet. A doctor or a physical or occupational therapist can help a patient get a splint and ensure that it fits properly. Other ways to reduce stress on joints include self-help devices (for example, zipper pullers, long-handled shoe horns); devices to help with getting on and off chairs, toilet seats, and beds; and changes in the ways that a person carries out daily activities.

Stress Reduction

People with rheumatoid arthritis face emotional challenges as well as physical ones. The emotions they feel because of the disease—fear, anger, frustration—combined with any pain and physical limitations can increase their stress level. Although there is no evidence that stress plays a role in causing rheumatoid arthritis, it can make living with the disease difficult at times. Stress may also affect the amount of pain a person feels. There are a number of successful techniques for coping with stress. Regular rest periods can help, as can relaxation, distraction, or visualization exercises. Exercise programs, participation in support groups, and good communication with the health care team are other ways to reduce stress.

Healthful Diet

There is little scientific evidence that any specific food or nutrient helps or harms most people with rheumatoid arthritis. However, an overall nutritious diet with enough—but not an excess of—calories, protein, and calcium is important. Some people may need to be careful about drinking alcoholic beverages because of the medications they take for rheumatoid arthritis. Those taking methotrexate may need to avoid alcohol altogether. Patients should ask their doctors for guidance on this issue.

Climate

Some people notice that their arthritis gets worse when there is a sudden change in the weather. However, there is no evidence that a specific climate can prevent or reduce the effects of rheumatoid arthritis. Moving to a new place with a different climate usually does not make a long-term difference in a person's rheumatoid arthritis.

Medications

Most people who have rheumatoid arthritis take medications. Some medications are used only for pain relief; others are used to reduce inflammation. Still others—often called disease-modifying antirheumatic drugs, or DMARDs—are used to try to slow the course of the disease. The person's general condition, the current and predicted severity of the illness, the length of time he or she will take the drug, and the drug's effectiveness and potential side effects are important considerations in prescribing drugs for rheumatoid arthritis.

Traditionally, rheumatoid arthritis therapy has involved an approach in which doctors prescribed aspirin or similar drugs, rest, and physical therapy first, and prescribed more powerful drugs later only if the disease became much worse. Recently, many doctors have changed their approach, especially for patients with severe, rapidly progressing rheumatoid arthritis. This change is based on the belief that early treatment with more powerful drugs, and the use of drug combinations in place of single drugs, may be more effective ways to halt the progression of the disease and reduce or prevent joint damage. Medications such as prednisone and methotrexate are commonly employed to reduce disease activity and prevent joint damage. However, these drugs are potentially toxic and cause immunosuppression (a weakened immune system), which increases the risk of serious infections.

Recently, a new generation of medications known as immunomodulators have become available for rheumatoid arthritis. These drugs are the result of an improved scientific understanding of the cellular events that lead to joint inflammation. Often, they dramatically improve disease activity, and prevent the progression of crippling arthritis. These drugs include adalimumab (Humira™), anakinra (Kineret™), etanercept (Enbrel™), infliximab (Remicade™), and leflunomide (Arava™). Many other drugs are under development.

Although these new drugs are the most promising therapies for rheumatoid arthritis so far, they do have a number of drawbacks. They must be given by injection and are extremely expensive. Because they work by blocking the action of specific chemicals produced by immune cells, they also cause some degree of immunosuppression. Still, for patients with more than mild rheumatoid arthritis, they present exciting new treatment options.

Surgery

Several types of surgery are available to patients with severe joint damage. The primary purpose of these procedures is to reduce pain, improve the affected joint's function, and improve the patient's ability to perform daily activities. Surgery is not for everyone, however, and the decision should be made only after careful consideration by patient and doctor. Together they should discuss the patient's overall health, the condition of the joint or tendon that will be operated on, and the reason for and the risks and benefits of, the surgical procedure. Cost may be another factor. Commonly performed surgical procedures include joint replacement, tendon reconstruction, and synovectomy.

Joint replacement. This is the most frequently performed surgery for rheumatoid arthritis, and it is done primarily to relieve pain and improve or preserve joint function. Artificial joints are not always permanent and may eventually have to be replaced. This may be an issue for younger people.

Tendon reconstruction. Rheumatoid arthritis can damage and even rupture tendons, the tissues that attach muscle to bone. This surgery, which is used most frequently on the hands, reconstructs the damaged tendon by attaching an intact tendon to it. This procedure can help to restore hand function, especially if the tendon is completely ruptured.

Synovectomy. In this surgery, the doctor actually removes the inflamed synovial tissue. Synovectomy by itself is seldom performed now because not all of the tissue can be removed, and it eventually grows back. Synovectomy is done as part of reconstructive surgery, especially tendon reconstruction.

Routine Monitoring and Ongoing Care

Regular medical care is important to monitor the course of the disease, determine the effectiveness and any negative effects of medications, and change therapies as needed. Monitoring typically includes regular visits to the doctor. It may also include blood, urine, and other laboratory tests and x-rays.

Osteoporosis prevention is one issue that patients may want to discuss with their doctors as part of their long-term, ongoing care. Osteoporosis is a condition in which bones lose calcium and become weakened and fragile. Many older women are at increased risk for osteoporosis, and their rheumatoid arthritis increases the risk further, particularly if they are taking corticosteroids such as prednisone. These patients may want to discuss with their doctors the potential benefits of calcium and vitamin D supplements, hormone replacement therapy, or other treatments for osteoporosis.

Alternative and Complementary Therapies

Special diets, vitamin supplements, and other alternative approaches have been suggested for the treatment of rheumatoid arthritis. However, none that have been scientifically studied have shown significant benefit. Some alternative or complementary approaches may help the patient cope or reduce some of the stress associated with living with a chronic illness. As with any therapy, patients should discuss the benefits and drawbacks with their doctors before beginning an alternative or new type of therapy. It is not safe to assume that a therapy "can't hurt." If the doctor feels the approach has value and will not be harmful, it can be incorporated into a patient's treatment plan. However, it is important not to neglect regular health care. The Arthritis Foundation publishes material on alternative therapies as well as established therapies, and patients may want to contact this organization for information.

For More Information

National Institute of Arthritis and Musculoskeletal and Skin Diseases
1 AMS Circle
Bethesda, MD 20892-3675
Toll-Free: (877) 22-NIAMS (226-4267)
Phone: (301) 495-4484
TTY: (301) 565-2966
Fax: (301) 718-6366
Website: http://www.niams.nih.gov
E-mail: niamsinfo@mail.nih.gov

Arthritis Foundation
1330 West Peachtree Street
Atlanta, GA 30309
Toll-Free: (800) 283-7800
Phone: (404) 872-7100
Website: http://www.arthritis.org

American College of Rheumatology
1800 Century Place, Suite 250
Atlanta, GA 30345-4300
Phone: (404) 633-3777
Fax: (404) 633-1870
Website: http://www.rheumatology.org

American Academy of Orthopaedic Surgeons (AAOS)
6300 North River Road
Rosemont, IL 60018-4262
Toll-Free: (800) 824-BONE (2663)
Phone: (847) 823-7186
Fax: (847) 823-8125
Website: http://www.aaos.org
E-mail: custserv@aaos.org

Chapter 8

Juvenile Rheumatoid Arthritis and Still Disease

Chapter Contents

Section 8.1

Questions and Answers about Juvenile Rheumatoid Arthritis

National Institute of Arthritis and Musculoskeletal and Skin Diseases (NIAMS), July 2001. Available online at http://www.niams.nih.gov; accessed December 2003.

What Is Arthritis?

Arthritis means joint inflammation and refers to a group of diseases that cause pain, swelling, stiffness, and loss of motion in the joints. Arthritis is often used as a more general term to refer to the more than 100 rheumatic diseases that may affect the joints but can also cause pain, swelling, and stiffness in other supporting structures of the body such as muscles, tendons, ligaments, and bones. Some rheumatic diseases can affect other parts of the body, including various internal organs. Children can develop almost all types of arthritis that affect adults, but the most common type that affects children is juvenile rheumatoid arthritis (JRA).

What Is Juvenile Rheumatoid Arthritis?

Juvenile rheumatoid arthritis is arthritis that causes joint inflammation and stiffness for more than 6 weeks in a child of 16 years of age or less. Inflammation causes redness, swelling, warmth, and soreness in the joints, although many children with JRA do not complain of joint pain. Any joint can be affected and inflammation may limit the mobility of affected joints. One type of JRA can also affect the internal organs. Doctors classify JRA into three types by the number of joints involved, the symptoms, and the presence or absence of certain antibodies found by a blood test. (Antibodies are special proteins made by the immune system.) These classifications help the doctor determine how the disease will progress and whether the internal organs or skin is affected.

120

Pauciarticular JRA

Pauciarticular means that four or fewer joints are affected. Pauciarticular is the most common form of JRA; about half of all children with JRA have this type. Pauciarticular disease typically affects large joints, such as the knees. Girls under age 8 are most likely to develop this type of JRA.

Some children have special kinds of antibodies in the blood. One is called antinuclear antibody (ANA) and one is called rheumatoid factor. Eye disease affects about 20 to 30 percent of children with pauciarticular JRA. Up to 80 percent of those with eye disease also test positive for ANA and the disease tends to develop at a particularly early age in these children. Regular examinations by an ophthalmologist (a doctor who specializes in eye diseases) are necessary to prevent serious eye problems such as iritis (inflammation of the iris, the colored part of the eye) or uveitis (inflammation of the uvea, or the inner eye). Some children with pauciarticular disease outgrow arthritis by adulthood, although eye problems can continue and joint symptoms may recur in some people.

Polyarticular JRA

About 30 percent of all children with JRA have polyarticular disease. In polyarticular disease, five or more joints are affected. The small joints, such as those in the hands and feet, are most commonly involved, but the disease may also affect large joints. Polyarticular JRA often is symmetrical; that is, it affects the same joint on both sides of the body. Some children with polyarticular disease have an antibody in their blood called IgM rheumatoid factor (RF). These children often have a more severe form of the disease, which doctors consider to be similar in many ways to adult rheumatoid arthritis.

Systemic JRA

Besides joint swelling, the systemic form of JRA is characterized by fever and a light skin rash, and may also affect internal organs such as the heart, liver, spleen, and lymph nodes. Doctors sometimes call it Still disease. Almost all children with this type of JRA test negative for both RF and ANA. The systemic form affects 20 percent of all children with JRA. A small percentage of these children develop arthritis in many joints and can have severe arthritis that continues into adulthood.

What Causes Juvenile Rheumatoid Arthritis?

JRA is an autoimmune disorder, which means that the body mistakenly identifies some of its own cells and tissues as foreign. The immune system, which normally helps to fight off harmful, foreign substances such as bacteria or viruses, begins to attack healthy cells and tissues.

The result is inflammation—marked by redness, heat, pain, and swelling. Doctors do not know why the immune system goes awry in children who develop JRA. Scientists suspect that it is a two-step process. First, something in a child's genetic makeup gives them a tendency to develop JRA; then an environmental factor, such as a virus, triggers the development of JRA.

What Are the Symptoms and Signs of Juvenile Rheumatoid Arthritis?

The most common symptom of all types of JRA is persistent joint swelling, pain, and stiffness that typically is worse in the morning or after a nap. The pain may limit movement of the affected joint although many children, especially younger ones, will not complain of pain. JRA commonly affects the knees and joints in the hands and feet. One of the earliest signs of JRA may be limping in the morning because of an affected knee. Besides joint symptoms, children with systemic JRA have a high fever and a light skin rash. The rash and fever may appear and disappear very quickly. Systemic JRA also may cause the lymph nodes located in the neck and other parts of the body to swell. In some cases (less than half), internal organs including the heart and, very rarely, the lungs may be involved.

Eye inflammation is a potentially severe complication that sometimes occurs in children with pauciarticular JRA. Eye diseases such as iritis and uveitis often are not present until some time after a child first develops JRA.

Typically, there are periods when the symptoms of JRA are better or disappear (remissions) and times when symptoms are worse (flare-ups). JRA is different in each child—some may have just one or two flare-ups and never have symptoms again, while others experience many flare-ups or even have symptoms that never go away.

Some children with JRA may have growth problems. Depending on the severity of the disease and the joints involved, growth in affected joints may be too fast or too slow, causing one leg or arm to be longer than the other. Overall growth may also be slowed. Doctors are exploring the use of growth hormones to treat this problem. JRA also may cause joints to grow unevenly or to one side.

How Is Juvenile Rheumatoid Arthritis Diagnosed?

Doctors usually suspect JRA, along with several other possible conditions, when they see children with persistent joint pain or swelling, unexplained skin rashes and fever, or swelling of lymph nodes or inflammation of internal organs. A diagnosis of JRA also is considered in children with an unexplained limp or excessive clumsiness.

No one test can be used to diagnose JRA. A doctor diagnoses JRA by carefully examining the patient and considering the patient's medical history, the results of laboratory tests, and x-rays that help rule out other conditions.

- Symptoms—One important consideration in diagnosing JRA is the length of time that symptoms have been present. Joint swelling or pain must last for at least 6 weeks for the doctor to consider a diagnosis of JRA. Because this factor is so important, it may be useful to keep a record of the symptoms, when they first appeared, and when they are worse or better.

- Laboratory tests—Laboratory tests, usually blood tests, cannot by themselves provide the doctor with a clear diagnosis. But these tests can be used to help rule out other conditions and to help classify the type of JRA that a patient has. Blood may be taken to test for RF and ANA, and to determine the erythrocyte sedimentation rate (ESR). ANA is found in the blood more often than RF, and both are found in only a small portion of JRA patients. The RF test helps the doctor tell the difference among the three types of JRA. ESR is a test that measures how quickly red blood cells fall to the bottom of a test tube. Some people with rheumatic disease have an elevated ESR or sed rate (cells fall quickly to the bottom of the test tube), showing that there is inflammation in the body. Not all children with active joint inflammation have an elevated ESR.

- X-rays—X-rays are needed if the doctor suspects injury to the bone or unusual bone development. Early in the disease, some x-rays can show cartilage damage. In general, x-rays are more useful later in the disease, when bones may be affected.

- Other diseases—Because there are many causes of joint pain and swelling, the doctor must rule out other conditions before diagnosing JRA. These include physical injury, bacterial or viral infection, Lyme disease, inflammatory bowel disease, lupus, dermatomyositis, and some forms of cancer. The doctor may use additional laboratory tests to help rule out these and other possible conditions.

Who Treats Juvenile Rheumatoid Arthritis? What Are the Treatments?

The special expertise of rheumatologists in caring for patients with JRA is extremely valuable. Pediatric rheumatologists are trained in both pediatrics and rheumatology and are best equipped to deal with the complex problems of children with arthritis and other rheumatic diseases. However, there are very few such specialists, and some areas of the country have none at all. In such circumstances, a team approach involving the child's pediatrician and a rheumatologist with experience in both adult and pediatric rheumatic disease provides optimal care for children with arthritis. Other important members of the team include physical therapists and occupational therapists.

The main goals of treatment are to preserve a high level of physical and social functioning and maintain a good quality of life. To achieve these goals, doctors recommend treatments to reduce swelling; maintain full movement in the affected joints; relieve pain; and identify, treat, and prevent complications. Most children with JRA need medication and physical therapy to reach these goals.

Several types of medication are available to treat JRA:

- **Nonsteroidal anti-inflammatory drugs (NSAIDs)**—Aspirin, ibuprofen (Motrin, Advil, Nuprin), and naproxen or naproxen sodium (Naprosyn, Aleve) are examples of NSAIDs. They often are the first type of medication used. Most doctors do not treat children with aspirin because of the possibility that it will cause bleeding problems, stomach upset, liver problems, or Reye syndrome. But for some children, aspirin in the correct dose (measured by blood test) can control JRA symptoms effectively with few serious side effects. If the doctor prefers not to use aspirin, other NSAIDs are available. For example, in addition to those mentioned above, diclofenac and tolmetin are available with a doctor's prescription. Studies show that these medications are as effective as aspirin with fewer side effects. An upset stomach is the most common complaint. Any side effects should be reported to the doctor, who may change the type or amount of medication.

- **Disease-modifying anti-rheumatic drugs (DMARDs)**—If NSAIDs do not relieve symptoms of JRA, the doctor is likely to prescribe this type of medication. DMARDs slow the progression of JRA, but because they take weeks or months to relieve symptoms, they often are taken with an NSAID. Various types of DMARDs are available. Doctors are likely to use one type of DMARD, methotrexate, for children with JRA. Researchers have learned that methotrexate is safe and effective for some children with rheumatoid arthritis whose symptoms are not relieved by other medications. Because only small doses of methotrexate are needed to relieve arthritis symptoms, potentially dangerous side effects rarely occur. The most serious complication is liver damage, but it can be avoided with regular blood screening tests and doctor followup. Careful monitoring for side effects is important for people taking methotrexate. When side effects are noticed early, the doctor can reduce the dose and eliminate side effects.

- **Corticosteroids**—In children with very severe JRA, stronger medicines may be needed to stop serious symptoms such as inflammation of the sac around the heart (pericarditis). Corticosteroids like prednisone may be added to the treatment plan to control severe symptoms. This medication can be given either intravenously (directly into the vein) or by mouth. Corticosteroids can interfere with a child's normal growth and can cause other side effects, such as a round face, weakened bones, and increased susceptibility to infections. Once the medication controls severe symptoms, the doctor may reduce the dose gradually and eventually stop it completely. Because it can be dangerous to stop taking corticosteroids suddenly, it is important that the patient carefully follow the doctor's instructions about how to take or reduce the dose.

- **Biologic agents**—Children with polyarticular JRA who have gotten little relief from other drugs may be given one of a new class of drug treatments called biologic agents. Etanercept (Enbrel), for example, is such an agent. It blocks the actions of tumor necrosis factor, a naturally occurring protein in the body that helps cause inflammation.

- **Physical therapy**—Exercise is an important part of a child's treatment plan. It can help to maintain muscle tone and preserve and recover the range of motion of the joints. A physiatrist

125

(rehabilitation specialist) or a physical therapist can design an appropriate exercise program for a person with JRA. The specialist also may recommend using splints and other devices to help maintain normal bone and joint growth.

- **Complementary and alternative medicine**—Many adults seek alternative ways of treating arthritis, such as special diets or supplements. Although these methods may not be harmful in and of themselves, no research to date shows that they help. Some people have tried acupuncture, in which thin needles are inserted at specific points in the body. Others have tried glucosamine and chondroitin sulfate, two natural substances found in osteoarthritis of the knee. Some alternative or complementary approaches may help a child to cope with or reduce some of the stress of living with a chronic illness. If the doctor feels the approach has value and will not harm the child, it can be incorporated into the treatment plan. However, it is important not to neglect regular health care or treatment of serious symptoms.

How Can the Family Help a Child Live Well with JRA?

JRA affects the entire family who must cope with the special challenges of this disease. JRA can strain a child's participation in social and after-school activities and make schoolwork more difficult. There are several things that family members can do to help the child do well physically and emotionally.

- Treat the child as normally as possible.

- Ensure that the child receives appropriate medical care and follows the doctor's instructions. Many treatment options are available, and because JRA is different in each child, what works for one may not work for another. If the medications that the doctor prescribes do not relieve symptoms or if they cause unpleasant side effects, patients and parents should discuss other choices with their doctor. A person with JRA can be more active when symptoms are controlled.

- Encourage exercise and physical therapy for the child. For many young people, exercise and physical therapy play important roles in managing JRA. Parents can arrange for children to participate in activities that the doctor recommends. During symptom-free periods, many doctors suggest playing team sports or doing other activities to help keep the joints strong

126

and flexible and to provide play time with other children and encourage appropriate social development.

- Work closely with the school to develop a suitable lesson plan for the child and to educate the teacher and the child's classmates about JRA. Some children with JRA may be absent from school for prolonged periods and need to have the teacher send assignments home. Some minor changes such as an extra set of books, or leaving class a few minutes early to get to the next class on time can be a great help. With proper attention, most children progress normally through school.

- Explain to the child that getting JRA is nobody's fault. Some children believe that JRA is a punishment for something they did.

- Consider joining a support group. The American Juvenile Arthritis Organization runs support groups for people with JRA and their families. Support group meetings provide the chance to talk to other young people and parents of children with JRA and may help a child and the family cope with the condition.

- Work with therapists or social workers to adapt more easily to the lifestyle change JRA may bring.

Do Children with Juvenile Rheumatoid Arthritis Have to Limit Activities?

Although pain sometimes limits physical activity, exercise is important to reduce the symptoms of JRA and maintain function and range of motion of the joints. Most children with JRA can take part fully in physical activities and sports when their symptoms are under control. During a disease flare-up, however, the doctor may advise limiting certain activities depending on the joints involved. Once the flare-up is over, a child can start regular activities again.

Swimming is particularly useful because it uses many joints and muscles without putting weight on the joints. A doctor or physical therapist can recommend exercises and activities.

What Are Researchers Trying to Learn about Juvenile Rheumatoid Arthritis?

Scientists are investigating the possible causes of JRA. Researchers suspect that both genetic and environmental factors are involved in development of the disease and they are studying these factors in detail. To help explore the role of genetics, the National Institute of Arthritis and Musculoskeletal and Skin Diseases (NIAMS) has established a research registry for families in which two or more siblings have JRA. NIAMS also funds a Multipurpose Arthritis and Musculoskeletal Diseases Center (MAMDC) that specializes in research on pediatric rheumatic diseases including JRA.

The research registry for JRA is located at Children's Hospital Medical Center at the University of Cincinnati College of Medicine in Ohio. The registry, established in 1994, continues to list new cases as well as be maintained and systematically updated. The focus of the registry is on families whose brothers and sisters have JRA, with emphasis on genetic susceptibility in those affected families.

Researchers are continuing to try to improve existing treatments and find new medicines that will work better with fewer side effects. For example, researchers are studying the long-term effects of the use of methotrexate in children. In addition, the Food and Drug Administration's Pediatric Rule requires manufacturers of new drugs and biologic agents, such as etanercept, that will be commonly used for children to provide specific information about safe pediatric use.

For More Information

National Institute of Arthritis and Musculoskeletal and Skin Diseases
1 AMS Circle
Bethesda, MD 20892-3675
Toll-Free: (877) 22-NIAMS (226-4267)
Phone: (301) 495-4484
TTY: (301) 565-2966
Fax: (301) 718-6366
Website: http://www.niams.nih.gov
E-mail: niamsinfo@mail.nih.gov

American Academy of Orthopaedic Surgeons (AAOS)
6300 North River Road
Rosemont, IL 60018-4262
Toll-Free: (800) 824-BONE (2663)
Phone: (847) 823-7186
Fax: (847) 823-8125
Website: http://www.aaos.org
E-mail: custserv@aaos.org

American College of Rheumatology
1800 Century Place, Suite 250
Atlanta, GA 30345-4300
Phone: (404) 633-3777
Fax: (404) 633-1870
Website: http://www.rheumatology.org

American Juvenile Arthritis Organization
1330 West Peachtree Street
Atlanta, GA 30309
Toll-Free: (800) 283-7800
Phone: (404) 872-7100
Website: http://www.arthritis.org

Kids on the Block, Inc.
9385-C Gerwig Lane
Columbia, MD 21046
Toll-Free: (800) 368-KIDS (5437)
Phone: (410) 290-9095
Fax: (410) 290-9358
Website: http://www.kotb.com
E-mail: kotb@kotb.com

Section 8.2

Pain of Juvenile Arthritis May Reduce School and Social Activity

National Institute of Arthritis and Musculoskeletal and Skin Diseases (NIAMS), August 2003. Available online at http://www.niams.nih.gov; accessed January 2004.

Scientists studying children with juvenile arthritis have found that increased pain and fatigue are linked to reduced participation in school and social activity. In addition, the researchers, led by Laura E. Schanberg, M.D., of Duke University Medical Center, noted that anxiety is also significantly associated with increased pain and fatigue. Physicians, conclude the authors, "should consider treating pain more aggressively in children with arthritis with standard pharmacologic therapies." The scientists also recommend "therapeutic interventions to treat anxiety, including psychotropic medication and cognitive-behavioral therapy."

The two-month study, supported by the National Institute of Arthritis and Musculoskeletal and Skin Diseases (NIAMS), the Office of Research on Women's Health (ORWH) and the private sector, involved 41 children with juvenile arthritis. Key components of the study were new assessment tools and a patient diary. Diary analysis in conjunction with standard clinical testing showed that increased anxiety—and, surprisingly, not depressed mood—was significantly associated with increased fatigue and pain frequency and intensity.

Juvenile arthritis is one of the most prevalent chronic diseases in children in the United States. While arthritis pain has been the focus of much research in adults, there is an increasing awareness of the need to focus on pain in children. Children with juvenile arthritis may have pain that can be intense and disabling, and comprehensive treatment optimizes their ability to fully participate in school and social activities.

Schanberg L, Anthony K, Gil K, and Maurin E. Daily pain and symptoms in children with polyarticular arthritis. *Arthritis and Rheumatism,* 2003; 48(5):1390–97.

Section 8.3

Systemic Juvenile Rheumatoid Arthritis (Still Disease) in Adults

Definition

Adult Still disease is an illness with fever, rash, and joint pain. It may lead to chronic arthritis.

Causes, Incidence, and Risk Factors

The cause of adult Still disease is unknown. The condition rarely occurs in adults. It is more common in children, where it is called systemic juvenile rheumatoid arthritis. No risk factors for the disease have been identified.

Symptoms

Almost all patients will have fever, joint pain, sore throat, and a rash. The fever usually comes on quickly once per day, most commonly in the afternoon or evening. The rash is typically salmon pink-colored and comes and goes with the fever.

Another common symptom is joint pain and inflammation (warmth and swelling of the joint). Usually, several joints are involved at the same time.

Additional symptoms include swollen lymph nodes (glands), pain with a deep breath (pleurisy), abdominal pain and swelling, and weight loss.

Signs and Tests

The physical exam may show the fever, rash, and arthritis. Other signs include enlargement of the lymph nodes, liver, or spleen. Also, the presence of changes in the sound of the heart or lungs may indicate pericarditis or pleurisy.

Blood tests that can be helpful in diagnosing adult Still disease include:

- elevation in the ESR (erythrocyte sedimentation rate)
- elevation in the white blood cell count
- elevation in liver function tests
- decrease in the red blood cell count
- very high elevation in the ferritin level
- negative rheumatoid factor and antinuclear antibodies (ANA) test

Other tests may include:

- joint x-rays
- chest x-ray that may show pericarditis or pleural effusion
- abdominal x-ray, computed tomography (CT) scan, or ultrasound for liver and spleen enlargement

Adult Still disease can only be diagnosed after other diseases are excluded. It may require many medical tests before a final diagnosis is made.

Treatment

The symptoms of arthritis are generally controlled with adequate doses of salicylates (aspirin) or nonsteroidal anti-inflammatory medications (NSAIDs) such as ibuprofen. Prednisone may be used for more severe cases. If the disease becomes chronic, immunosuppressive medications might be needed. These may include methotrexate or new biologic therapies.

Expectations (Prognosis)

Studies show that about 20% of patients have all of the symptoms go away in a year and never come back. About 30% of patients have all of the symptoms go away, but they come back several times over the next years. The rest of the patients (about 50%) will develop chronic arthritis.

Complications

- arthritis

- liver disease
- spleen enlargement
- pericarditis
- pleural effusion

Calling Your Health Care Provider

Call for an appointment with your health care provider if symptoms are present that are suggestive of adult Still disease.

Call your health care provider if cough, difficulty breathing, or other symptoms develop in a person with adult Still disease.

Chapter 9

Infectious and Reactive Arthritis

Chapter Contents

135

Section 9.1

Understanding Infectious Arthritis

What Is It?

Septic arthritis, also called infectious or bacterial arthritis, is not as common as some of the other types of arthritis. However, it needs to be diagnosed and treated quickly because it can destroy joints in a short period of time. Septic arthritis occurs most often following direct injury, such as in an accident, in persons with artificial joints, and in persons with bacteremia due to certain infections, such as a skin infection. Additional risk factors include age (older than 80 years), having diabetes or rheumatoid arthritis, and recent joint surgery. The knee and the hip are the most commonly infected joints. The acute form of septic arthritis is usually caused by organisms, such as *staphylococcus, streptococcus (pneumoniae)*, and *group B streptococcus*; the chronic form, although more rare, is often caused by *Mycobacterium tuberculosis* and *Candida albicans*.

What Tests Are Used?

The following are common tests used to diagnose septic arthritis:

- Blood culture;
- Culture of joint fluid or synovial fluid analysis; and
- X-ray of joint(s).

What Treatments Exist?

Treatment is with antibiotics. The exact antibiotic used will depend on the causative bacteria, which can be identified from a culture. Then, the antibiotic therapy can be adjusted depending on the results of antibiotic susceptibility tests, which determine what specific antibiotics the bacterium is most sensitive to.

In some cases, the build up of synovial fluid in the joint that occurs because of the infection requires aspiration (using a needle and suction to remove the liquid); in more severe cases, surgery may be needed to drain the fluid.

Section 9.2

Reiter Syndrome (Reactive Arthritis)

"Questions and Answers about Reactive Arthritis," National Institute of Arthritis and Musculoskeletal and Skin Diseases (NIAMS), August 2002. Available online at http://www.niams.nih.gov; accessed February 2004.

What Is Reactive Arthritis?

Reactive arthritis is a form of arthritis, or joint inflammation, that occurs as a reaction to an infection elsewhere in the body. Inflammation is a characteristic reaction of tissues to injury or disease and is marked by swelling, redness, heat, and pain. Besides this joint inflammation, reactive arthritis is associated with two other symptoms: redness and inflammation of the eyes (conjunctivitis) and inflammation of the urinary tract (urethritis). These symptoms may occur alone, together, or not at all.

Reactive arthritis is also known as Reiter syndrome, and your doctor may refer to it by yet another term, as a seronegative spondyloarthropathy. The seronegative spondyloarthropathies are a group of disorders that can cause inflammation throughout the body, especially in the spine. (Examples of other disorders in this group include psoriatic arthritis, ankylosing spondylitis, and the kind of arthritis that sometimes accompanies inflammatory bowel disease.)

In many patients, reactive arthritis is triggered by a venereal infection in the bladder, the urethra, or, in women, the vagina (the urogenital tract) that is often transmitted through sexual contact. This form of the disorder is sometimes called genitourinary or urogenital reactive arthritis. Another form of reactive arthritis is caused by an infection in the intestinal tract from eating food or handling substances that are contaminated with bacteria. This form of arthritis is sometimes called enteric or gastrointestinal reactive arthritis.

The symptoms of reactive arthritis usually last 3 to 12 months, although symptoms can return or develop into a long-term disease in a small percentage of people.

What Causes Reactive Arthritis?

Reactive arthritis typically begins about 1 to 3 weeks after infection. The bacterium most often associated with reactive arthritis is *Chlamydia trachomatis,* commonly known as chlamydia. It is usually acquired through sexual contact. Some evidence also shows that respiratory infections with *Chlamydia pneumoniae* may trigger reactive arthritis.

Infections in the digestive tract that may trigger reactive arthritis include *Salmonella, Shigella, Yersinia,* and *Campylobacter*. People may become infected with these bacteria after eating or handling improperly prepared food, such as meats that are not stored at the proper temperature.

Doctors do not know exactly why some people exposed to these bacteria develop reactive arthritis and others do not, but they have identified a genetic factor, human leukocyte antigen (HLA) B27, that increases a person's chance of developing reactive arthritis. Approximately 80 percent of people with reactive arthritis test positive for HLA-B27. However, inheriting the HLA-B27 gene does not necessarily mean you will get reactive arthritis. Eight percent of healthy people have the HLA-B27 gene, and only about one fifth of them will develop reactive arthritis if they contract the triggering infections.

Is Reactive Arthritis Contagious?

Reactive arthritis is not contagious; that is, a person with the disorder cannot pass the arthritis on to someone else. However, the bacteria that can trigger reactive arthritis can be passed from person to person.

Who Gets Reactive Arthritis?

Overall, men between the ages of 20 and 40 are most likely to develop reactive arthritis. However, evidence shows that although men are nine times more likely than women to develop reactive arthritis due to venereally acquired infections, women and men are equally likely to develop reactive arthritis as a result of food-borne infections. Women with reactive arthritis often have milder symptoms than men.

What Are the Symptoms of Reactive Arthritis?

Reactive arthritis most typically results in inflammation of the urogenital tract, the joints, and the eyes. Less common symptoms are mouth ulcers and skin rashes. Any of these symptoms may be so mild that patients do not notice them. They usually come and go over a period of several weeks to several months.

Urogenital Tract Symptoms

Reactive arthritis often affects the urogenital tract, including the prostate or urethra in men and the urethra, uterus, or vagina in women. Men may notice an increased need to urinate, a burning sensation when urinating, and a fluid discharge from the penis. Some men with reactive arthritis develop prostatitis (inflammation of the prostate gland). Symptoms of prostatitis can include fever and chills, as well as an increased need to urinate and a burning sensation when urinating.

Women with reactive arthritis may develop problems in the urogenital tract, such as cervicitis (inflammation of the cervix) or urethritis (inflammation of the urethra), which can cause a burning sensation during urination. In addition, some women also develop salpingitis (inflammation of the fallopian tubes) or vulvovaginitis (inflammation of the vulva and vagina). These conditions may or may not cause any arthritic symptoms.

Joint Symptoms

The arthritis associated with reactive arthritis typically involves pain and swelling in the knees, ankles, and feet. Wrists, fingers, and other joints are affected less often. People with reactive arthritis commonly develop inflammation of the tendons (tendinitis) or at places where tendons attach to the bone (enthesitis). In many people with reactive arthritis, this results in heel pain or irritation of the Achilles tendon at the back of the ankle. Some people with reactive arthritis also develop heel spurs, which are bony growths in the heel that may cause chronic (long-lasting) foot pain. Approximately half of people with reactive arthritis report low back and buttock pain.

Reactive arthritis also can cause spondylitis (inflammation of the vertebrae in the spinal column) or sacroiliitis (inflammation of the joints in the lower back that connect the spine to the pelvis). People with reactive arthritis who have the HLA-B27 gene are even more likely to develop spondylitis and/or sacroiliitis.

Eye Involvement

Conjunctivitis, an inflammation of the mucous membrane that covers the eyeball and eyelid, develops in approximately half of people with reactive arthritis. Some people may develop uveitis, which is an inflammation of the inner eye. Conjunctivitis and uveitis can cause redness of the eyes, eye pain and irritation, and blurred vision. Eye involvement typically occurs early in the course of reactive arthritis, and symptoms may come and go.

Other Symptoms

Between 20 and 40 percent of men with reactive arthritis develop small, shallow, painless sores (ulcers) on the end of the penis. A small percentage of men and women develop rashes or small, hard nodules on the soles of the feet and, less often, on the palms of their hands or elsewhere. In addition, some people with reactive arthritis develop mouth ulcers that come and go. In some cases, these ulcers are painless and go unnoticed.

How Is Reactive Arthritis Diagnosed?

Doctors sometimes find it difficult to diagnose reactive arthritis because there is no specific laboratory test to confirm that a person has it. A doctor may order a blood test to detect the genetic factor HLA-B27, but even if the result is positive, the presence of HLA-B27 does not always mean that a person has the disorder.

At the beginning of an examination, the doctor will probably take a complete medical history and note current symptoms as well as any previous medical problems or infections. Before and after seeing the doctor, it is sometimes useful for the patient to keep a record of the symptoms that occur, when they occur, and how long they last. It is especially important to report any flu-like symptoms, such as fever, vomiting, or diarrhea, because they may be evidence of a bacterial infection.

The doctor may use various blood tests besides the HLA-B27 test to help rule out other conditions and confirm a suspected diagnosis of reactive arthritis. For example, the doctor may order rheumatoid factor or antinuclear antibody tests to rule out reactive arthritis. Most people who have reactive arthritis will have negative results on these tests. If a patient's test results are positive, he or she may have some other form of arthritis, such as rheumatoid arthritis or lupus. Doctors also may order a blood test to determine the erythrocyte sedimentation rate (sed rate), which is the rate at which red blood cells settle to the bottom of a test tube of blood. A high sed rate often indicates inflammation somewhere in the body. Typically, people with rheumatic diseases, including reactive arthritis, have an elevated sed rate.

The doctor also is likely to perform tests for infections that might be associated with reactive arthritis. Patients generally are tested for a *Chlamydia* infection because recent studies have shown that early treatment of *Chlamydia*-induced reactive arthritis may reduce the progression of the disease. The doctor may look for bacterial infections by testing cell samples taken from the patient's throat as well as the urethra in men or cervix in women. Urine and stool samples also may be tested. A sample of synovial fluid (the fluid that lubricates the joints) may be removed from the arthritic joint. Studies of synovial fluid can help the doctor rule out infection in the joint.

Doctors sometimes use x-rays to help diagnose reactive arthritis and to rule out other causes of arthritis. X-rays can detect some of the symptoms of reactive arthritis, including spondylitis, sacroiliitis, swelling of soft tissues, damage to cartilage or bone margins of the joint, and calcium deposits where the tendon attaches to the bone.

What Type of Doctor Treats Reactive Arthritis?

A person with reactive arthritis probably will need to see several different types of doctors because reactive arthritis affects different parts of the body. However, it may be helpful to the doctors and the patient for one doctor, usually a rheumatologist (a doctor specializing in arthritis), to manage the complete treatment plan. This doctor can coordinate treatments and monitor the side effects from the various medicines the patient may take. The following specialists treat other features that affect different parts of the body.

- Ophthalmologist—treats eye disease
- Gynecologist—treats genital symptoms in women
- Urologist—treats genital symptoms in men and women
- Dermatologist—treats skin symptoms
- Orthopaedist—performs surgery on severely damaged joints

- Physiatrist—supervises exercise regimens

How Is Reactive Arthritis Treated?

Although there is no cure for reactive arthritis, some treatments relieve symptoms of the disorder. The doctor is likely to use one or more of the following treatments:

- **Nonsteroidal anti-inflammatory drugs (NSAIDs)**—NSAIDs reduce joint inflammation and are commonly used to treat patients with reactive arthritis. Some traditional NSAIDs, such as aspirin and ibuprofen, are available without a prescription, but others that are more effective for reactive arthritis, such as indomethacin and tolmetin, must be prescribed by a doctor. Less is known about whether a new class of NSAIDs, called COX-2 inhibitors, is effective for reactive arthritis, but they may reduce the risk of gastrointestinal complications associated with traditional NSAIDs.

- **Corticosteroid injections**—For people with severe joint inflammation, injections of corticosteroids directly into the affected joint may reduce inflammation. Doctors usually prescribe these injections only after trying unsuccessfully to control arthritis with NSAIDs.

- **Topical corticosteroids**—These corticosteroids come in a cream or lotion and can be applied directly on the skin lesions, such as ulcers, associated with reactive arthritis. Topical corticosteroids reduce inflammation and promote healing.

- **Antibiotics**—The doctor may prescribe antibiotics to eliminate the bacterial infection that triggered reactive arthritis. The specific antibiotic prescribed depends on the type of bacterial infection present. It is important to follow instructions about how much medicine to take and for how long; otherwise the infection may persist. Typically, an antibiotic is taken for 7 to 10 days or longer. Some doctors may recommend a person with reactive arthritis take antibiotics for a long period of time (up to 3 months). Current research shows that in most cases, this practice is necessary.

- **Immunosuppressive medicines**—A small percentage of patients with reactive arthritis have severe symptoms that cannot be controlled with any of the above treatments. For these people, medicine that suppresses the immune system, such as sulfasalazine or methotrexate, may be effective.

- **Tumor necrosis factor (TNF) inhibitors**—Several relatively new treatments that suppress TNF, a protein involved in the body's inflammatory response, may be effective for reactive arthritis and other spondyloarthropathies. They include etanercept and infliximab. These treatments were first used to treat rheumatoid arthritis.

- **Exercise**—Exercise, when introduced gradually, may help improve joint function. In particular, strengthening and range-of-motion exercises will maintain or improve joint function. Strengthening exercises build up the muscles around the joint to better support it. Muscle-tightening exercises that do not move any joints can be done even when a person has inflammation and pain. Range-of-motion exercises improve movement and flexibility and reduce stiffness in the affected joint. For patients with spine pain or inflammation, exercises to stretch and extend the back can be particularly helpful in preventing long-term disability. Aquatic exercise also may be helpful. Before beginning an exercise program, patients should talk to a health professional who can recommend appropriate exercises.

What Is the Prognosis for People Who Have Reactive Arthritis?

Most people with reactive arthritis recover fully from the initial flare of symptoms and are able to return to regular activities 2 to 6 months after the first symptoms appear. In such cases, the symptoms of arthritis may last up to 12 months, although these are usually very mild and do not interfere with daily activities. Approximately 20 percent of people with reactive arthritis will have chronic (long-term) arthritis, which usually is mild. Studies show that between 15 and 50 percent of patients will develop symptoms again some time after the initial flare has disappeared. It is possible that such relapses may be due to reinfection. Back pain and arthritis are the symptoms that most commonly reappear. A small percentage of patients will have chronic, severe arthritis that is difficult to control with treatment and may cause joint deformity.

What Are Researchers Learning about Reactive Arthritis?

Researchers continue to investigate the causes of reactive arthritis and study treatments for the condition. For example:

- Researchers are trying to better understand the relationship between infection and reactive arthritis. In particular, they are trying to determine why an infection triggers arthritis and why some people who develop infections get reactive arthritis whereas others do not.

- Scientists also are studying why people with the genetic factor HLA-B27 are more at risk than others.

- Researchers are developing methods to detect the location of the triggering bacteria in the body. Some scientists suspect that after the bacteria enter the body, they are transported to the joints, where they can remain in small amounts indefinitely.

- Researchers are testing combination treatments for reactive arthritis. In particular, they are testing the use of antibiotics in combination with TNF inhibitors and with other immunosuppressant medicines, such as methotrexate and sulfasalazine.

Chapter 10

Ankylosing Spondylitis

Chapter Contents

Section 10.1

Overview of Ankylosing Spondylitis

"What Is Ankylosing Spondylitis," is reprinted with permission from the Spondylitis Association of America, www.spondylitis.org. © 2003 Spondylitis Association of America. All rights reserved.

Ankylosing spondylitis (AS) is the main rheumatic disease in a group of conditions called the spondyloarthropathies (SpA). Collectively, they are referred to as spondylitis.

Although AS primarily affects the mobility of the spine, it rarely affects the entire spine. Sometimes other areas of the body such as the eyes and or small joints of the hands and feet can be involved, but there are treatments available to reduce symptoms.

It is helpful to remember that even if you have mild symptoms, which you are able to manage quite well, it is important to see your rheumatologist once a year to ensure that the condition is not progressing.

Symptoms

The early symptoms of ankylosing spondylitis (AS) can vary from person to person. Most often, the symptoms begin slowly over the course of several months, however, some people describe the pain and muscle spasms as suddenly appearing, almost overnight. Many people notice that the fatigue, muscle spasms, and poor sleep quality when symptoms first appear can cause activities that were once enjoyable and easy to suddenly become exhausting and difficult to accomplish. Early diagnosis is essential. Here are important telltale symptoms to look out for: Symptoms include:

- Gradual onset of back pain and stiffness over a period of weeks or months

- Duration of symptoms longer than 3 months

- Early morning stiffness, which is improved by a warm shower or light exercise

- Sometimes the pain is located in other areas of the body, such as the buttocks or the neck.

- Average age, 26 years; gender, male or female

The pain is usually first felt in the low back, but may eventually be present throughout the whole spine or felt down the back of the buttocks and thighs (sciatic-like pain). Areas of the body where inflammation is most likely to develop are the central parts of the skeleton, i.e., the spine and pelvis. Anecdotally, the pain in women can first show in places other than the lower back. The neck is reported to be vulnerable to the first signs of pain and stiffness in some women. In children, the symptoms almost never appear first in the spine, but pain is usually felt in the heel or knee.

Iritis is an inflammation that can sometimes show up as a first symptoms of AS.

Diagnosis

Clues to Diagnosis

X-ray changes are considered to be important in the definitive diagnosis of AS. However, this poses a problem in that plain x-rays don't show anything for many years after the first symptoms are felt. That is why it is important for your rheumatologist to be very astute in recognizing clues that can quickly lead to a diagnosis of AS before x-rays of the pelvic area show any changes.

Detailed Clinical History of Symptoms and Physical Examination

Rheumatologists are trained to recognize the symptoms of AS. Typically, early morning stiffness that gets better after a warm shower, deep buttock pain in the night, possibly bouts of iritis (inflammation of the eye), and other clues should tip your doctor off to a possible diagnosis of AS.

HLA-B27 Gene Test Is Not Diagnostic of AS

A very high percentage of people with AS test positive for this gene—depending upon ethnicity. HLA-B27 is a perfectly normal gene found in 8% of the general population. Generally speaking, no more than 2% of people born with this gene will eventually get spondylitis.

The gene itself does not cause spondylitis, but people with HLA-B27 are more susceptible to getting it. Occasionally, a test for HLA-B27 will be done, particularly if your doctor isn't quite sure that you have AS.

Treatment

If you, a family member, or friend has been diagnosed with ankylosing spondylitis (AS), it is important to know that there is a lot that can be done to reduce its effects. As with other chronic conditions, the more you learn, the better off you will be. It is also helpful to build a good relationship with your medical team. Even those people with mild symptoms can benefit from seeing a rheumatologist at least annually, so that he or she can check to make sure that you are doing well. Complications can sometimes occur and it is better to catch them early on.

What Is Important?

A treatment plan includes medications to help reduce the pain and stiffness caused by AS; this paves the way so that a daily exercise program can be adopted. Some people do not need to take medication, but this is not usually the norm. Good posture techniques are critical to put less strain on the body.

Additional Aids to Improved Quality of Life

Additional symptom management tools include: heat for stiffness, ice for swelling, hot baths and warm showers, ultrasound or gentle massage therapy, electrical stimulators for pain (transcutaneous electrical nerve stimulation [TENS]), and avoiding excess calories and obesity to lessen body weight stress on joints. Much can be done to help.

Medications

Many types of medications are effective in managing the symptoms of ankylosing spondylitis (AS) and related diseases (spondyloarthropathies or SpA), sometimes collectively called spondylitis.

Recent Developments

The United States Food and Drug Administration (FDA) recently approved the Tumor-Necrosis-Factor alpha (TNF) blocker etanercept (brand name Enbrel), the first biological medicine approved for the treatment of ankylosing spondylitis in the U.S.. The FDA based its decision on a study conducted at California-based Stanford University, which showed that at 24 weeks, 58 percent of those treated with twice-weekly etanercept injections maintained a significant improvement in measures of pain, function, and inflammation (greater than 20 percent improvement), as compared 23 percent of those patients on the placebo. The study's principal investigator, John Davis, MD, noted that this is the first treatment to show improvement in range of motion in ankylosing spondylitis patients.

Non-Steroidal Anti-Inflammatories (NSAIDs)

Non-steroidal anti-inflammatories (NSAIDs) are the most commonly used medications to treat AS. For many people they can be effective in reducing the pain and stiffness associated with these conditions. However, they can sometimes cause heartburn, gastritis, and even bleeding. It is important to talk to your doctor about the possible side effects of any medication that you are being prescribed. Sometimes is it necessary to take medication that is designed to neutralize or prevent the production of gastric acid when you are taking NSAIDs. Some of these are called antacids or H2 blockers.

There are also medications that can coat the stomach, such as Carafate. Another type of medication can help to restore the lost gastric mucus caused by NSAIDs. They may also cause less common additional side effects that include: fluid retention, headaches, dizziness, and even confusion. Increasing evidence suggests that the new class of NSAIDs, the cyclooxygenase-2 specific inhibitors, or COX-2 inhibitors, sold under various brand names, may reduce the risk of these gastrointestinal problems. There is still some controversy among medical experts as to whether these drugs reduce gastrointestinal complications, but evidence seems to point in this direction.

When NSAIDs Are Not Enough

In severe spondylitis when NSAIDs do not sufficiently control the pain and stiffness and other symptoms, additional medications can be tried. However, it is important to give the NSAIDs sufficient time to be effective—this can take up to several weeks for some NSAIDs. If you are considering changing medications, remember to ask your doctor about the potential benefits and side effects before you and your doctor decide whether the change in treatment is right for you.

Sulfasalazine

Sulfasalazine is one type of medication that can be helpful to some people with severe disease. It is known to effectively control not only pain and joint swelling from arthritis of the small joints, but also the intestinal lesions in inflammatory bowel disease. Side effects can include headaches, abdominal bloating, nausea, and oral ulcers. Rarely, someone being prescribed this medication can develop bone marrow suppression, which is why it is important for your doctor to regularly monitor your blood count.

Methotrexate

Methotrexate can also be effective in controlling the symptoms of severe spondylitis in some people, particularly those with psoriatic arthritis and reactive arthritis (Reiter syndrome). It has the added benefit of controlling the skin rash of psoriasis. Side effects include bone marrow suppression, with lowering of the blood counts, oral ulcers, nausea, gastritis or peptic laceration, and liver toxicity. Use of this medication requires frequent monitoring of the blood counts and liver profile. The vitamin folic acid is often prescribed to combat the thinning hair and mouth ulcers associated with methotrexate.

Corticosteroids

Corticosteroids, such as prednisone, can be effective in relieving the inflammation associated with spondyloarthropathies, but the side effects of long-term use (weight gain, osteoporosis, etc.) can be very severe. They are sometimes prescribed for short periods of time. The use of corticosteroid injections into inflamed joints can also provide temporary relief of the pain and swelling of arthritis or bursitis. But because of the concern of rupture of the Achilles tendon, such injections are rarely, if ever used to treat Achilles tendonitis. Similarly, their usefulness in plantar fasciitis (inflamed heels) is not clear.

Section 10.2

Genetically Engineered Protein Approved to Treat Ankylosing Spondylitis

"FDA Approves Enbrel to Treat Ankylosing Spondylitis," U.S. Food and Drug Administration, July 24, 2003. Available online at http://www.fda.gov; accessed December 2003.

FDA today approved an application for etanercept (trade name Enbrel), a genetically engineered protein, for a new indication for treatment of patients with active ankylosing spondylitis (AS), a chronic inflammatory disease affecting primarily the lower back and joints. The product is manufactured by Immunex Corporation, Thousand Oaks, California, and marketed by Amgen and Wyeth Pharmaceuticals. Etanercept is also licensed for treatment of patients with rheumatoid arthritis, juvenile rheumatoid arthritis, and psoriatic arthritis.

Approximately 350,000 patients in the United States have AS. The disease affects men more often than women. Symptoms of the disease may start in adolescence and are usually present by age 30. Patients often have lower back pain and stiffness, chest pain, joint pain and swelling, and tenderness due to the inflammation. In some patients the disease can cause significant pain and disability for many years.

Currently approved drugs for AS include some non-steroidal anti-inflammatory drugs (NSAIDs), which are approved to treat the symptoms of AS. Disease Modifying Anti-Rheumatic Drugs (DMARDs) that are approved for use in other inflammatory joint diseases are sometimes used when NSAIDs are ineffective, but none is FDA approved for use in the treatment of AS.

Etanercept binds to tumor necrosis factor (TNF), a naturally occurring protein in the body, and inhibits its action. TNF, which promotes inflammation in the body, is found at elevated levels in the blood and certain tissues of patients with AS. It is believed that interference with TNF plays a role in the beneficial effects of etanercept for AS.

The major efficacy trial of etanercept for AS was a randomized, double-blind, placebo-controlled study of 277 patients. The study excluded patients with the most severe forms of AS. After six months of twice-weekly treatments, 58% of patients who received etanercept showed significant improvement on a scale that measured pain, function, and inflammation compared to 23% who received a placebo.

The main side effects of etanercept in the study were similar to those previously seen for this drug for other indications, including injection site reactions and upper respiratory infections. The approved labeling warns physicians about post-marketing reports of serious infections. The labeling says that Enbrel should not be given to patients with any active infection, including chronic or localized infections. It also recommends that patients who develop a new infection while being treated with Enbrel should be monitored closely.

Amgen will continue to follow patients in the trial to evaluate the long-term safety of etanercept in patients with AS.

Chapter 11

Polymyalgia Rheumatica and Giant Cell Arteritis

What Are Polymyalgia Rheumatica and Giant Cell Arteritis?

Polymyalgia rheumatica is a rheumatic disorder that is associated with moderate to severe muscle pain and stiffness in the neck, shoulder, and hip area. Stiffness is most noticeable in the morning. This disorder may develop rapidly—in some patients, overnight. In other people, polymyalgia rheumatica develops more gradually. The cause of polymyalgia rheumatica is not known; however, possibilities include immune system abnormalities and genetic factors. The fact that polymyalgia rheumatica is rare in people under the age of 50 suggests it may be linked to the aging process.

Polymyalgia rheumatica may go away without treatment in 1 to several years. With treatment, the symptoms of polymyalgia rheumatica are quickly controlled, but a person may relapse if treatment is stopped too early.

Giant cell arteritis, also known as temporal arteritis and cranial arteritis, is a disorder that results in swelling of arteries in the head (most often the temporal arteries, which are located on the temples on each side of the head), neck, and arms. This swelling causes the

"Questions and Answers about Polymyalgia Rheumatica and Giant Cell Arteritis," National Institute of Arthritis and Musculoskeletal and Skin Diseases (NIAMS), February 2001. Available online at http://www.niams.nih.gov; accessed February 2004.

arteries to narrow, reducing blood flow. Early treatment is critical for good prognosis.

How Are Polymyalgia Rheumatica and Giant Cell Arteritis Related?

It is unclear how or why polymyalgia rheumatica and giant cell arteritis are related, but an estimated 15 percent of people in the United States with polymyalgia rheumatica also develop giant cell arteritis. Patients can develop giant cell arteritis either at the same time as polymyalgia rheumatica or after the polymyalgia symptoms disappear. About half of the people affected by giant cell arteritis also have polymyalgia rheumatica.

When a person is diagnosed with polymyalgia rheumatica, the doctor also should look for symptoms of giant cell arteritis because of the risk of blindness. With proper treatment, the disease is not threatening. Untreated, however, giant cell arteritis can lead to serious complications including permanent vision loss and stroke. Patients must learn to recognize the signs of giant cell arteritis, because they can develop even after the symptoms of polymyalgia rheumatica disappear. Patients should report any symptoms to the doctor immediately.

Who Is at Risk?

White women over the age of 50 are most at risk of developing polymyalgia rheumatica and giant cell arteritis. Women are twice as likely as men to develop the conditions. Both conditions almost exclusively affect people over the age of 50. The average age at onset is 70 years. Polymyalgia rheumatica and giant cell arteritis are quite common. In the United States, it is estimated that 700 per 100,000 people in the general population over 50 years of age develop polymyalgia rheumatica. An estimated 200 per 100,000 people over the age of 50 develop giant cell arteritis.

What Are the Symptoms?

The primary symptoms of polymyalgia rheumatica are moderate to severe stiffness and muscle pain near the neck, shoulders, or hips. The stiffness is more severe upon waking or after a period of inactivity, and typically lasts longer than 30 minutes. People with this condition also may have flu-like symptoms, including fever, weakness, and weight loss.

154

Early symptoms of giant cell arteritis also may resemble the flu. People are likely to experience headaches, pain in the temples, and blurred or double vision. Pain may also affect the jaw and tongue.

How Are Polymyalgia Rheumatica and Giant Cell Arteritis Diagnosed?

No single test is available to definitively diagnose polymyalgia rheumatica. To diagnose the condition, a physician considers the patient's medical history, including symptoms that the patient reports, and results of laboratory tests that can rule out other possible diagnoses.

The most typical laboratory finding in people with polymyalgia rheumatica is an elevated erythrocyte sedimentation rate, commonly referred to as the sed rate. This test measures how quickly red blood cells fall to the bottom of a test tube of unclotted blood. Rapidly descending cells (an elevated sed rate) indicate inflammation in the body. Although the sed rate measurement is a helpful diagnostic tool, it alone does not confirm polymyalgia rheumatica. An abnormal result indicates only that tissue is inflamed, which also is a symptom of many forms of arthritis and/ or other rheumatic diseases. Before making a diagnosis of polymyalgia rheumatica, the doctor may perform additional tests to rule out other conditions, including rheumatoid arthritis, because symptoms of polymyalgia rheumatica and rheumatoid arthritis can be similar.

The doctor may recommend a test for rheumatoid factor (RF). RF is an antibody sometimes found in the blood. (An antibody is a special protein made by the immune system.) People with rheumatoid arthritis are likely to have RF in their blood, but most people with polymyalgia rheumatica do not. If the diagnosis still is unclear, a physician may conduct additional tests to rule out other disorders.

Doctors and patients both need to be aware of the risk of giant cell arteritis in people with polymyalgia rheumatica and should be on the lookout for symptoms of the disorder. Severe headaches, jaw pain, and vision problems are typical symptoms of giant cell arteritis. In addition, physical examination may reveal an abnormal temporal artery: tender to the touch, inflamed, and with reduced pulse. Because of the possibility of permanent blindness, a temporal artery biopsy is recommended if there is any suspicion of giant cell arteritis.

In a person with giant cell arteritis, the biopsy will show abnormal cells in the artery walls. Some patients showing symptoms of giant cell arteritis will have negative biopsy results. In such cases the doctor may suggest a second biopsy.

What Are the Treatments?

Polymyalgia rheumatica usually disappears without treatment in 1 to several years. With treatment, however, symptoms disappear quickly, usually in 24 to 48 hours. If there is no improvement, the doctor is likely to consider other possible diagnoses.

The treatment of choice is corticosteroid medication, usually prednisone. Polymyalgia rheumatica responds to a low daily dose of prednisone. The dose is increased as needed until symptoms disappear.

Once symptoms disappear, the doctor may gradually reduce the dosage to determine the lowest amount needed to alleviate symptoms. The amount of time that treatment is needed is different for each patient. Most patients can discontinue medication after 6 months to 2 years. If symptoms recur, prednisone treatment is required again.

Nonsteroidal anti-inflammatory drugs (NSAIDs) such as aspirin and ibuprofen also may be used to treat polymyalgia rheumatica. The medication must be taken daily, and long-term use may cause stomach irritation. For most patients, NSAIDs alone are not enough to relieve symptoms.

Giant cell arteritis carries a small but definite risk of blindness. The blindness is permanent once it happens. A high dose of prednisone is needed to prevent blindness and should be started as soon as possible, perhaps even before the diagnosis is confirmed with a temporal artery biopsy. When treated, symptoms quickly disappear. Typically, people with giant cell arteritis must continue taking a high dose of prednisone for 1 month. Once symptoms disappear and the sed rate is normal and there is no longer a risk of blindness, the doctor can begin to gradually reduce the dose. When treated properly, giant cell arteritis rarely recurs.

People taking low doses of prednisone rarely experience side effects. Side effects are more common among people taking higher doses. But all patients should be aware of potential effects, which include:

- fluid retention and weight gain
- rounding of the face
- delayed wound healing
- bruising easily
- diabetes
- myopathy (muscle wasting)
- glaucoma

- increased blood pressure
- decreased calcium absorption in the bones, which can lead to osteoporosis
- irritation of the stomach

People taking corticosteroids may have some side effects or none at all. A patient should report any side effects to the doctor. When the medication is stopped, the side effects disappear. Because prednisone and other corticosteroid drugs change the body's natural production of corticosteroid hormones, the patient should not stop taking the medication unless instructed by the doctor. The patient and doctor must work together to gradually reduce the medication.

What Is the Outlook?

Most people with polymyalgia rheumatica and giant cell arteritis lead productive, active lives. The duration of drug treatment differs by patient. Once treatment is discontinued, polymyalgia may recur; but once again, symptoms respond rapidly to prednisone. When properly treated, giant cell arteritis rarely recurs.

What Research Is Being Conducted to Help People Who Have Polymyalgia Rheumatica and Giant Cell Arteritis?

Researchers studying possible causes of polymyalgia rheumatica and giant cell arteritis are investigating the role of genetic predisposition, immune system abnormalities, and environmental factors. Scientists also are looking for markers of the diseases, exploring treatments, and studying why the two disorders often occur together.

With funding from the National Eye Institute, a new mouse model of giant cell arteritis is being used to examine interactions between the immune system and blood vessels to explain tissue damage.

Where Can People Get More Information about Polymyalgia Rheumatica and Giant Cell Arteritis?

National Institute of Arthritis and Musculoskeletal and Skin Diseases
1 AMS Circle
Bethesda, MD 20892-3675
Toll-Free: (877) 22-NIAMS (226-4267)

157

Phone: (301) 495-4484
TTY: (301) 565-2966
Fax: (301) 718-6366
Website: http://www.niams.nih.gov
E-mail: niamsinfo@mail.nih.gov

National Eye Institute Information Clearinghouse
2020 Vision Place
Bethesda, MD 20892-3655
Phone: (301) 496-5248
Fax: (301) 402-1065
Website: http://www.nei.nih.gov

National Heart, Lung, and Blood Institute
Building 31, Room 5A52
31 Center Drive, MSC 2486
Bethesda, MD 20892-2480
Phone: (301) 592-8573
Fax: (301) 592-8563
TTY: (240) 629-3255
Website: http://www.nhlbi.nih.gov
E-mail: nhlbiinfo@nhlbi.nih.gov

American College of Rheumatology
1800 Century Place, Suite 250
Atlanta, GA 30345-4300
Phone: (404) 633-3777
Fax: (404) 633-1870
Website: http://www.rheumatology.org

Arthritis Foundation
1330 West Peachtree Street
Atlanta, GA 30309
Toll-Free: (800) 283-7800
Phone: (404) 872-7100
Website: http://www.arthritis.org

Part Three

Disorders with Symptoms Linked to Arthritis

Chapter 12

Behçet Disease

What Is Behçet Disease?

The disease was first described in 1937 by Dr. Helusi Behçet, a professor of dermatology in Istanbul. Behçet disease is now recognized as a chronic condition that causes sores or ulcers in the mouth and on the genitals and inflammation in parts of the eye. In some people, the disease also results in arthritis (swollen, painful, stiff joints) and inflammation of the digestive tract, brain, and spinal cord.

Who Gets Behçet Disease?

Behçet disease is common in the Middle East, Asia, and Japan, but rare in the United States. In Middle Eastern and Asian countries, the disease affects more men than women. In the United States, the opposite is true. Behçet disease tends to develop in people in their twenties or thirties, but people of all ages can develop it.

What Causes Behçet Disease?

The exact cause of Behçet disease is unknown. Most of the symptoms are caused by inflammation of the blood vessels, particularly

"Questions and Answers About Behçet's Disease," National Institute of Arthritis and Musculoskeletal and Skin Diseases (NIAMS), January 1999. Available online at http://www.niams.nih.gov; accessed November 2003. Reviewed and revised by David A. Cooke, M.D. on November 27, 2003.

veins. Inflammation is the body's characteristic reaction to injury or disease and is marked by four signs: swelling, redness, heat, and pain. Doctors think that an autoimmune reaction may cause blood vessels to become inflamed, but they do not know what triggers this reaction. In an autoimmune reaction, the immune system mistakenly attacks and harms the body's own tissues. Under normal conditions, the immune system protects the body from diseases and infections by killing harmful foreign substances, such as germs, that enter the body.

Behçet disease is not contagious and does not spread from one person to another. Researchers think that two factors are probably important in its development. First, it is believed that abnormalities of the immune system make some people susceptible to the disease. Researchers think that this problem may be inherited; that is, it may be due to one or more specific genes. Second, something in the environment, possibly a bacterium or virus, might trigger or activate the disease in susceptible people. Researchers have found that people who have frequent strep infections (caused by *Streptococcus* bacteria) are more likely to develop Behçet disease.

What Are the Symptoms of Behçet Disease?

Behçet disease affects each person differently. Some people have only mild symptoms, such as skin sores or ulcers in the mouth or on the genitals. Others have more severe disease, such as meningitis or inflammation of the membranes that cover the brain and spinal cord. Meningitis can cause fever, a stiff neck, and headaches. More severe symptoms usually appear months or years after a person notices the first signs of Behçet disease. Symptoms can last for a long time or can come and go in a few weeks. Typically, symptoms appear, disappear, then reappear. The times when a person is having symptoms are called flares. To help the doctor diagnose Behçet disease and monitor its course, patients may want to keep a record of the symptoms that occur and when they occur. Because many conditions mimic Behçet disease, physicians must observe symptoms to make an accurate diagnosis. The four most common symptoms of Behçet disease are mouth sores, genital sores, inflammation of parts of the eye, and arthritis.

- **Mouth sores**—Mouth sores (known as oral aphthosis and aphthous stomatitis) affect almost all patients with Behçet disease. They are often the first symptom that a person notices and may occur long before any other symptoms appear. The sores usually have a red border and several may appear at the same time. They can be painful and make eating difficult. Mouth sores go away in 10 to 14 days but often come back. Small sores usually heal without scarring, but larger ones may scar.

- **Genital sores**—Affecting more that half of all people with Behçet disease, most genital sores appear on the scrotum in men and vulva in women. The sores look similar to mouth sores and may be painful. After several outbreaks, they may cause scarring.

- **Uveitis**—Inflammation of the middle part of the eye (the uvea), including the iris, occurs in more than half of all people with Behçet disease. This symptom is more common among men than women and typically begins within 2 years of the first symptoms. Eye inflammation can cause blurred vision and, rarely, pain and redness. Because partial loss of vision or blindness can result if the eye frequently becomes inflamed, patients should report these symptoms to their doctor immediately.

- **Arthritis**—Inflammation of the joints occurs in more than half of all patients with Behçet disease. Arthritis causes pain, swelling, and stiffness in the joints, especially the knees, ankles, wrists, and elbows. Arthritis that results from Behçet disease usually lasts a few weeks and does not cause permanent damage to the joints.

In addition to mouth and genital sores, eye inflammation, and arthritis, Behçet disease may cause other skin problems, blood clots, and inflammation in the central nervous system and digestive organs.

Skin Problems

Behçet disease causes various skin sores that look like red bumps on a black-and-blue mark. The sores are red, raised, and typically appear on the legs and upper torso. In some people, sores or lesions may appear when the skin is scratched or pricked. When doctors suspect that a person may have Behçet disease, they may perform a test called pathergy in which they prick the skin with a small needle; 1 to 2 days after the test, people with Behçet disease may develop a bump where the doctor pricked the skin. Doctors disagree about the usefulness of a pathergy test because Behçet patients in the United States rarely have a skin reaction. However, more than half of the patients in Middle Eastern countries and Japan do have a reaction.

Blood Clots

About 10 percent of patients with Behçet disease have blood clots resulting from inflammation in the veins (thrombophlebitis), usually in the legs. Symptoms include pain and tenderness in the affected area, which may also be swollen and warm. Because thrombophlebitis can have severe complications, people should report symptoms to their doctor immediately. A few patients may experience artery problems such as aneurysms (a stretching or expanding of a weakened blood vessel).

Central Nervous System

Behçet disease affects the central nervous system in about 10 percent of all patients with the disease. The central nervous system includes the brain and spinal cord and helps the body to coordinate movements and process information. Behçet disease can cause meningoencephalitis—inflammation of the brain and the thin membrane that covers and protects it. People with meningoencephalitis may have fever, headache, stiff neck, and difficulty coordinating movement, and should report any of these symptoms to their doctor immediately. If this condition is left untreated, a stroke can result.

Digestive Tract

Only rarely does Behçet disease cause inflammation and ulceration (sores) in the digestive tract and lead to stomach pain, diarrhea, constipation, and vomiting. Because these symptoms are very similar to symptoms of other diseases of the digestive tract, such as a peptic ulcer, ulcerative colitis, and especially Crohn disease, careful evaluation is essential.

How Is Behçet Disease Diagnosed?

Diagnosing Behçet disease is very difficult because no specific test confirms it. Less than half of the patients initially thought to have Behçet disease actually have it. The doctor must examine a patient with symptoms and rule out other conditions with similar symptoms. Because it may take several months or even years for all the common symptoms to appear, the diagnosis may not be made for a long time. A patient may even visit several different kinds of doctors before the diagnosis is made.

These symptoms are key to diagnosing Behçet disease:

- Mouth sores at least three times in 12 months
- Any two of the following symptoms: recurring genital sores, eye inflammation with loss of vision, skin lesions, or positive pathergy (skin prick test).

Besides finding these signs, the doctor must rule out other conditions with similar symptoms, such as Crohn disease and Reiter syndrome. The doctor may also recommend that the patient see an eye specialist to identify possible complications related to eye inflammation.

What Kind of Doctor Treats a Patient with Behçet Disease?

Because the disease affects different parts of the body, a patient will probably see several different doctors. It may be helpful to both the doctors and the patient for one doctor to manage the complete treatment plan. This doctor can coordinate treatment and monitor any side effects from the various medications the patient takes.

A rheumatologist (a doctor specializing in arthritis) often manages the patient's overall treatment and treats joint disease. The following specialists treat other symptoms that affect different body systems:

- Gynecologist—treats genital sores in women.
- Urologist—treats genital sores in men.
- Dermatologist—treats genital sores in men, and skin and mucous membrane problems.
- Ophthalmologist—treats eye inflammation.
- Gastroenterologist—treats digestive tract symptoms.
- Neurologist—treats central nervous system symptoms.

How Is Behçet Disease Treated?

Although there is no cure for Behçet disease, people can usually control their symptoms with proper medication, rest, and exercise. Treatment goals are to reduce discomfort and prevent serious complications such as disability from arthritis or blindness. The type of medicine and the length of treatment depend on the person's symptoms and their severity.

It is likely that a combination of treatments will be needed to relieve specific symptoms. Patients should tell each of their doctors about all of the medicines they are taking so that the doctors can coordinate treatment.

Topical Medicine

Topical medicine is applied directly on the sores to relieve pain and discomfort. For example, doctors prescribe rinses to treat mouth sores. Creams are used to treat skin and genital sores. The medicine usually contains corticosteroids, which reduce inflammation, or an anesthetic, which relieves pain.

Oral Medicine

Doctors also prescribe medicines taken by mouth to reduce inflammation throughout the body, suppress the overactive immune system, and relieve symptoms. Doctors may prescribe one or more of the medicines described below to treat the various symptoms of Behçet disease.

- Corticosteroids—Prednisone is a corticosteroid prescribed to reduce pain and swelling throughout the body in people with severe joint pain and inflammation, skin sores, eye disease, or central nervous system symptoms. Patients must carefully follow the doctor's instructions about when to take prednisone and how much to take. It is also important not to stop taking the medicine suddenly because it alters the body's production of the natural corticosteroid hormones. Long-term use of prednisone can have side effects such as osteoporosis, weight gain, delayed wound healing, persistent heartburn, and elevated blood pressure. However, these side effects are rare when prednisone is taken at low doses for a short time. It is important that patients see their doctor regularly to monitor possible side effects.

- Immunosuppressive drugs—Medicines (including corticosteroids) that help control an overactive immune system, such as is the case in people with Behçet disease, reduce inflammation throughout the body and can lessen the number of flares. Doctors may use immunosuppressive drugs when a person has eye disease or central nervous system involvement. These medicines are very strong and can have serious side effects. Patients must see their doctor regularly for blood tests to detect and monitor side effects.

Depending on the person's specific symptoms, doctors may use one or more of the following immunosuppressive drugs:

- Azathioprine—Most commonly prescribed for people with organ transplants because it suppresses the immune system, azathioprine is now used to treat uveitis and central nervous system involvement in Behçet disease. This medicine can upset the stomach and may reduce the production of new blood cells by the bone marrow.

- Chlorambucil—Doctors use chlorambucil to treat uveitis and meningoencephalitis. People taking chlorambucil must see their doctor frequently because it can have serious side effects, such as permanent sterility and cancers of the blood. Patients need regular blood tests to monitor blood counts of white cells and platelets.

- Cyclosporine—Like azathioprine, doctors prescribe this medicine for people with organ transplants. When used by patients with Behçet disease, cyclosporine reduces uveitis and central nervous system involvement. To reduce the risk of side effects, such as kidney and liver disease, the doctor can adjust the dose. Patients must tell their doctor if they take any other medicines, because some affect the way the body uses cyclosporine.

- Colchicine—Commonly used to treat gout, which is a form of arthritis, colchicine reduces inflammation throughout the body. The medicine is sometimes used to treat eye inflammation and skin symptoms in patients with Behçet disease. Common side effects of colchicine include nausea, vomiting, and diarrhea. The doctor can decrease the dose to relieve these side effects.

- Thalidomide—This medication is well known because of the severe deformities it caused in the children of women who took the drug while pregnant. Recently, it has proven useful for treating several inflammatory diseases, including Behçet disease. However, potential toxicity and the strict measures needed to avoid pregnancy in patients taking it can limit its use.

- Interferon alfa-2b—This is a synthetic version of a natural hormone active in the immune system. Some studies have found it useful in treating Behçet disease. However, it can have significant side effects, and it is immunosuppressive (which means it weakens the immune system).

If these medicines do not reduce symptoms, doctors may use other drugs such as cyclophosphamide and methotrexate. Cyclophosphamide is similar to chlorambucil. Methotrexate, which is also used to treat various kinds of cancer as well as rheumatoid arthritis, can relieve Behçet symptoms because it suppresses the immune system and reduces inflammation throughout the body.

Rest and Exercise

Although rest is important during flares, doctors usually recommend moderate exercise, such as swimming or walking, when the symptoms have improved or disappeared. Exercise can help people with Behçet disease keep their joints strong and flexible.

What Is the Prognosis for a Person with Behçet Disease?

Most people with Behçet disease can lead normal lives and control their symptoms with proper medicine, rest, and exercise. Doctors can use many medicines to relieve pain, treat symptoms, and prevent complications. When treatment is effective, flares usually become less frequent after 1 or 2 years. Many patients eventually enter a period of remission. In some people, however, treatment does not relieve symptoms, and gradually more serious symptoms such as eye disease may occur. Serious symptoms may appear months or years after the first signs of Behçet disease.

What Are Researchers Trying to Learn about Behçet Disease?

Researchers are exploring possible genetic, bacterial, and viral causes of Behçet disease, as well as improved drug treatment. Researchers hope to identify genes that increase a person's chance of developing the disease. Studying these genes and how they work may lead to a new understanding of the disease and possibly new treatments.

Researchers are also investigating factors in the environment, such as a bacterium or virus, which could trigger Behçet disease. They are particularly interested in whether *Streptococcus*, the bacterium that causes strep throat, is associated with the disease. Many people with Behçet disease have had several strep infections. In addition, researchers suspect that herpes virus type I, a virus that causes cold sores, may be associated with the disease.

Finally, researchers are identifying other medicines to better treat Behçet disease. Thalidomide, for example, appears effective in treating severe mouth sores, but its use is experimental and very limited. Thalidomide is not used in women of childbearing age because it causes severe birth defects.

Where Can People Get More Information about Behçet Disease?

Arthritis Foundation
1330 West Peachtree Street
Atlanta, GA 30309
Toll-Free: (800) 283-7800
Phone: (404) 872-7100
Website: http://www.arthritis.org

American Behçet's Disease Association
P.O. Box 19952
Amarillo, TX 78114
Toll-Free: (800) 723-4238
Website: http://www.behcets.com

National Institute of Arthritis and Musculoskeletal and Skin Diseases
1 AMS Circle
Bethesda, MD 20892-3675
Toll-Free: (877) 22-NIAMS (226-4267)
Phone: (301) 495-4484
TTY: (301) 565-2966
Fax: (301) 718-6366
Website: http://www.niams.nih.gov
E-mail: niamsinfo@mail.nih.gov

Chapter 13

Bursitis and Tendinitis

This chapter first answers general questions about the shoulder and shoulder problems. It then answers questions about specific shoulder problems (tendinitis and bursitis) as well as shoulder pain caused by arthritis of the shoulder.

How Common Are Shoulder Problems?

According to the American Academy of Orthopaedic Surgeons, about 4 million people in the United States seek medical care each year for shoulder sprain, strain, dislocation, or other problems. Each year, shoulder problems account for about 1.5 million visits to orthopaedic surgeons—doctors who treat disorders of the bones, muscles, and related structures.

What Are the Structures of the Shoulder and How Does the Shoulder Function?

The shoulder joint is composed of three bones: the clavicle (collarbone), the scapula (shoulder blade), and the humerus (upper arm bone). Two joints facilitate shoulder movement. The acromioclavicular (AC) joint is located between the acromion (part of the scapula that forms the highest point of the shoulder) and the clavicle. The glenohumeral

"Questions and Answers about Shoulder Problems," National Institute of Arthritis and Musculoskeletal and Skin Diseases (NIAMS), May 2001. Available online at http://www.niams.nih.gov; accessed February 2004.

joint, commonly called the shoulder joint, is a ball-and-socket type joint that helps move the shoulder forward and backward and allows the arm to rotate in a circular fashion or hinge out and up away from the body. (The ball is the top, rounded portion of the upper arm bone or humerus; the socket, or glenoid, is a dish-shaped part of the outer edge of the scapula into which the ball fits.) The capsule is a soft tissue envelope that encircles the glenohumeral joint. It is lined by a thin, smooth synovial membrane.

The bones of the shoulder are held in place by muscles, tendons, and ligaments. Tendons are tough cords of tissue that attach the shoulder muscles to bone and assist the muscles in moving the shoulder. Ligaments attach shoulder bones to each other, providing stability. For example, the front of the joint capsule is anchored by three glenohumeral ligaments.

The rotator cuff is a structure composed of tendons that, with associated muscles, holds the ball at the top of the humerus in the glenoid socket and provides mobility and strength to the shoulder joint.

Two filmy sac-like structures called bursae permit smooth gliding between bone, muscle, and tendon. They cushion and protect the rotator cuff from the bony arch of the acromion.

What Are the Origin and Causes of Shoulder Problems?

The shoulder is the most movable joint in the body. However, it is an unstable joint because of the range of motion allowed. It is easily subject to injury because the ball of the upper arm is larger than the shoulder socket that holds it. To remain stable, the shoulder must be anchored by its muscles, tendons, and ligaments. Some shoulder problems arise from the disruption of these soft tissues as a result of injury or from overuse or underuse of the shoulder. Other problems arise from a degenerative process in which tissues break down and no longer function well.

Shoulder pain may be localized or may be referred to areas around the shoulder or down the arm. Disease within the body (such as gallbladder, liver, or heart disease, or disease of the cervical spine of the neck) also may generate pain that travels along nerves to the shoulder.

How Are Shoulder Problems Diagnosed?

Following are some of the ways doctors diagnose shoulder problems:

- Medical history (the patient tells the doctor about an injury or other condition that might be causing the pain).

- Physical examination to feel for injury and discover the limits of movement, location of pain, and extent of joint instability.

- Tests to confirm the diagnosis of certain conditions. Some of these tests include:

  - x-ray

  - arthrogram– Diagnostic record that can be seen on an x-ray after injection of a contrast fluid into the shoulder joint to outline structures such as the rotator cuff. In disease or injury, this contrast fluid may either leak into an area where it does not belong, indicating a tear or opening, or be blocked from entering an area where there normally is an opening.

  - MRI (magnetic resonance imaging)—A non-invasive procedure in which a machine produces a series of cross-sectional images of the shoulder.

  - Other diagnostic tests, such as injection of an anesthetic into and around the shoulder joint.

Tendinitis, Bursitis, and Impingement Syndrome of the Shoulder

What Are Tendinitis, Bursitis, and Impingement Syndrome of the Shoulder?

These conditions are closely related and may occur alone or in combination. If the rotator cuff and bursa are irritated, inflamed, and swollen, they may become squeezed between the head of the humerus and the acromion. Repeated motion involving the arms or the aging process involving shoulder motion over many years may also irritate and wear down the tendons, muscles, and surrounding structures.

Tendinitis is inflammation (redness, soreness, and swelling) of a tendon. In tendinitis of the shoulder, the rotator cuff and/or biceps tendon become inflamed, usually as a result of being pinched by surrounding structures. The injury may vary from mild inflammation to involvement of most of the rotator cuff. When the rotator cuff tendon becomes inflamed and thickened, it may get trapped under the acromion. Squeezing of the rotator cuff is called impingement syndrome.

Tendinitis and impingement syndrome are often accompanied by inflammation of the bursa sacs that protect the shoulder. An inflamed bursa is called bursitis. Inflammation caused by a disease such as rheumatoid arthritis may cause rotator cuff tendinitis and bursitis. Sports involving overuse of the shoulder and occupations requiring frequent overhead reaching are other potential causes of irritation to the rotator cuff or bursa and may lead to inflammation and impingement.

What Are the Signs of Tendinitis and Bursitis?

Signs of these conditions include the slow onset of discomfort and pain in the upper shoulder or upper third of the arm and/or difficulty sleeping on the shoulder. Tendinitis and bursitis also cause pain when the arm is lifted away from the body or overhead. If tendinitis involves the biceps tendon (the tendon located in front of the shoulder that helps bend the elbow and turn the forearm), pain will occur in the front or side of the shoulder and may travel down to the elbow and forearm. Pain may also occur when the arm is forcefully pushed upward overhead.

How Are These Conditions Diagnosed?

Diagnosis of tendinitis and bursitis begins with a medical history and physical examination. X-rays do not show tendons or the bursae but may be helpful in ruling out bony abnormalities or arthritis. The doctor may remove and test fluid from the inflamed area to rule out infection. Impingement syndrome may be confirmed when injection of a small amount of anesthetic (lidocaine hydrochloride) into the space under the acromion relieves pain.

How Are Tendinitis, Bursitis, and Impingement Syndrome Treated?

The first step in treating these conditions is to reduce pain and inflammation with rest, ice, and anti-inflammatory medicines such as aspirin, naproxen (Naprosyn), ibuprofen (Advil, Motrin, or Nuprin), or cox-2 inhibitors (Celebrex or Vioxx). In some cases the doctor or therapist will use ultrasound (gentle sound-wave vibrations) to warm deep tissues and improve blood flow. Gentle stretching and strengthening exercises are added gradually. These may be preceded or followed by use of an ice pack. If there is no improvement, the doctor may inject a corticosteroid medicine into the space under the acromion. Although steroid injections are a common treatment, they must be used with caution because they may lead to tendon rupture. If there is still no improvement after 6 to 12 months, the doctor may perform either arthroscopic or open surgery to repair damage and relieve pressure on the tendons and bursae.

Arthritis of the Shoulder

What Is Arthritis of the Shoulder?

Arthritis is a degenerative disease caused by either wear and tear of the cartilage (osteoarthritis) or an inflammation (rheumatoid arthritis) of one or more joints. Arthritis not only affects joints; it may also affect supporting structures such as muscles, tendons, and ligaments.

What Are the Signs of Shoulder Arthritis and How Is It Diagnosed?

The usual signs of arthritis of the shoulder are pain, particularly over the AC joint, and a decrease in shoulder motion. A doctor may suspect the patient has arthritis when there is both pain and swelling in the joint. The diagnosis may be confirmed by a physical examination and x-rays. Blood tests may be helpful for diagnosing rheumatoid arthritis, but other tests may be needed as well. Analysis of synovial fluid from the shoulder joint may be helpful in diagnosing some kinds of arthritis. Although arthroscopy permits direct visualization of damage to cartilage, tendons, and ligaments, and may confirm a diagnosis, it is usually done only if a repair procedure is to be performed.

How Is Arthritis of the Shoulder Treated?

Most often osteoarthritis of the shoulder is treated with nonsteroidal anti-inflammatory drugs, such as aspirin, ibuprofen, or cox-2 inhibitors. (Rheumatoid arthritis of the shoulder may require physical therapy and additional medicine, such as corticosteroids.) When nonoperative treatment of arthritis of the shoulder fails to relieve pain or improve function, or when there is severe wear and tear of the joint causing parts to loosen and move out of place, shoulder joint replacement (arthroplasty) may provide better results. In this operation, a surgeon replaces the shoulder joint with an artificial ball for the top of the humerus and a cap (glenoid) for the scapula. Passive shoulder exercises (where someone else moves the arm to rotate the shoulder joint) are started soon after surgery. Patients begin exercising on their own about 3 to 6 weeks after surgery. Eventually, stretching and strengthening exercises become a major part of the rehabilitation program. The success of the operation often depends on the condition of rotator cuff muscles prior to surgery and the degree to which the patient follows the exercise program.

Where Can People Get Additional Information about Shoulder Problems?

National Institute of Arthritis and Musculoskeletal and Skin Diseases
1 AMS Circle
Bethesda, MD 20892-3675
Toll-Free: (877) 22-NIAMS (226-4267)
Phone: (301) 495-4484
TTY: (301) 565-2966
Fax: (301) 718-6366
Website: http://www.niams.nih.gov
E-mail: niamsinfo@mail.nih.gov

American Academy of Orthopaedic Surgeons (AAOS)
6300 North River Road
Rosemont, IL 60018-4262
Toll-Free: (800) 824-BONE (2663)
Phone: (847) 823-7186
Fax: (847) 823-8125
Website: http://www.aaos.org
E-mail: custserv@aaos.org

American College of Rheumatology
1800 Century Place, Suite 250
Atlanta, GA 30345-4300
Phone: (404) 633-3777
Fax: (404) 633-1870
Website: http://www.rheumatology.org

American Physical Therapy Association
1111 North Fairfax Street
Alexandria, VA 22314-1488
Toll-Free: (800) 999-2782, X3395
Phone: (703) 684-2782
Fax: (703) 684-7343

TDD: (703) 683-6748
Website: http://www.apta.org

Arthritis Foundation
1330 West Peachtree Street
Atlanta, GA 30309
Toll-Free: (800) 283-7800
Phone: (404) 872-7100
Website: http://www.arthritis.org
E-mail: arthritis@finelinesolutions.com

Chapter 14

Fibromyalgia

What Is Fibromyalgia?

Fibromyalgia is a chronic disorder characterized by widespread musculoskeletal pain, fatigue, and multiple tender points. Tender points refer to tenderness that occurs in precise, localized areas, particularly in the neck, spine, shoulders, and hips. People with this syndrome may also experience sleep disturbances, morning stiffness, irritable bowel syndrome, anxiety, and other symptoms.

How Many People Have Fibromyalgia?

According to the American College of Rheumatology, fibromyalgia affects 3 to 6 million Americans. It primarily occurs in women of childbearing age, but children, the elderly, and men can also be affected.

What Causes Fibromyalgia?

The cause and triggers of fibromyalgia remain unknown. Many theories about the disease have been explored, including muscle injury, changes in muscle metabolism, hormonal disorders, infectious agents, and autoimmune disease. Although none of these ideas have

"Questions and Answers about Fibromyalgia," National Institute of Arthritis and Musculoskeletal and Skin Diseases (NIAMS), December 1999. Available online at http://www.niams.nih.gov; accessed November 2003. Reviewed and revised by David A. Cooke, M.D. on November 27, 2003.

been completely ruled out, research has generally not supported them. Current evidence strongly suggests fibromyalgia is a disorder of the central nervous system. For unknown reasons, people with fibromyalgia appear to have increased sensitivity to pain. As a result, even ordinary activity and sensations may be painful. This disorder of pain processing in the brain also appears to affect nearby regions, which may explain the sleep and psychological symptoms that often accompany fibromyalgia.

How Is Fibromyalgia Diagnosed?

Fibromyalgia is difficult to diagnose because many of the symptoms mimic those of other disorders. The physician reviews the patient's medical history and makes a diagnosis of fibromyalgia based on a history of chronic widespread pain that persists for more than 3 months. The American College of Rheumatology (ACR) has developed criteria for fibromyalgia that physicians can use in diagnosing the disorder. According to ACR criteria, a person is considered to have fibromyalgia if he or she has widespread pain in combination with tenderness in at least 11 of 18 specific tender point sites.

How Is Fibromyalgia Treated?

Treatment of fibromyalgia requires a comprehensive approach. The physician, physical therapist, and patient may all play an active role in the management of fibromyalgia. Studies have shown that aerobic exercise, such as swimming and walking, improves muscle fitness and reduces muscle pain and tenderness. Heat and massage may also give short-term relief. Antidepressant medications may help elevate mood, improve quality of sleep, and relax muscles. Patients with fibromyalgia may benefit from a combination of exercise, medication, physical therapy, and relaxation.

What Research Is Being Conducted on Fibromyalgia?

The NIAMS is sponsoring research that will increase understanding of the specific abnormalities that cause and accompany fibromyalgia with the hope of developing better ways to diagnose, treat, and prevent this disorder.

Multiple avenues of research are currently being explored. Several research groups are examining brain activity in fibromyalgia patients to look for insights into neurologic abnormalities than may cause the condition. Others are examining interplay between the brain and production of certain key hormones such as cortisol, which might play a role in the condition. Still other groups are searching for medications that alter pain perception to help relieve the symptoms of fibromyalgia. Studies of psychological and exercise interventions to treat fibromyalgia have also been fruitful in recent years.

The NIAMS supports and encourages outstanding basic and clinical research that increases the understanding of fibromyalgia. However, much more research needs to be done before fibromyalgia can be successfully treated or prevented.

The Federal Government, in collaboration with researchers, physicians, and private voluntary health organizations, is committed to research efforts that are directed at significantly improving the health of all Americans afflicted with fibromyalgia.

Where Can People Get More Information about Fibromyalgia?

Arthritis Foundation
1330 West Peachtree Street
Atlanta, GA 30309
Toll-Free: (800) 283-7800
Phone: (404) 872-7100
Website: http://www.arthritis.org

National Fibromyalgia Association
2200 Glassell Street, Suite A
Orange, CA 92865
Phone: (714) 921-0150
Fax: (714) 921-6920
Website: http://fmaware.org
E-mail: NFA@fmaware.org

Chapter 15

Gout and Pseudogout

Chapter Contents

Section 15.1

Gout

"Questions and Answers About Gout," National Institute of Arthritis and Musculoskeletal and Skin Diseases (NIAMS), April 2002. Available online at http://www.niams.nih.gov; accessed February 2004.

This section contains general information about gout. It describes what gout is and how it develops. It also explains how gout is diagnosed and treated. If you have additional questions after reading this section, you may wish to discuss them with your doctor.

What Is Gout?

Gout is one of the most painful rheumatic diseases. It results from deposits of needle-like crystals of uric acid in connective tissue, in the joint space between two bones, or in both. These deposits lead to inflammatory arthritis, which causes swelling, redness, heat, pain, and stiffness in the joints. The term arthritis refers to more than 100 different rheumatic diseases that affect the joints, muscles, and bones, as well as other tissues and structures. Gout accounts for approximately 5 percent of all cases of arthritis.

Pseudogout is sometimes confused with gout because it produces similar symptoms of inflammation. However, in this condition, also called chondrocalcinosis, deposits are made up of calcium phosphate crystals, not uric acid. Therefore, pseudogout is treated somewhat differently and is not reviewed in this section.

Uric acid is a substance that results from the breakdown of purines, which are part of all human tissue and are found in many foods. Normally, uric acid is dissolved in the blood and passed through the kidneys into the urine, where it is eliminated. If the body increases its production of uric acid or if the kidneys do not eliminate enough uric acid from the body, levels of it build up in the blood (a condition called hyperuricemia). Hyperuricemia also may result when a person eats too many high-purine foods, such as liver, dried beans and peas, anchovies, and gravies. Hyperuricemia is not a disease and by itself is not dangerous. However, if excess uric acid crystals form as a result

184

of hyperuricemia, gout can develop. The excess crystals build up in the joint spaces, causing inflammation. Deposits of uric acid, called tophi (singular: tophus), can appear as lumps under the skin around the joints and at the rim of the ear. In addition, uric acid crystals can collect in the kidneys and cause kidney stones.

For many people, gout initially affects the joints in the big toe. Some time during the course of the disease, gout will affect the big toe in about 75 percent of patients. It also can affect the instep, ankles, heels, knees, wrists, fingers, and elbows. The disease can progress through four stages:

- **Asymptomatic (without symptoms) hyperuricemia**—In this stage, a person has elevated levels of uric acid in the blood but no other symptoms. A person in this stage does not usually require treatment.

- **Acute gout or acute gouty arthritis**—In this stage, hyperuricemia has caused the deposit of uric acid crystals in joint spaces. This leads to a sudden onset of intense pain and swelling in the joints, which also may be warm and very tender. An acute attack commonly occurs at night and can be triggered by stressful events, alcohol or drugs, or the presence of another illness. Early attacks usually subside within 3 to 10 days, even without treatment, and the next attack may not occur for months or even years. Over time, however, attacks can last longer and occur more frequently.

- **Interval or intercritical gout**—This is the period between acute attacks. In this stage, a person does not have any symptoms and has normal joint function.

- **Chronic tophaceous gout**—This is the most disabling stage of gout and usually develops over a long period, such as 10 years. In this stage, the disease has caused permanent damage to the affected joints and sometimes to the kidneys. With proper treatment, most people with gout do not progress to this advanced stage.

What Causes Gout?

A number of risk factors are related to the development of hyperuricemia and gout:

- Genetics may play a role in determining a person's risk, since up to 18 percent of people with gout have a family history of the disease.

- Gender and age are related to the risk of developing gout; it is more common in men than in women and more common in adults than in children.

- Being overweight increases the risk of developing hyperuricemia and gout because there is more tissue available for turnover or breakdown, which leads to excess uric acid production.

- Drinking too much alcohol can lead to hyperuricemia because it interferes with the removal of uric acid from the body.

- Eating too many foods rich in purines can cause or aggravate gout in some people.

- An enzyme defect that interferes with the way the body breaks down purines causes gout in a small number of people, many of whom have a family history of gout.

- Exposure to lead in the environment can cause gout.

Some people who take certain medicines or have certain conditions are at risk for having high levels of uric acid in their body fluids. For example, the following types of medicines can lead to hyperuricemia because they reduce the body's ability to remove uric acid:

- Diuretics, which are taken to eliminate excess fluid from the body in conditions like hypertension, edema, and heart disease, and which decrease the amount of uric acid passed in the urine.

- Salicylates, or anti-inflammatory medicines made from salicylic acid, such as aspirin.

- The vitamin niacin, also called nicotinic acid.

- Cyclosporine, a medicine used to suppress the body's immune system (the system that protects the body from infection and disease) and control the body's rejection of transplanted organs.

- Levodopa, a medicine used to support communication along nerve pathways in the treatment of Parkinson's disease.

Who Is Likely to Develop Gout?

Gout occurs in approximately 840 out of every 100,000 people. It is rare in children and young adults. Adult men, particularly those between the ages of 40 and 50, are more likely to develop gout than women, who rarely develop the disorder before menopause. People who have had an organ transplant are more susceptible to gout.

Signs and Symptoms of Gout

- Hyperuricemia
- Presence of uric acid crystals in joint fluid
- More than one attack of acute arthritis
- Arthritis that develops in 1 day, producing a swollen, red, and warm joint
- Attack of arthritis in only one joint, usually the toe, ankle, or knee

How Is Gout Diagnosed?

Gout may be difficult for doctors to diagnose because the symptoms may be vague, and they often mimic other conditions. Although most people with gout have hyperuricemia at some time during the course of their disease, it may not be present during an acute attack. In addition, having hyperuricemia alone does not mean that a person will get gout. In fact, most people with hyperuricemia do not develop the disease.

To confirm a diagnosis of gout, a doctor may insert a needle into an inflamed joint and draw a sample of synovial fluid, the substance that lubricates a joint. A laboratory technician places some of the fluid on a slide and looks for monosodium urate crystals under a microscope.

Their absence, however, does not completely rule out the diagnosis. The doctor also may find it helpful to examine chalky, sodium urate deposits (tophi) around joints to diagnose gout. Gout attacks may mimic joint infections, and a doctor who suspects a joint infection (rather than gout) may check for the presence of bacteria.

How Is Gout Treated?

With proper treatment, most people with gout are able to control their symptoms and live productive lives. Gout can be treated with one or a combination of therapies. The goals of treatment are to ease the pain associated with acute attacks, to prevent future attacks, and to avoid the formation of tophi and kidney stones. Successful treatment can reduce both the discomfort caused by the symptoms of gout and long-term damage of the affected joints. Treatment will help to prevent disability due to gout.

The most common treatments for an acute attack of gout are high doses of nonsteroidal anti-inflammatory drugs (NSAIDs) taken orally (by mouth) or corticosteroids, which are taken orally or injected into the affected joint. NSAIDs reduce the inflammation caused by deposits of uric acid crystals but have no effect on the amount of uric acid in the body. The NSAIDs most commonly prescribed for gout are indomethacin (Indocin) and naproxen (Anaprox and Naprosyn), which are taken orally every day. Corticosteroids are strong anti-inflammatory hormones. The most commonly prescribed corticosteroid is prednisone. Patients often begin to improve within a few hours of treatment with a corticosteroid, and the attack usually goes away completely within a week or so.

When NSAIDs or corticosteroids do not control symptoms, the doctor may consider using colchicine. This drug is most effective when taken within the first 12 hours of an acute attack. Doctors may ask patients to take oral colchicine as often as every hour until joint symptoms begin to improve or side effects such as nausea, vomiting, abdominal cramps, or diarrhea make it uncomfortable to continue the drug.

For some patients, the doctor may prescribe either NSAIDs or oral colchicine in small daily doses to prevent future attacks. The doctor also may consider prescribing medicine such as allopurinol (Zyloprim) or probenecid (Benemid) to treat hyperuricemia and reduce the frequency of sudden attacks and the development of tophi.

What Can People with Gout Do to Stay Healthy?

- To help prevent future attacks, take the medicines your doctor prescribes. Carefully follow instructions about how much medicine to take and when to take it. Acute gout is best treated when symptoms first occur.

- Tell your doctor about all the medicines and vitamins you take. He or she can tell you if any of them increase your risk of hyperuricemia.

- Plan follow-up visits with your doctor to evaluate your progress.

- Maintain a healthy, balanced diet; avoid foods that are high in purines; and drink plenty of fluids, especially water. Fluids help remove uric acid from the body.

- Exercise regularly and maintain a healthy body weight. Lose weight if you are overweight, but do not go on diets designed for quick or extreme loss of weight because they increase uric acid levels in the blood.

What Research Is Being Conducted to Help People with Gout?

Scientists are studying which NSAIDs are the most effective gout treatments, and they are analyzing new compounds to develop safe, effective medicines to lower the level of uric acid in the blood and to treat symptoms. They also are studying the structure of the enzymes that break down purines in the body to achieve a better understanding of the enzyme defects that can cause gout.

Scientists are studying the effect of crystal deposits on cartilage cells for clues to treatment. They also are looking at the role of calcium deposits in pseudogout in the hope of developing new treatments. The role genetics and environmental factors play in hyperuricemia also is being investigated.

Where Can People Find More Information about Gout?

National Institute of Arthritis and Musculoskeletal and Skin Diseases
1 AMS Circle
Bethesda, MD 20892-3675
Toll-Free: (877) 22-NIAMS (226-4267)
Phone: (301) 495-4484
TTY: (301) 565-2966
Fax: (301) 718-6366
Website: http://www.niams.nih.gov
E-mail: niamsinfo@mail.nih.gov

American College of Rheumatology
1800 Century Place, Suite 250
Atlanta, GA 30345-4300
Phone: (404) 633-3777
Fax: (404) 633-1870
Website: http://www.rheumatology.org

Arthritis Foundation
1330 West Peachtree Street
Atlanta, GA 30309
Toll-Free: (800) 283-7800
Phone: (404) 872-7100
Website: http://www.arthritis.org

Section 15.2

Pseudogout

Definition

Pseudogout is a joint disease that may include intermittent attacks of arthritis.

Causes, Incidence, and Risk Factors

Pseudogout is caused by the collection of calcium pyrophosphate crystals in joints. There may be attacks of joint swelling and pain in the knees, wrists, ankles, and other joints.

This condition primarily affects the elderly and usually has no known cause. However, it can sometimes affect younger patients who have conditions such as acromegaly, ochronosis, thyroid disease, hemochromatosis, Wilson disease, and parathyroid disease, which are known to increase risk.

Pseudogout can be initially be misdiagnosed as gouty arthritis, rheumatoid arthritis, or osteoarthritis because the symptoms are similar to those of these conditions.

Careful workup, with analysis of crystals found in joints, should ultimately lead to the correct diagnosis. Fortunately, because most conditions involving joint pain are treated by the same medicines, early misdiagnosis does not necessarily result in inappropriate treatment. Such treatment often includes steroids and nonsteroidal anti-inflammatory drugs (NSAIDs).

Symptoms

- Attacks of joint pain and fluid accumulation in the joint, leading to joint swelling

- No symptoms between attacks

- Chronic arthritis

Signs and Tests

- Culture of joint fluid reveals white blood cells and calcium pyrophosphate crystals.

- Joint x-rays may show joint damage, calcification of cartilage, and chondrocalcinosis (calcium deposits in joint spaces).

Treatment

Treatment may involve joint aspiration to relieve pressure within the joint caused by fluid buildup. A needle is placed into the joint and fluid is removed (aspirated).

Steroid injections may be helpful to treat severely inflamed joints. A course of oral steroids is sometimes used when multiple joints are inflamed.

Nonsteroidal anti-inflammatory medications (NSAIDs) may help ease the pain of acute attacks. Colchicine may be useful in some people.

Expectations (Prognosis)

The probable outcome is good with treatment.

Complications

Permanent joint damage can occur without treatment.

Calling Your Health Care Provider

Call for an appointment with your health care provider if you have attacks of joint swelling and joint pain.

Prevention

There is no known way to prevent this disorder. However, treatment of a known predisposing condition may reduce the severity of pseudogout and may in effect prevent it from developing in unaffected patients.

Chapter 16

Lyme Disease

In the early 1970s, a mysterious clustering of arthritis cases occurred among children in Lyme, Connecticut, and surrounding towns. Medical experts soon recognized the illness as a distinct disease, which they called Lyme disease. They subsequently described the signs and symptoms of Lyme disease, established the usefulness of antibiotics for treating it, identified the deer tick as the key to its spread, and isolated the bacterium that caused it.

Lyme disease is still mistaken for other ailments, and it continues to pose many other challenges, including the following:

- It can be difficult to diagnose.

- It can be troublesome to treat in its later phases.

- A number of different ticks can transmit diseases with symptoms similar to Lyme disease.

- Deer ticks can transmit diseases other than Lyme disease.

This chapter presents the most recently available information on the diagnosis, treatment, and prevention of Lyme disease.

"Lyme Disease: The Facts, The Challenge," National Institute of Arthritis and Musculoskeletal and Skin Diseases (NIAMS), National Institute of Allergy and Infectious Diseases (NIAID), April 2003. Available online at http://www.niaid.nih.gov; accessed February 2004.

How Lyme Disease Became Known

Lyme disease was first recognized in 1975 after researchers investigated why unusually large numbers of children were being diagnosed with juvenile rheumatoid arthritis in Lyme, Connecticut, and two neighboring towns. The researchers discovered that most of the affected children lived and played near wooded areas where ticks live. They also found that the children's first symptoms typically started in the summer months, the height of the tick season. Several of the patients interviewed reported having a skin rash just before developing their arthritis, and many also recalled being bitten by a tick at the rash site.

Further investigations discovered that tiny deer ticks infected with a spiral-shaped bacterium or spirochete (which was later named *Borrelia burgdorferi*) were responsible for the outbreak of arthritis in Lyme.

In Europe, a skin rash similar to that of Lyme disease had been described in medical literature dating back to the turn of the twentieth century. Lyme disease may have spread from Europe to the United States in the early 1900s, but health experts only recently recognized it as a distinct illness.

The number of reported cases of Lyme disease as well as the number of geographic areas in which it is found have been increasing. Lyme disease has been reported in nearly all states in the United States, although more than 98 percent of all reported cases are concentrated in the coastal Northeast, mid-Atlantic states, Wisconsin and Minnesota, and northern California. Lyme disease is also found in large areas of Asia and Europe.

Symptoms of Lyme Disease

Erythema Migrans

Usually, the first symptom of Lyme disease is a red rash known as erythema migrans (EM). The telltale rash starts as a small red spot at the site of the tick bite. The spot expands over a period of days or weeks, forming a circular or oval-shaped rash. Sometimes the rash resembles a bull's eye, appearing as a red ring surrounding a clear area with a red center. The rash, which can range in size from that of a dime to the width of a person's back, appears within a few weeks of a tick bite and usually at the site of the bite. As infection spreads, rashes can appear at different sites on the body.

Erythema migrans is often accompanied by symptoms such as fever, headache, stiff neck, body aches, and fatigue. Although these flu-like symptoms may resemble those of common viral infections, Lyme disease symptoms tend to persist or may come and go.

Arthritis

After several months of *B. burgdorferi* infection, slightly more than half of people not treated with antibiotics develop recurrent attacks of painful and swollen joints that last a few days to a few months. The arthritis can shift from one joint to another. The knee is most commonly affected. About 10 to 20 percent of untreated people will go on to develop chronic (long-lasting) arthritis.

Neurological Symptoms

Lyme disease can also affect the nervous system, causing symptoms such as:

- Stiff neck and severe headache (meningitis)
- Temporary paralysis of facial muscles (Bell's palsy)
- Numbness, pain, or weakness in the limbs
- Poor muscle movement

More subtle changes such as memory loss, difficulty concentrating, and a change in mood or sleeping habits have also been associated with Lyme disease.

Nervous system problems usually develop several weeks, months, or even years following an untreated infection. These symptoms often last for weeks or months and may return.

Long-Term Problems

Less commonly, untreated people may develop other problems weeks, months, or even years after infection. These include:

Heart Problems

Fewer than 1 out of 10 people with Lyme disease develop heart problems, such as an irregular heartbeat, which can start with dizziness or shortness of breath. These symptoms rarely last more than a few days or weeks. Such heart problems generally show up several weeks after infection.

Other Symptoms

Less commonly, Lyme disease can result in eye inflammation, hepatitis (liver disease), and severe fatigue, although none of these problems is likely to appear without other Lyme disease symptoms being present.

How Lyme Disease Is Diagnosed

Doctors or other health care workers may have difficulty diagnosing Lyme disease because many of its symptoms are similar to those of other disorders. In addition, the only distinctive sign unique to Lyme disease is the erythema migrans rash, which is absent in at least one-fourth of the people who become infected.

The results of recent research studies show that an infected tick must be attached to a person's skin for at least 2 days to transmit Lyme bacteria. Although a tick bite is an important clue for diagnosis, many people cannot recall having been bitten recently by a tick. This is not surprising because the deer tick is tiny and a tick bite is usually painless.

When a person with possible Lyme disease symptoms does not develop the distinctive rash, a doctor will rely on a detailed medical history and a careful physical examination for clues to diagnose it, with laboratory tests to support the diagnosis.

How Lyme Disease Is Treated

Using antibiotics appropriately, health care workers can effectively treat nearly anyone with Lyme disease. In general, the sooner treatment is begun following infection, the quicker and more complete the recovery.

Antibiotics such as doxycycline, cefuroxime axetil, or amoxicillin, taken orally for a few weeks, can speed the healing of the EM rash and usually prevent subsequent symptoms such as arthritis or neurological problems. Doxycycline will also effectively treat most other tickborne diseases.

When Lyme disease occurs in children younger than 9 years or in pregnant or breastfeeding women, they are usually treated with amoxicillin, cefuroxime axetil, or penicillin because doxycycline can stain the permanent teeth developing in young children or unborn babies. People allergic to penicillin are given erythromycin or related drugs.

Arthritis

People with Lyme arthritis may be treated with oral antibiotics. People with severe arthritis may be treated with ceftriaxone or penicillin given intravenously. To ease discomfort and to further healing, the doctor might also give anti-inflammatory drugs, draw fluid from affected joints, or surgically remove the inflamed lining of the joints.

Lyme arthritis goes away in most people within a few weeks or months following antibiotic treatment. In some, however, it can take years to disappear completely. Some people with Lyme disease who are untreated for several years may be cured of their arthritis with the proper antibiotic treatment. If the disease has persisted long enough, however, it may permanently damage the structure of the joints.

Neurological Problems

Doctors usually treat people who have neurological symptoms with the antibiotic ceftriaxone given intravenously once a day for a month or less. Most people recover completely.

Heart Problems

Doctors prefer to treat people with Lyme disease who have heart symptoms with antibiotics such as ceftriaxone or penicillin given intravenously for about 2 weeks. If these symptoms persist or are severe enough, they may also be given a temporary internal cardiac pacemaker. People with Lyme disease rarely have long-term heart damage.

Following treatment for Lyme disease, some people still have muscle achiness, neurological symptoms such as problems with memory and concentration, and fatigue. NIH-sponsored researchers are conducting studies to determine the cause of these symptoms and how to best treat them. Studies suggest that people who suffer from chronic Lyme disease may be genetically predisposed to develop an autoimmune response that contributes to their symptoms. Researchers are now examining the significance of this finding in great detail.

Researchers are also currently conducting studies to find out the best length of time to give antibiotics for the various signs and symptoms of Lyme disease.

Unfortunately, a bout with Lyme disease is no guarantee that the illness will not return. The disease can strike more than once in the same person if he or she is reinfected with Lyme disease bacteria.

Lyme Disease Prevention

Avoid Ticks

At present, the best way to avoid Lyme disease is to avoid deer ticks. Although generally only about 1 percent of all deer ticks are infected with Lyme disease bacteria, in some areas more than half of them harbor the germs.

Most people with Lyme disease become infected during the summer, when immature ticks are most prevalent. In warm climates, deer ticks thrive and bite during the winter months.

Deer ticks are most often found in wooded areas and nearby shady grasslands, and are especially common where the two areas merge. Because the adult ticks feed on deer, areas where deer are frequently seen are likely to harbor large numbers of deer ticks.

Pregnant women should be especially careful to avoid ticks in Lyme disease areas because infection can be transferred to an unborn child. Although rare, such a prenatal infection may make the woman more likely to miscarry or deliver a stillborn baby.

Here are some tips to prevent exposure to the ticks that carry Lyme disease:

- To help prevent contact with ticks, walk in the center of trails to avoid picking up ticks from overhanging grass and brush.

- To minimize skin exposure to ticks, wear long pants and long-sleeved shirts that fit tightly at the ankles and wrists. As a further safeguard wear a hat, tuck pant legs into socks, and wear shoes that leave no part of the feet exposed.

- To make it easy to find ticks on clothes, wear light-colored clothing.

- To keep ticks away, spray clothing with the insecticide permethrin, commonly found in insect lawn and garden stores.

- To repel ticks, spray clothing or the skin with repellents that contain a chemical called DEET (N, N-diethyl-M-toluamide).

Although highly effective, these repellents can cause some serious side effects, particularly when high concentrations are used repeatedly on the skin. Infants and children especially may suffer from bad reactions to DEET. If you repeatedly apply insect repellants with concentrations of DEET higher than 15 percent, you should wash your skin with soap and water as well as any clothing.

Check for Ticks

The immature deer ticks most likely to cause Lyme disease are only about the size of a poppy seed, so they are easily mistaken for a freckle or a speck of dirt. Once indoors:

- Check for ticks, particularly in the hairy regions of the body.
- Wash all clothing.
- Check pets for ticks before letting them in the house. A pet can carry ticks into the house.

These ticks could fall off without biting the animal and then attach to and bite people. In addition, pets can develop symptoms of Lyme disease.

If a tick is attached to the skin:

- Pull it out gently with tweezers, taking care not to squeeze the tick's body.
- Apply an antiseptic to the bite.

Studies by NIH-supported researchers suggest that a tick must be attached for at least 48 hours to transmit Lyme disease bacteria, so removing the tick promptly could keep you from getting infected.

The risk of developing Lyme disease from a tick bite is small, even in heavily infested areas, and most doctors prefer not to use antibiotics to treat people bitten by ticks unless they develop symptoms of Lyme disease.

Get Rid of Ticks

Deer provide a safe haven for ticks that transmit *B. burgdorferi* and other disease-causing microbes. You can reduce the number of ticks, which can spread diseases in your area, by clearing trees and removing yard litter and excess brush that attract deer and rodents.

In the meantime, researchers are trying to develop an effective strategy for ridding areas of deer ticks. Studies show that spraying pesticide in wooded areas in the spring and fall can substantially reduce for more than a year the number of adult deer ticks living there. Spraying on a large scale, however, may not be economically feasible and may prompt environmental or health concerns.

Researchers are also testing pesticide-treated deer and rodent feeders, which may offer an environmentally safer alternative. One product, the Maxforce Tick Management System, tested by the U.S. Centers for Disease Control and Prevention, reduces the number of ticks in the landscape by 80 percent the first year and 97 percent by year two.

Successful control of deer ticks will probably depend on a combination of tactics. Before wide-scale tick control strategies can be put into practice, there need to be more definitive studies.

Chapter 17

Myositis

What Is Myositis?

Myositis is the general term used to describe swelling of the muscles. Injury, infection, and even exercise can cause muscle swelling. The swelling will go away once the injury or infection is treated, or once you rest your muscles from exercise. Certain medicines can also cause some muscle swelling that goes away once you stop taking the medicine.

Often people who have temporary myositis from one of these causes become concerned when they read about the serious, chronic form of myositis. When we talk about myositis, we mean the inflammatory myopathies.

What Are Inflammatory Myopathies?

Myositis is used in the medical terms of dermatomyositis (DM), polymyositis (PM), inclusion-body myositis (IBM), and juvenile forms of myositis (JM or JPM). These are all considered inflammatory myopathies. Inflammatory myopathies are diseases of the muscle where there is swelling and loss of muscle.

Inflammatory myopathies are thought to be autoimmune diseases, meaning the body's immune system, which normally fights infections and viruses, does not stop fighting once the infection or virus is gone.

The immune system then attacks the body's own normal, healthy tissue through inflammation, or swelling. All of these diseases can cause muscle weakness, but each type is different.

Some early signs of myositis include:

- trouble rising from a chair, climbing stairs, or lifting arms
- tired feeling after standing or walking
- trouble swallowing or breathing

Your doctor may run some tests, including a physical examination, blood tests, electromyogram (EMG), and a muscle biopsy.

A myositis diagnosis is often confirmed by the muscle biopsy.

If you think you or someone you know may have DM, PM, IBM, JM, or JPM, talk to your doctor right away. It is important to start treatment as soon as possible.

Getting Diagnosed

Your doctor may first ask you questions about your health in general, including your health history. The doctor will want to know when you first saw signs of the skin rash or muscle weakness. He or she will then look at your skin and muscles.

Finally, the doctor may ask the hospital's lab to run one or more of the following tests:

- blood tests for muscle enzymes (including CPK and aldolase tests)
- muscle biopsy
- magnetic resonance imaging (MRI)
- electromyogram (EMG)

There may be other tests to rule out another type of disease or condition. If you have questions about any test, be sure to talk with your doctor or lab technician.

Treatment

Because myositis varies so much from patient to patient, no one treatment works for everyone. That's why it is so very important that you communicate well with your doctor about what is working for you and any side effects you may have. Over the years, doctors have identified some standard treatments, with careful attention to the sometimes serious complications of myositis.

To move forward with effective myositis treatments, researchers use clinical trials to test drugs that have already proved to be safe on actual patients.

Research articles pertaining to a variety of myositis related issues will help you further understand your condition and treatment options. Please share this material with your doctor.

What Type of Doctor Should I See?

Many new patients don't know where to find a doctor who knows about myositis. There are many types of doctors, so which one do you see?

You should find a doctor who makes you feel comfortable and who knows about myositis. Most patients see a rheumatologist, neurologist, or dermatologist. Some patients see two or three different types of doctors, using a team of doctors to get the best care possible.

How Do I Find a Doctor in My Area?

To find a doctor in your area, there are a number of places to look.

- The Bulletin Board section of The Myositis Association website (http://www.myositis.org) is a good place to start. Post a message to other patients, telling them where you live and what type of myositis you have. Many patients will give you the name of their own doctor and let you know how they feel about the care they receive.

- Find a major medical center or university/teaching hospital in your area. Since these hospitals are used for teaching about most medical conditions, many doctors will know about myositis and how to treat it.

- The American College of Rheumatology website, at http://www .rheumatology.org, lists doctors by city and state, so you can locate a doctor in your area or within reasonable traveling distance.

- The Muscular Dystrophy Association has clinics across the United States, and you can find one by visiting their website at http://www.mdausa.org or by calling (800) 572-1717.

- Mayo Clinics are located in Jacksonville, Florida; Scottsdale, Arizona; and Rochester, MN. These clinics are known for their understanding of a wide range of medical problems.

- The American Academy of Neurology website offers a "Find a Neurologist" search at http://www.aan.com/public/find.cfm. Enter your city and state for more information on doctors in your area.

- Some of The Myositis Association's Medical Advisors also see patients. To find one near you, visit the Medical Advisory Board section of the TMA website at http://www.myositis.org.

How Do I Set up an Appointment to See a New Doctor about Myositis?

Often, your family doctor or general practitioner (GP) will tell you to see a specialist (rheumatologist, neurologist or dermatologist) to order more tests for myositis. How you set up the appointment with the specialist depends on what type of insurance you have (PPO, HMO, etc.).

Your family doctor may recommend a particular doctor, or you can find a doctor using one of the ways listed above. If your doctor refers you to a clinic, your tests and follow-up care may be free of charge.

It may take weeks or months to set up an appointment with a specialist, so call the doctor's office as soon as you can. Ask to be put on a waiting list so if another patient cancels, you can see the doctor earlier.

Chapter 18

Osteoporosis

Chapter Contents

Section 18.1

Osteoporosis and Arthritis: Two Different but Common Conditions

National Institutes of Health Osteoporosis and Related Bone Diseases-National Resource Center, January 2003. Available online at http://www.osteo.org; accessed February 2004.

Many people confuse osteoporosis and some types of arthritis. This section will discuss the similarities and differences between osteoporosis and arthritis.

Osteoporosis

Osteoporosis is a major health threat for 44 million Americans, 68% of whom are women. In osteoporosis, there is a loss of bone tissue that leaves bones less dense and prone to fracture. It can result in a loss of height, severe back pain, and deformity. Osteoporosis can impair a person's ability to walk and can cause prolonged or permanent disability.

Risk factors for developing osteoporosis include: thinness or small frame; family history of osteoporosis; being postmenopausal or having had early menopause; abnormal absence of menstrual periods; prolonged use of certain medications, such as those used to treat diseases like systemic lupus erythematosus, asthma, thyroid deficiencies, and seizures; low calcium intake; physical inactivity; smoking; and excessive alcohol intake.

Osteoporosis is a silent disease that can often be prevented. However, if undetected, it can progress for many years without symptoms until a fracture occurs. Osteoporosis is diagnosed by a bone mineral density (BMD) test, a safe and painless way to detect low bone density.

Although there is no cure for the disease, several medications have been approved by the Food and Drug Administration for the prevention and treatment of osteoporosis. In addition, a diet rich in calcium and vitamin D, regular weight-bearing exercise, and a healthy lifestyle can prevent or lessen the effects of the disease.

Arthritis

Arthritis is a general term for conditions that affect the joints and surrounding tissues. Joints are places in the body where bones come together, such as the knee, wrist, fingers, toes, and hips. The two most common types of arthritis are osteoarthritis and rheumatoid arthritis.

Osteoarthritis (OA) is a painful, degenerative joint disease that often involves the hips, knees, neck, lower back, or the small joints of the hands. OA usually develops in joints that are injured by repeated overuse in the performance of a particular job or a favorite sport or from carrying around excess body weight.

Eventually this injury or repeated impact thins or wears away the cartilage that cushions the ends of the bones in the joint so that the bones rub together, causing a grating sensation. Joint flexibility is reduced, bony spurs develop, and the joint swells.

Usually, the first symptom a person has with OA is pain that worsens following exercise or immobility. Treatment usually includes analgesics, topical creams, or non-steroidal anti-inflammatory medications (known as NSAIDs); appropriate exercises or physical therapy; joint splinting; or joint replacement surgery for seriously damaged larger joints, such as the knee or hip.

Rheumatoid arthritis (RA) is an autoimmune inflammatory disease that usually involves the hands, wrists, elbows, shoulders, knees, feet, or ankles. An autoimmune disease is one in which the body releases enzymes that attack its own healthy tissues. In RA, these enzymes destroy the linings of joints causing pain, swelling, stiffness, deformity, and reduced movement and function. People with RA also may have systemic symptoms, such as fatigue, fever, weight loss, eye inflammation, anemia, subcutaneous nodules (bumps under the skin), or pleurisy (a lung inflammation).

While osteoporosis and osteoarthritis are two very different medical conditions with little in common, the similarity of their names causes great confusion. These conditions develop differently, have different symptoms, are diagnosed differently, and are treated differently. While it is possible to have both osteoporosis and arthritis, studies show that people with osteoarthritis are less likely to develop osteoporosis. On the other hand, people with rheumatoid arthritis may be more likely to develop osteoporosis, especially as a secondary condition from medications used to treat RA.

Osteoporosis and arthritis do share many coping strategies. With either or both conditions, people benefit from exercise programs that

Table 18.1. Similarities between Osteoporosis, Osteoarthritis, and Rheumatoid Arthritis (*continued on next page*)

	Osteoporosis	Osteoarthritis	Rheumatoid Arthritis
Risk Factors			
Age-related	X	X	
Menopause	X		
Family History	X	X	X
Use of certain medications, such as glucocorticoids and seizure medications	X		
Calcium deficiency and inadequate vitamin D	X		
Inactivity	X		
Overuse of joints		X	
Smoking	X		
Excessive alcohol	X		
Anorexia nervosa	X		
Excessive weight		X	
Physical Effects			
Affects entire skeleton	X		
Affects joints		X	X
Is an autoimmune disease			X
Bony spurs		X	X
Enlarged or deformed joints		X	X
Height loss	X		
Treatment Options			
Raloxifene	X		
Alendronate and risedronate	X		
Calcitonin	X		
Teriparatide	X		
Calcium and Vitamin D	X		
Weight management		X	
Glucocorticoids			X
NSAIDs	X	X	X

Treatment Options are continued on the next page.

Table 18.1. Similarities between Osteoporosis, Osteoarthritis, and Rheumatoid Arthritis (*continued from previous page*)

	Osteoporosis	Osteoarthritis	Rheumatoid Arthritis
Treatment Options (continued)			
Methotrexate			X
Disease modifying antirheumatic drugs (hydroxychloroquine, gold salts, sulfasalazine, azathioprine, D-penicillamine)			X
Pain Management			
Pain medication (NSAIDs, narcotics, muscle relaxers)	X	X	X
Rehabilitation	X	X	X
Support groups	X	X	X
Exercises-postural	X	X	X
Exercises (isometric, isotonic, isokinetic)	X	X	X
Joint splinting		X	X
Physical therapy	X	X	X
Passive exercises		X	X
Hip fracture surgical repair (may include hip replacement depending on type of hip fracture)	X		
Joint replacement surgery (usually for pain, deformity, or impaired mobility)		X	X
Heat and cold	X		X
Massage therapy	X	X	X
Acupuncture	X	X	X
Psychological approaches (relaxation, visualization, biofeedback)	X	X	X
Tai chi	X	X	X
Low stress yoga	X	X	X

may include physical therapy and rehabilitation. In general, exercises that emphasize stretching, strengthening, posture, and range of motion are appropriate, such as low impact aerobics, swimming, tai chi, and low stress yoga.

However, people with osteoporosis must take care to avoid activities that include bending forward from the waist, twisting the spine, or lifting heavy weights. People with arthritis must compensate for limited movement in arthritic joints. Always check with your physician to determine if a certain exercise or exercise program is safe for your specific medical situation.

Everyone with arthritis will use pain management strategies at some time. This is not always true for people with osteoporosis. Usually, people with osteoporosis need pain relief when they are recovering from a fracture. In cases of severe osteoporosis with multiple spine fractures, pain control also may become part of daily life. Regardless of the cause, pain management strategies are similar for people with osteoporosis, OA, and RA. Table 18.1 provides an overview of some of the similarities and differences between osteoporosis, osteoarthritis, and rheumatoid arthritis. Some individuals with these conditions may have a different experience or may require a different medical approach to manage their disorder.

Section 18.2

What People with Rheumatoid Arthritis Need to Know about Osteoporosis

National Institutes of Health Osteoporosis and Related Bone Diseases-National Resource Center, January 2003. Available online at http://www.osteo.org; accessed February 2004.

What Is Rheumatoid Arthritis?

Rheumatoid arthritis (RA) is an autoimmune disease, a disorder in which the body attacks its own healthy cells and tissues. In rheumatoid arthritis the membranes surrounding the joints become inflamed and release enzymes that cause the surrounding cartilage and bone to wear away. In severe cases, other tissues and body organs also can be affected.

Individuals with rheumatoid arthritis often experience pain, swelling, and stiffness in their joints, especially those in the hands and feet. Limited motion of the affected joints can also occur, curtailing one's ability to accomplish even the most basic everyday tasks. About one quarter of those with rheumatoid arthritis develop nodules (bumps) that grow under the skin, usually close to the joints. Fatigue, anemia (low blood cell count), neck pain, and dry eyes and mouth can also occur in individuals with the disease.

According to the National Institute of Arthritis and Musculoskeletal and Skin Diseases, it is estimated that about 2.1 million people in the United States have rheumatoid arthritis. The disease occurs in all racial and ethnic groups, but affects two to three times as many women as men. Rheumatoid arthritis is more commonly found in older individuals, though the disease typically begins in middle age. Children and young adults can also be affected.

What Is Osteoporosis?

Osteoporosis is a condition in which the bones become less dense and more likely to fracture. Fractures from osteoporosis can result in significant pain and disability. It is a major health threat for an estimated 44 million Americans, 80% of whom are women.

211

Risk factors for developing osteoporosis include: thinness or small frame; family history of the disease; being postmenopausal or having had early menopause; abnormal absence of menstrual periods; prolonged use of certain medications, such as glucocorticoids; low calcium intake; physical inactivity; smoking; and excessive alcohol intake.

Osteoporosis is a silent disease that can often be prevented. However, if undetected, it can progress for many years without symptoms until a fracture occurs.

The Rheumatoid Arthritis—Osteoporosis Link

Studies have found an increased risk of bone loss and fracture in individuals with rheumatoid arthritis. People with rheumatoid arthritis are at increased risk for osteoporosis for many reasons. To begin with, the glucocorticoid medications often prescribed for the treatment of RA can trigger significant bone loss. In addition, pain and loss of joint function caused by the disease can result in inactivity, further increasing osteoporosis risk. Studies also show that bone loss in rheumatoid arthritis may occur as a direct result of the disease. The bone loss is most pronounced in areas immediately surrounding the affected joints. Of concern is the fact that women, a group already at increased osteoporosis risk, are two to three times more likely than men to suffer from RA as well.

Osteoporosis Management Strategies

Strategies for the prevention and treatment of osteoporosis in people with rheumatoid arthritis are not significantly different from the strategies for those who do not have the disease.

Nutrition and Exercise. A diet rich in calcium and vitamin D is important for healthy bones. Good sources of calcium include low-fat dairy products, dark green, leafy vegetables, and calcium fortified foods and beverages. Also, supplements can help ensure that the calcium requirement is met each day.

Vitamin D plays an important role in calcium absorption and bone health. It is synthesized in the skin through exposure to sunlight. Although many people are able to obtain enough vitamin D naturally, older individuals are often deficient in this vitamin due, in part, to limited time spent outdoors. Such individuals may require vitamin D supplements to ensure an adequate daily intake.

Like muscle, bone is living tissue that responds to exercise by becoming stronger. The best exercise for your bones is weight-bearing exercise that forces you to work against gravity. Some examples include walking, stair climbing, and dancing.

Exercising can be challenging for people with rheumatoid arthritis and needs to be balanced with rest when the disease is active. However, regular exercises such as walking can help prevent bone loss and, by enhancing balance and flexibility, can reduce the likelihood of falling and breaking a bone. Exercise is also important for preserving joint mobility.

Healthy Lifestyle. Smoking is bad for bones as well as the heart and lungs. Women who smoke tend to go through menopause earlier, triggering earlier bone loss. In addition, smokers may absorb less calcium from their diets. Alcohol can also negatively affect bone health. Those who drink heavily are more prone to bone loss and fracture, both because of poor nutrition as well as increased risk of falling.

Bone Density Test. Specialized tests known as bone mineral density (BMD) tests measure bone density at various sites of the body. These tests can detect osteoporosis before a fracture occurs and predict one's chances of fracturing in the future. RA patients, particularly those receiving glucocorticoid therapy for two months or more, should talk to their doctors about whether they might be a candidate for a bone density test.

Medication. Like rheumatoid arthritis, there is no cure for osteoporosis. However, there are medications available for the prevention and treatment of osteoporosis. Several medications (alendronate, risedronate, raloxifene, calcitonin, teriparatide, and estrogen/hormone therapy) are approved by the Food and Drug Administration (FDA) for the prevention and/or treatment of osteoporosis in postmenopausal women. Alendronate is also approved for use in men. For RA patients on glucocorticoid therapy, alendronate (for treatment) and risedronate (for prevention and treatment) are approved for glucocorticoid-induced osteoporosis.

Juvenile Rheumatoid Arthritis

Juvenile rheumatoid arthritis (JRA) occurs in children sixteen years of age or younger. Children with severe JRA may be candidates for glucocorticoid medication, the use of which has been linked to bone loss in children as well as adults. Physical activity can be challenging in children with JRA because it may cause pain. Incorporating physical activities recommended by the child's physician and a diet rich in calcium and vitamin D are especially important for these children to help optimize peak bone mass and reduce the risk of future fracture.

Section 18.3

Did You Know Osteoporosis Can Be Prevented?

National Institute of Arthritis and Musculoskeletal and Skin Diseases (NIAMS), 2004. Available online at http://www.niams.nih.gov; accessed March 2004.

Osteoporosis means thin bones, and it is caused by the loss of bone material, which leads to fragile bones and fractures. Many men, as well as women, suffer from osteoporosis, but it is a disease that can be prevented before it occurs or treated after it happens.

What Is Bone?

Bone is living, growing tissue made mostly of two components: a protein called collagen, which provides a soft framework for bone, and a mineral, calcium phosphate, which strengthens and hardens the framework. This combination makes bone strong, yet flexible.

Throughout a person's lifetime, old bone is removed (called resorption) and new bone is added to the skeleton (called formation). During childhood and the teenage years, new bone is added faster than old bone is removed, making bones grow larger and denser. Bone formation outpaces resorption until bone reaches its greatest density and strength sometime before age 30. With natural aging, bone resorption may slowly outpace formation. Osteoporosis develops when bone resorption occurs too quickly and/or when bone replacement occurs too slowly.

Facts and Figures

- In the United States, more than 10 million people have osteoporosis and 34 million more are at increased risk for the disease.

- One out of every two women and one in four men older than age 50 will have an osteoporosis-related fracture in his or her lifetime.

- Each year, 80,000 men suffer a hip fracture and one third of these men die within a year.

Risk Factors

Certain risk factors are linked to the development of osteoporosis or to an individual's likelihood of developing the disease. Some risk factors can be changed, but others cannot.

What You Can't Change

- Gender—Women have smaller bones and lose bone more rapidly than men because of hormone changes associated with menopause, so women are at higher risk for osteoporosis.

- Age—The older you are, the greater your risk of osteoporosis because bones become less dense with age.

- Ethnicity—Caucasian and Asian women are at the highest risk for osteoporosis. African American and Latino women have a lower, but still significant, risk.

- History of fracture—Having had a fracture is one of the most important risk factors for future fractures. Anyone who has fractured a bone after age 45 or who has had several fractures before that age should see a physician to be screened for osteoporosis.

- Family history—Susceptibility to bone loss and fractures may be partly hereditary.

What You Can Change

You can lower your risk of developing osteoporosis. To reach optimal bone mass and continue building new bone tissue, consider the following recommendations.

215

- Calcium—Researchers think getting too little calcium over a lifetime may contribute to osteoporosis. The most concentrated dietary sources of calcium include dairy products, such as milk, yogurt, cheese and ice cream. A typical American diet supplies approximately 300 milligrams of calcium from nondairy foods, such as dark green, leafy vegetables (including broccoli, collard greens and bok choy), sardines and salmon with bones, tofu, almonds and foods fortified with calcium. Recent guidelines suggest that adults need between 1,000 and 1,200 milligrams daily. If you're not getting enough calcium each day in the food you eat, you also may need to take a supplement that contains calcium.

- Vitamin D—Vitamin D helps the body absorb calcium. The body makes vitamin D in the skin when it is exposed to sunlight, and many people obtain enough of it. Studies show, however, that vitamin D production decreases in the elderly, in the housebound, and during the winter. Milk (in liquid form) is supplemented with vitamin D; fish such as salmon and tuna also are good sources of vitamin D. Some people, especially the elderly, may need to take a supplement containing vitamin D to ensure that each day they get 200 to 600 IU (international units, the standard of measurement used for many nutritional supplements).

- Exercise—Like muscle, bone responds to exercise by becoming stronger. The best kind of exercise for your bones is weight-bearing exercise, which forces you to work against gravity. Such exercise includes walking, jogging, stair climbing, weight training, and dancing.

- Smoking—It is easier said than done, but quitting smoking can reduce your risk of developing osteoporosis, not to mention heart disease and a number of types of cancer. Smokers may absorb less calcium from their diets. Women who smoke have lower levels of estrogen than nonsmokers and frequently go through menopause earlier.

- Medications—Long-term use of glucocorticoids (commonly called steroids, although these are not the same type of steroids abused by some athletes) can lead to a loss of bone density and fractures. Other medications that increase osteoporosis risk include certain antiseizure drugs, such as phenytoin and barbiturates; gonadotropin releasing hormone (GnRH) analogs used to treat endometriosis; and excessive use of aluminum-containing

216

antacids. It is important to discuss these medications with your physician and to consult him or her before you stop taking them or alter your dosage.

Treatment

Osteoporosis is a treatable disease. A person over age 65 or at high risk of developing osteoporosis for other reasons may wish to see a physician to have a bone mineral density test. Such a screening can lead to steps to reduce the risk of fracture. The Food and Drug Administration has approved several medications for the prevention and treatment of osteoporosis. A comprehensive treatment program often includes exercise, proper nutrition, safety precautions to prevent falls that may result in fractures, and sometimes medications.

Chapter 19

Paget Disease of Bone

What Is Paget Disease of Bone?

Paget disease is a chronic disorder that typically results in enlarged and deformed bones. The excessive breakdown and formation of bone tissue that occurs with Paget disease can cause bone to weaken, resulting in bone pain, arthritis, deformities, and fractures. Paget disease may be caused by a slow virus infection, which is present for many years before symptoms appear. There is also a hereditary factor because the disease may appear in more than one family member.

Who Is Affected?

Paget disease is rarely diagnosed in people under 40 years of age. Men and women are affected equally. Prevalence of Paget disease ranges from 1.5 to 8 percent depending on age and country of residence. Prevalence of familial Paget disease (where more than one family member has the disease) ranges from 10 to 40 percent in different parts of the world. Because early diagnosis and treatment is important, after age 40, siblings and children of someone with Paget disease may wish to have an alkaline phosphatase blood test every 2 or 3 years. If the alkaline phosphatase level is above normal, other tests such as a bone-specific alkaline phosphatase test, bone scan, or x-ray can be performed.

"Information for Patients about Paget's Disease of Bone," National Institutes of Health Osteoporosis and Related Bone Diseases-National Resource Center, May 2000. Available online at http://www.osteo.org; accessed January 2004.

Symptoms

Many patients do not know they have Paget disease because they have a mild case of the disease with no symptoms. Sometimes, symptoms may be confused with those of arthritis or other disorders. In other cases, the diagnosis is made only after complications have developed. Symptoms can include:

- Bone pain—the most common symptom. Bone pain can occur in any bone affected by Paget disease. It often localizes to areas adjacent to the joints.

- Headaches and hearing loss—may occur when Paget disease affects the skull.

- Pressure on nerves—may occur when Paget disease affects the skull or spine.

- Increased head size, bowing of limb, or curvature of spine—may occur in advanced cases.

- Hip pain—may occur when Paget disease affects the pelvis or thighbone.

- Damage to cartilage of joints—may lead to arthritis.

Diagnosis

Paget disease may be diagnosed using one or more of the following tests:

- X-rays—Pagetic bone has a characteristic appearance on x-rays.

- Alkaline phosphatase blood test—An elevated level of alkaline phosphatase in the blood can be suggestive of Paget disease.

- Bone scans—Useful in determining the extent and activity of the condition. If a bone scan suggests Paget disease, the affected bones should be x-rayed to confirm the diagnosis.

Prognosis

The outlook is generally good, particularly if treatment is given before major changes in the affected bones have occurred. Any bone or bones can be affected, but Paget disease occurs most frequently in the spine, skull, pelvis, thighs, and lower legs. In general, symptoms progress slowly, and the disease does not spread to normal bones.

Treatment can control Paget disease and lessen symptoms but is not a cure. Osteogenic sarcoma, a form of bone cancer, is an extremely rare complication that occurs in less than one percent of all patients.

Other Medical Conditions

Paget disease may lead to other medical conditions, including:

- Arthritis—Long bones in the leg may bow, distorting alignment and increasing pressure on nearby joints. In addition, Pagetic bone may enlarge, causing joint surfaces to undergo excessive wear and tear. In these cases, pain may be due to a combination of Paget disease and osteoarthritis.

- Hearing problems—Loss of hearing in one or both ears may occur when Paget disease affects the skull and the bone that surrounds the inner ear. Treating the Paget disease may slow or stop hearing loss. Hearing aids may also help.

- Heart disease—In severe Paget disease, the heart works harder to pump blood to affected bones. This usually does not result in heart failure except in some people who also have hardening of the arteries.

- Kidney stones—Kidney stones are somewhat more common in patients with Paget disease.

- Nervous system problems—Pagetic bone can cause pressure on the brain, spinal cord, or nerves, and reduced blood flow to the brain and spinal cord.

- Sarcoma—Rarely, Paget disease is associated with the development of a malignant tumor of bone. When there is a sudden onset or worsening of pain, sarcoma should be considered.

- Dental problems—When Paget disease affects the facial bones, the teeth may become loose. Disturbance in chewing may occur.

- Vision problems—Rarely, when the skull is involved, the nerves to the eye may be affected, causing some loss of vision.

Paget disease is not associated with the following disorder:

- Osteoporosis—Although Paget disease and osteoporosis can occur in the same patient, they are completely different disorders. Despite their marked differences, many treatments for Paget disease can also be used to treat osteoporosis.

221

Treatment

Types of Physicians

The following types of medical specialists are generally knowledge-able about treating Paget disease.

- Endocrinologists—Internists who specialize in hormonal and metabolic disorders.

- Rheumatologists—Internists who specialize in joint and muscle disorders.

- Specialists—Orthopedic surgeons, neurologists, and otolaryngologists (physicians who specialize in ear, nose, and throat disorders) may be called upon to evaluate specialized symptoms.

Drug Therapy

The goal of treatment is to control Paget disease activity for as long a period of time as possible. The U.S. Food and Drug Administration (FDA) has approved the following treatments for Paget disease.

Bisphosphonates

Five bisphosphonates are currently available. As a rule, bisphosphonate tablets should be taken with 6 to 8 ounces of tap water on an empty stomach. None of these drugs should be used by people with severe kidney disease.

- Didronel® (etidronate disodium)—Tablet; approved regimen is 200 to 400 mg once daily for 6 months; the higher dose (400 mg) is more commonly used; no food, beverages, or medications for 2 hours before and after taking; course should not exceed 6 months, but repeat courses can be given after rest periods, preferably of 3 to 6 months duration.

- Aredia® (pamidronate disodium)—Intravenous; approved regimen 30 mg infusion over 4 hours on 3 consecutive days; more commonly used regimen 60 mg over 2 to 4 hours for 2 or more consecutive or non-consecutive days.

- Fosamax® (alendronate sodium)—Tablet; 40 mg once daily for 6 months; patients should wait at least 30 minutes after taking before eating any food, drinking anything other than tap water, taking any medication, or lying down (patient may sit).

- Skelid® (tiludronate disodium)—Tablet; 400 mg (two 200 mg tablets) once daily for 3 months; may be taken any time of day, as long as there is a period of 2 hours before and after resuming food, beverages, and medications.

- Actonel® (risedronate sodium)—Tablet; 30 mg once daily for 2 months; patients should wait at least 30 minutes after taking before eating any food, drinking anything other than tap water, taking any medication, or lying down (patient may sit).

Calcitonin

Miacalcin® is administered by injection; 50 to 100 units daily or 3 times per week for 6 to 18 months.

Surgery

Medical therapy prior to surgery helps to decrease bleeding and other complications. Patients who are having surgery should discuss pre-treatment with their physician. There are generally three major complications of Paget disease for which surgery may be recommended.

- Fractures—Surgery may allow fractures to heal in better position.

- Severe degenerative arthritis—If disability is severe and medication and physical therapy are no longer helpful, joint replacement of the hips and knees may be considered.

- Bone deformity—Cutting and realignment of Pagetic bone (osteotomy) may help painful weight-bearing joints, especially the knees.

Complications resulting from enlargement of the skull or spine may injure the nervous system. However, most neurologic symptoms, even those that are moderately severe, can be treated with medication and do not require neurosurgery.

Diet and Exercise

In general, patients with Paget disease should receive 1,000 to 1,500 mg of calcium, adequate sunshine, and at least 400 units of vitamin D daily. This is especially important in patients being treated with bisphosphonates. Patients with a history of kidney stones should discuss calcium and vitamin D intake with their physician.

Exercise is very important in maintaining skeletal health, avoiding weight gain, and maintaining joint mobility. Since undue stress on affected bones should be avoided, patients should discuss any exercise program with their physician before beginning.

For more information about Paget disease, contact:

The Paget Foundation for Paget's Disease of Bone and Related Disorders

120 Wall Street
Suite 1602
New York, NY 10005-4001
Toll-Free: (800) 23-PAGET
Phone: (212) 509-5335
Fax: (212) 509-8492
Website: http://www.paget.org
E-mail: PagetFdn@aol.com

Chapter 20

Psoriasis and Arthritis

Chapter Contents

Section 20.1

Questions and Answers about Psoriasis

National Institute of Arthritis and Musculoskeletal and Skin Diseases (NIAMS), May 2003. Available online at http://www.niams.nih.gov; accessed March 2004.

This section contains general information about psoriasis. It describes what psoriasis is, what causes it, and what the treatment options are. If you have further questions after reading this information you may wish to discuss them with your doctor.

What Is Psoriasis?

Psoriasis is a chronic (long-lasting) skin disease of scaling and inflammation that affects 2 to 2.6 percent of the United States population, or between 5.8 and 7.5 million people. Although the disease occurs in all age groups, it primarily affects adults. It appears about equally in males and females. Psoriasis occurs when skin cells quickly rise from their origin below the surface of the skin and pile up on the surface before they have a chance to mature. Usually this movement (also called turnover) takes about a month, but in psoriasis it may occur in only a few days. In its typical form, psoriasis results in patches of thick, red (inflamed) skin covered with silvery scales. These patches, which are sometimes referred to as plaques, usually itch or feel sore. They most often occur on the elbows, knees, other parts of the legs, scalp, lower back, face, palms, and soles of the feet, but they can occur on skin anywhere on the body.

The disease may also affect the fingernails, the toenails, and the soft tissues of the genitals and inside the mouth. While it is not unusual for the skin around affected joints to crack, approximately 1 million people with psoriasis experience joint inflammation that produces symptoms of arthritis. This condition is called psoriatic arthritis.

How Does Psoriasis Affect Quality of Life?

Individuals with psoriasis may experience significant physical discomfort and some disability. Itching and pain can interfere with basic functions, such as self-care, walking, and sleep. Plaques on hands and feet can prevent individuals from working at certain occupations, playing some sports, and caring for family members or a home. The frequency of medical care is costly and can interfere with an employment or school schedule. People with moderate to severe psoriasis may feel self-conscious about their appearance and have a poor self-image that stems from fear of public rejection and psychosexual concerns. Psychological distress can lead to significant depression and social isolation.

What Causes Psoriasis?

Psoriasis is a skin disorder driven by the immune system, especially involving a type of white blood cell called a T cell. Normally, T cells help protect the body against infection and disease. In the case of psoriasis, T cells are put into action by mistake and become so active that they trigger other immune responses, which lead to inflammation and to rapid turnover of skin cells. In about one third of the cases, there is a family history of psoriasis. Researchers have studied a large number of families affected by psoriasis and identified genes linked to the disease. (Genes govern every bodily function and determine the inherited traits passed from parent to child.) People with psoriasis may notice that there are times when their skin worsens, then improves. Conditions that may cause flare-ups include infections, stress, and changes in climate that dry the skin. Also, certain medicines, including lithium and beta blockers, which are prescribed for high blood pressure, may trigger an outbreak or worsen the disease.

How Is Psoriasis Diagnosed?

Occasionally, doctors may find it difficult to diagnose psoriasis, because it often looks like other skin diseases. It may be necessary to confirm a diagnosis by examining a small skin sample under a microscope. There are several forms of psoriasis. Some of these include:

- Plaque psoriasis—Skin lesions are red at the base and covered by silvery scales.

- Guttate psoriasis—Small, drop-shaped lesions appear on the trunk, limbs, and scalp. Guttate psoriasis is most often triggered by upper respiratory infections (for example, a sore throat caused by streptococcal bacteria).

- Pustular psoriasis—Blisters of noninfectious pus appear on the skin. Attacks of pustular psoriasis may be triggered by medications, infections, stress, or exposure to certain chemicals.

- Inverse psoriasis—Smooth, red patches occur in the folds of the skin near the genitals, under the breasts, or in the armpits. The symptoms may be worsened by friction and sweating.

- Erythrodermic psoriasis—Widespread reddening and scaling of the skin may be a reaction to severe sunburn or to taking corticosteroids (cortisone) or other medications. It can also be caused by a prolonged period of increased activity of psoriasis that is poorly controlled.

- Psoriatic arthritis—Joint inflammation that produces symptoms of arthritis in patients who have or will develop psoriasis.

How Is Psoriasis Treated?

Doctors generally treat psoriasis in steps based on the severity of the disease, size of the areas involved, type of psoriasis, and the patient's response to initial treatments. This is sometimes called the "1-2-3" approach. In step 1, medicines are applied to the skin (topical treatment). Step 2 uses light treatments (phototherapy). Step 3 involves taking medicines by mouth or injection that treat the whole immune system (called systemic therapy).

Over time, affected skin can become resistant to treatment, especially when topical corticosteroids are used. Also, a treatment that works very well in one person may have little effect in another. Thus, doctors often use a trial-and-error approach to find a treatment that works, and they may switch treatments periodically (for example, every 12 to 24 months) if a treatment does not work or if adverse reactions occur.

Topical Treatment

Treatments applied directly to the skin may improve its condition. Doctors find that some patients respond well to ointment or cream forms of corticosteroids, vitamin D3, retinoids, coal tar, or anthralin. Bath solutions and moisturizers may be soothing, but they are seldom strong enough to improve the condition of the skin. Therefore, they usually are combined with stronger remedies.

- **Corticosteroids**—These drugs reduce inflammation and the turnover of skin cells, and they suppress the immune system.

Available in different strengths, topical corticosteroids (cortisone) are usually applied to the skin twice a day. Short-term treatment is often effective in improving, but not completely eliminating, psoriasis. Long-term use or overuse of highly potent (strong) corticosteroids can cause thinning of the skin, internal side effects, and resistance to the treatment's benefits. If less than 10 percent of the skin is involved, some doctors will prescribe a high-potency corticosteroid ointment. High-potency corticosteroids may also be prescribed for plaques that don't improve with other treatment, particularly those on the hands or feet. In situations where the objective of treatment is comfort, medium-potency corticosteroids may be prescribed for the broader skin areas of the torso or limbs. Low-potency preparations are used on delicate skin areas.

- **Calcipotriene**—This drug is a synthetic form of vitamin D3 that can be applied to the skin. Applying calcipotriene ointment (for example, Dovonex) twice a day controls the speed of turnover of skin cells. Because calcipotriene can irritate the skin, however, it is not recommended for use on the face or genitals. It is sometimes combined with topical corticosteroids to reduce irritation. Use of more than 100 grams of calcipotriene per week may raise the amount of calcium in the body to unhealthy levels.

- **Retinoid**—Topical retinoids are synthetic forms of vitamin A. The retinoid tazarotene (Tazorac) is available as a gel or cream that is applied to the skin. If used alone, this preparation does not act as quickly as topical corticosteroids, but it does not cause thinning of the skin or other side effects associated with steroids. However, it can irritate the skin, particularly in skin folds and the normal skin surrounding a patch of psoriasis. It is less irritating and sometimes more effective when combined with a corticosteroid. Because of the risk of birth defects, women of childbearing age must take measures to prevent pregnancy when using tazarotene.

- **Coal tar**—Preparations containing coal tar (gels and ointments) may be applied directly to the skin, added (as a liquid) to the bath, or used on the scalp as a shampoo. Coal tar products are available in different strengths, and many are sold over the counter (not requiring a prescription). Coal tar is less effective than corticosteroids and many other treatments and, therefore, is sometimes combined with ultraviolet B (UVB) phototherapy for a better result. The most potent form of coal tar may irritate the skin, is messy, has a strong odor, and may stain the skin or clothing. Thus, it is not popular with many patients.

- **Anthralin**—Anthralin reduces the increase in skin cells and inflammation. Doctors sometimes prescribe a 15- to 30-minute application of anthralin ointment, cream, or paste once each day to treat chronic psoriasis lesions. Afterward, anthralin must be washed off the skin to prevent irritation. This treatment often fails to adequately improve the skin, and it stains skin, bathtub, sink, and clothing brown or purple. In addition, the risk of skin irritation makes anthralin unsuitable for acute or actively inflamed eruptions.

- **Salicylic acid**—This peeling agent, which is available in many forms such as ointments, creams, gels, and shampoos, can be applied to reduce scaling of the skin or scalp. Often, it is more effective when combined with topical corticosteroids, anthralin, or coal tar.

- **Clobetasol propionate**—This is a foam topical medication (Olux), which has been approved for the treatment of scalp and body psoriasis. The foam penetrates the skin very well, is easy to use, and is not as messy as many other topical medications.

- **Bath solutions**—People with psoriasis may find that adding oil when bathing, then applying a moisturizer, soothes their skin. Also, individuals can remove scales and reduce itching by soaking for 15 minutes in water containing a coal tar solution, oiled oatmeal, Epsom salts, or Dead Sea salts.

- **Moisturizers**—When applied regularly over a long period, moisturizers have a soothing effect. Preparations that are thick and greasy usually work best because they seal water in the skin, reducing scaling and itching.

Light Therapy

Natural ultraviolet light from the sun and controlled delivery of artificial ultraviolet light are used in treating psoriasis.

- **Sunlight**—Much of sunlight is composed of bands of different wavelengths of ultraviolet (UV) light. When absorbed into the skin, UV light suppresses the process leading to disease, causing activated T cells in the skin to die. This process reduces inflammation and slows the turnover of skin cells that causes scaling. Daily, short, nonburning exposure to sunlight clears or improves psoriasis in many people. Therefore, exposing affected skin to sunlight is one initial treatment for the disease.

- **Ultraviolet B (UVB) phototherapy**—UVB is light with a short wavelength that is absorbed in the skin's epidermis. An artificial source can be used to treat mild and moderate psoriasis. Some physicians will start treating patients with UVB instead of topical agents. A UVB phototherapy, called broadband UVB, can be used for a few small lesions, to treat widespread psoriasis, or for lesions that resist topical treatment. This type of phototherapy is normally given in a doctor's office by using a light panel or light box. Some patients use UVB light boxes at home under a doctor's guidance. A newer type of UVB, called narrowband UVB, emits the part of the ultraviolet light spectrum band that is most helpful for psoriasis. Narrowband UVB treatment is superior to broadband UVB, but it is less effective than PUVA treatment (see next paragraph). It is gaining in popularity because it does help and is more convenient than PUVA. At first, patients may require several treatments of narrowband UVB spaced close together to improve their skin. Once the skin has shown improvement, a maintenance treatment once each week may be all that is necessary. However, narrowband UVB treatment is not without risk. It can cause more severe and longer lasting burns than broadband treatment.

- **Psoralen and ultraviolet A phototherapy (PUVA)**—This treatment combines oral or topical administration of a medicine called psoralen with exposure to ultraviolet A (UVA) light. UVA has a long wavelength that penetrates deeper into the skin than UVB. Psoralen makes the skin more sensitive to this light. PUVA is normally used when more than 10 percent of the skin is affected or when the disease interferes with a person's occupation (for example, when a teacher's face or a salesperson's hands are involved). Compared with broadband UVB treatment, PUVA treatment taken two to three times a week clears psoriasis more consistently and in fewer treatments. However, it is associated with more short-term side effects, including nausea, headache, fatigue, burning, and itching. Care must be taken to avoid sunlight after ingesting psoralen to avoid severe sunburns, and the eyes must be protected for one to two days with

UVA-absorbing glasses. Long-term treatment is associated with an increased risk of squamous-cell and, possibly, melanoma skin cancers. Simultaneous use of drugs that suppress the immune system, such as cyclosporine, have little beneficial effect and increase the risk of cancer.

- **Light therapy combined with other therapies**—Studies have shown that combining ultraviolet light treatment and a retinoid, like acitretin, adds to the effectiveness of UV light for psoriasis. For this reason, if patients are not responding to light therapy, retinoids may be added. UVB phototherapy, for example, may be combined with retinoids and other treatments. One combined therapy program, referred to as the Ingram regime, involves a coal tar bath, UVB phototherapy, and application of an anthralin-salicylic acid paste that is left on the skin for 6 to 24 hours. A similar regime, the Goeckerman treatment, combines coal tar ointment with UVB phototherapy. Also, PUVA can be combined with some oral medications (such as retinoids) to increase its effectiveness.

Systemic Treatment

For more severe forms of psoriasis, doctors sometimes prescribe medicines that are taken internally by pill or injection. This is called systemic treatment. Recently, attention has been given to a group of drugs called biologics (for example, alefacept and etanercept), which are made from proteins produced by living cells instead of chemicals. They interfere with specific immune system processes.

- **Methotrexate**—Like cyclosporine, methotrexate slows cell turnover by suppressing the immune system. It can be taken by pill or injection. Patients taking methotrexate must be closely monitored because it can cause liver damage and/or decrease the production of oxygen-carrying red blood cells, infection-fighting white blood cells, and clot-enhancing platelets. As a precaution, doctors do not prescribe the drug for people who have had liver disease or anemia (an illness characterized by weakness or tiredness due to a reduction in the number or volume of red blood cells that carry oxygen to the tissues). It is sometimes combined with PUVA or UVB treatments. Methotrexate should not be used by pregnant women, or by women who are planning to get pregnant, because it may cause birth defects.

- **Retinoids**—A retinoid, such as acitretin (Soriatane), is a compound with vitamin A-like properties that may be prescribed for severe cases of psoriasis that do not respond to other therapies. Because this treatment also may cause birth defects, women must protect themselves from pregnancy beginning 1 month before through 3 years after treatment with acitretin. Most patients experience a recurrence of psoriasis after these products are discontinued.

- **Cyclosporine**—Taken orally, cyclosporine acts by suppressing the immune system to slow the rapid turnover of skin cells. It may provide quick relief of symptoms, but the improvement stops when treatment is discontinued. The best candidates for this therapy are those with severe psoriasis who have not responded to, or cannot tolerate, other systemic therapies. Its rapid onset of action is helpful in avoiding hospitalization of patients whose psoriasis is rapidly progressing. Cyclosporine may impair kidney function or cause high blood pressure (hypertension). Therefore, patients must be carefully monitored by a doctor. Also, cyclosporine is not recommended for patients who have a weak immune system or those who have had skin cancers as a result of PUVA treatments in the past. It should not be given with phototherapy.

- **6-Thioguanine**—This drug is nearly as effective as methotrexate and cyclosporine. It has fewer side effects, but there is a greater likelihood of anemia. This drug must also be avoided by pregnant women and by women who are planning to become pregnant, because it may cause birth defects.

- **Hydroxyurea (Hydrea)**—Compared with methotrexate and cyclosporine, hydroxyurea is somewhat less effective. It is sometimes combined with PUVA or UVB treatments. Possible side effects include anemia and a decrease in white blood cells and platelets. Like methotrexate and retinoids, hydroxyurea must be avoided by pregnant women or those who are planning to become pregnant, because it may cause birth defects.

- **Alefacept (Amevive)**—This is the first biologic drug approved specifically to treat moderate to severe plaque psoriasis. It is administered by a doctor, who injects the drug once a week for 12 weeks. The drug is then stopped for a period of time while changes in the skin are observed and a decision is made regarding the need or further treatment. Because alefacept suppresses the immune system, the skin often improves, but there is also an increased risk of infection or other problems, possibly including cancer. Monitoring by a doctor is required, and a patient's blood must be tested weekly around the time of each injection to make certain that T cells and other immune system cells are not overly depressed.

- **Etanercept (Enbrel)**—This drug is an approved treatment for psoriatic arthritis where the joints swell and become inflamed. Like alefacept, it is a biologic response modifier, which after injection blocks interactions between certain cells in the immune system. Etanercept limits the action of a specific protein that is overproduced in the lubricating fluid of the joints and surrounding tissues, causing inflammation. Because this same protein is overproduced in the skin of people with psoriatic arthritis, patients receiving etanercept also may notice an improvement in their skin. Individuals should not receive etanercept treatment if they have an active infection, a history of recurring infections, or an underlying condition, such as diabetes, that increases their risk of infection. Those who have psoriasis and certain neurological conditions, such as multiple sclerosis, cannot be treated with this drug. Added caution is needed for psoriasis patients who have rheumatoid arthritis; these patients should follow the advice of a rheumatologist regarding this treatment.

- **Antibiotics**—These medications are not indicated in routine treatment of psoriasis. However, antibiotics may be employed when an infection, such as that caused by the bacteria *Streptococcus,* triggers an outbreak of psoriasis, as in certain cases of guttate psoriasis.

Combination Therapy

There are many approaches for treating psoriasis. Combining various topical, light, and systemic treatments often permits lower doses of each and can result in increased effectiveness. Therefore, doctors are paying more attention to combination therapy.

Psychological Support

Some individuals with moderate to severe psoriasis may benefit from counseling or participation in a support group to reduce self-consciousness about their appearance or relieve psychological distress resulting from fear of social rejection.

What Are Some Promising Areas of Psoriasis Research?

Significant progress has been made in understanding the inheritance of psoriasis. A number of genes involved in psoriasis are already known or suspected. In a multifactor disease (involving genes, environment, and other factors), variations in one or more genes may produce a greater likelihood of getting the disease. Researchers are continuing to study the genetic aspects of psoriasis. Since discovering that inflammation in psoriasis is triggered by T cells, researchers have been studying new treatments that quiet immune system reactions in the skin. Among these are treatments that block the activity of T cells or block cytokines (proteins that promote inflammation). Several of these drugs are awaiting approval by the U.S. Food and Drug Administration (FDA).

Advances in laser technology are making it possible for doctors to experiment with laser light treatment of localized plaques. A UVB laser was recently tested in a study that was conducted at several medical centers. Although improvements in the skin were noted, this treatment is not without possible side effects. In some patients, the skin became inflamed, blistered, or discolored following treatment.

Where Can People Find More Information about Psoriasis?

National Institute of Arthritis and Musculoskeletal and Skin Diseases
1 AMS Circle
Bethesda, MD 20892-3675
Toll-Free: (877) 22-NIAMS (226-4267)
Phone: (301) 495-4484
TTY: (301) 565-2966
Fax: (301) 718-6366
Website: http://www.niams.nih.gov
E-mail: niamsinfo@mail.nih.gov

American Academy of Dermatology
930 N. Meacham Road
P.O. Box 4014
Schaumburg, IL 60168-4014
Toll-Free: (888) 462-DERM (3376)
Fax: (947) 330-0050
Website: http://www.aad.org

National Psoriasis Foundation
6600 SW 92nd Avenue, Suite 300
Portland, OR 97223-7195
Toll-Free: (800) 723-9166
Phone: (503) 244-7404
Fax: (503) 245-0626
Website: http://www.psoriasis.org
E-mail: getinfo@psoriasis.org

Section 20.2

Psoriatic Arthritis

Psoriatic arthritis is a specific type of arthritis. It causes inflammation in and around the joints, usually the wrists, knees, ankles, lower back, and neck.

Psoriatic arthritis is a specific type of arthritis that has been diagnosed in approximately 23 percent of people who have psoriasis, according to the Psoriasis Foundation's 2001 Benchmark Survey.

It commonly affects the ends of the fingers and toes. It can also affect the spine. The disease can be difficult to diagnose, particularly in its milder forms and earlier stages. Early diagnosis, however, is important for preventing long-term damage to joints and tissue.

Most people with psoriatic arthritis also have psoriasis. Rarely, a person can have psoriatic arthritis without having psoriasis.

What Are the Symptoms?

- Stiffness, pain, swelling and tenderness of the joints, and surrounding soft tissue

- Reduced range of motion

- Morning stiffness and tiredness

- Nail changes, including pitting (small indentations in the nail) or lifting of the nail—found in 80 percent of people with psoriatic arthritis

- Redness and pain of the eye, similar to conjunctivitis

How Does It Develop?

Psoriatic arthritis can develop at any time. On average, it appears about 10 years after the first signs of psoriasis. For most people it appears between the ages of 30 and 50. It affects men and women equally. In about one of seven people with psoriatic arthritis, arthritis symptoms occur before any skin lesions.

Like rheumatoid arthritis, psoriatic arthritis is thought to be caused by a malfunctioning immune system. Psoriatic arthritis is usually milder than rheumatoid arthritis, but some patients with psoriatic arthritis have as severe a disease as patients with rheumatoid arthritis.

Psoriatic arthritis can start slowly with mild symptoms, or it can develop quickly. It is very important to have as early and accurate a diagnosis as possible. Left untreated, psoriatic arthritis can be a progressively disabling disease. In fact, half of those with psoriatic arthritis already have bone loss by the time the disease is diagnosed.

How Is It Diagnosed?

There is no definitive test for psoriatic arthritis, but the following steps are usually involved:

- A person with psoriatic arthritis talks to physician.

- A physician may refer the person to a rheumatologist, who specializes in arthritis.

- Diagnosis is done by process of elimination using medical history, physical examination, blood tests to rule out other diseases, and x-rays of the affected joints.

Chapter 21

Scleroderma

What Is Scleroderma?

Derived from the Greek words *sklerosis,* meaning hardness, and *derma,* meaning skin, scleroderma literally means hard skin. Though it is often referred to as if it were a single disease, scleroderma is really a symptom of a group of diseases that involve the abnormal growth of connective tissue, which supports the skin and internal organs. It is sometimes used, therefore, as an umbrella term for these disorders. In some forms of scleroderma, hard, tight skin is the extent of this abnormal process. In other forms, however, the problem goes much deeper, affecting blood vessels and internal organs, such as the heart, lungs, and kidneys.

Scleroderma is called both a rheumatic disease and a connective tissue disease. The term rheumatic disease refers to a group of conditions characterized by inflammation and/or pain in the muscles, joints, or fibrous tissue. A connective tissue disease is one that affects the major substances in the skin, tendons, and bones.

In this chapter we'll discuss the forms of scleroderma and the problems with each of them as well as diagnosis and disease management. We'll also take a look at what research is telling us about their possible causes, most effective treatments, and ways to help people with scleroderma live longer, healthier, and more productive lives.

"Handout on Health: Scleroderma," National Institute of Arthritis and Musculoskeletal and Skin Diseases (NIAMS), July 2001. Available online at http://www.niams.nih.gov; accessed February 2004.

What Are the Different Types of Scleroderma?

The group of diseases we call scleroderma falls into two main classes: localized scleroderma and systemic sclerosis. (Localized diseases affect only certain parts of the body; systemic diseases can affect the whole body.) Both groups include subgroups. Although there are different ways these groups and subgroups may be broken down or referred to (and your doctor may use different terms from what you see here), the following is a common way of classifying these diseases:

Localized Scleroderma

Localized types of scleroderma are those limited to the skin and related tissues and, in some cases, the muscle below. Internal organs are not affected by localized scleroderma, and localized scleroderma can never progress to the systemic form of the disease. Often, localized conditions improve or go away on their own over time, but the skin changes and damage that occur when the disease is active can be permanent. For some people, localized scleroderma is serious and disabling.

There are two generally recognized types of localized scleroderma:

Morphea

Morphea comes from a Greek word that means form or structure. The word refers to local patches of scleroderma. The first signs of the disease are reddish patches of skin that thicken into firm, oval-shaped areas. The center of each patch becomes ivory colored with violet borders. These patches sweat very little and have little hair growth. Patches appear most often on the chest, stomach, and back. Sometimes they appear on the face, arms, and legs.

Morphea can be either localized or generalized. Localized morphea limits itself to one or several patches, ranging in size from a half-inch to 12 inches in diameter. The condition sometimes appears on areas treated by radiation therapy. Some people have both morphea and linear scleroderma. The disease is referred to as generalized morphea when the skin patches become very hard and dark and spread over larger areas of the body.

Regardless of the type, morphea generally fades out in 3 to 5 years; however, people are often left with darkened skin patches and, in rare cases, muscle weakness.

Linear Scleroderma

As suggested by its name, the disease has a single line or band of thickened and/or abnormally colored skin. Usually, the line runs down an arm or leg, but in some people it runs down the forehead. People sometimes use the French term *en coup de sabre*, or sword stroke, to describe this highly visible line.

Systemic Scleroderma (Systemic Sclerosis)

Systemic scleroderma, or systemic sclerosis, is the term for the disease that not only includes the skin, but also involves the tissues beneath to the blood vessels and major organs. Systemic sclerosis is typically broken down into diffuse and limited disease. People with systemic sclerosis often have all or some of the symptoms that some doctors call CREST, which stands for the following:

- **Calcinosis:** the formation of calcium deposits in the connective tissues, which can be detected by x-ray. They are typically found on the fingers, hands, face, and trunk and on the skin above elbows and knees. When the deposits break through the skin, painful ulcers can result.

- **Raynaud phenomenon:** a condition in which the small blood vessels of the hands and/or feet contract in response to cold or anxiety. As the vessels contract, the hands or feet turn white and cold, then blue. As blood flow returns, they become red. Fingertip tissues may suffer damage, leading to ulcers, scars, or gangrene.

- **Esophageal dysfunction:** impaired function of the esophagus (the tube connecting the throat and the stomach) that occurs when smooth muscles in the esophagus lose normal movement. In the upper esophagus, the result can be swallowing difficulties; in the lower esophagus, the problem can cause chronic heartburn or inflammation.

- **Sclerodactyly:** thick and tight skin on the fingers, resulting from deposits of excess collagen within skin layers. The condition makes it harder to bend or straighten the fingers. The skin may also appear shiny and darkened, with hair loss.

- **Telangiectasias:** small red spots on the hands and face that are caused by the swelling of tiny blood vessels. Although not painful, these red spots can create cosmetic problems.

Limited Scleroderma

Limited scleroderma typically comes on gradually and affects the skin only in certain areas: the fingers, hands, face, lower arms, and legs. Many people with limited disease have Raynaud phenomenon for years before skin thickening starts. Others start out with skin problems over much of the body, which improves over time, leaving only the face and hands with tight, thickened skin. Telangiectasias and calcinosis often follow. Because of the predominance of CREST in people with limited disease, some doctors refer to limited disease as the CREST syndrome.

Diffuse Scleroderma

Diffuse scleroderma typically comes on suddenly. Skin thickening occurs quickly and over much of the body, affecting the hands, face, upper arms, upper legs, chest, and stomach in a symmetrical fashion (for example, if one arm or one side of the trunk is affected, the other is also affected). Some people may have more area of their skin affected than others. Internally, it can damage key organs such as the heart, lungs, and kidneys.

People with diffuse disease are often tired, lose appetite and weight, and have joint swelling and/or pain. Skin changes can cause the skin to swell, appear shiny, and feel tight and itchy.

The damage of diffuse scleroderma typically occurs over a few years. After the first 3 to 5 years, people with diffuse disease often enter a stable phase lasting for varying lengths of time. During this phase, skin thickness and appearance stay about the same. Damage to internal organs progresses little, if at all. Symptoms also subside: joint pain eases, fatigue lessens, and appetite returns.

Gradually, however, the skin starts to change again. Less collagen is made and the body seems to get rid of the excess collagen. This process, called softening, tends to occur in reverse order of the thickening process: the last areas thickened are the first to begin softening. Some patients' skin returns to a somewhat normal state, whereas other patients are left with thin, fragile skin without hair or sweat glands. More serious damage to heart, lungs, or kidneys is unlikely to occur unless previous damage leads to more advanced deterioration.

People with diffuse scleroderma face the most serious long-term outlook if they develop severe kidney, lung, digestive, or heart problems. Fortunately, less than one third of patients with diffuse disease develop these problems. Early diagnosis and continual and careful monitoring are important.

Sine Scleroderma

Some doctors break systemic sclerosis down into a third subset called systemic sclerosis sine scleroderma. Sine may resemble either limited or diffuse systemic sclerosis, causing changes in the lungs, kidneys, and blood vessels. However, there is one key difference between sine and other forms of systemic sclerosis: it does not affect the skin.

What Causes Scleroderma?

Although scientists don't know exactly what causes scleroderma, they are certain that people cannot catch it from or transmit it to others. Studies of twins suggest it is also not inherited. Scientists suspect that scleroderma comes from several factors that may include:

Abnormal immune or inflammatory activity: Like many other rheumatic disorders, scleroderma is believed to be an autoimmune disease. An autoimmune disease is one in which the immune system, for unknown reasons, turns against one's own body.

In scleroderma, the immune system is thought to stimulate cells called fibroblasts to produce too much collagen. In scleroderma, collagen forms thick connective tissue that builds up around the cells of the skin and internal organs. In milder forms, the effects of this buildup are limited to the skin and blood vessels. In more serious forms, it also can interfere with normal functioning of skin, blood vessels, joints, and internal organs.

Genetic makeup: While genes seem to put certain people at risk for scleroderma and play a role in its course, the disease is not passed from parent to child like some genetic diseases.

However, some research suggests that having children may increase a woman's risk of scleroderma. Scientists have learned that when a woman is pregnant, cells from her baby can pass through the placenta, enter her bloodstream, and linger in her body—in some cases, for many years after the child's birth. Recently, scientists have found fetal cells from pregnancies of years past in the skin lesions of some women with scleroderma. They think that these cells, which are different from the woman's own cells, may either begin an immune reaction to the woman's own tissues or trigger a response by the woman's immune system to rid her body of those cells. Either way, the woman's healthy tissues may be damaged in the process. Further studies are needed to find out if fetal cells play a role in the disease.

Environmental triggers: Research suggests that exposure to some environmental factors may trigger the disease in people who are genetically predisposed to it. Suspected triggers include viral infections, certain adhesive and coating materials, and organic solvents such as vinyl chloride or trichloroethylene. In the past, some people believed that silicone breast implants might have been a factor in developing connective tissue diseases such as scleroderma. But several studies have not shown evidence of a connection.

Hormones: By the middle to late childbearing years (ages 30 to 55), women develop scleroderma at a rate 7 to 12 times higher than men. Because of female predominance at this and all ages, scientists suspect that something distinctly feminine, such as the hormone estrogen, plays a role in the disease. So far, the role of estrogen or other female hormones has not been proven.

Who Gets Scleroderma?

Although scleroderma is more common in women, the disease also occurs in men and children. It affects people of all races and ethnic groups. However, there are some patterns by disease type. For example:

- Localized forms of scleroderma are more common in people of European descent than in African Americans.

- Morphea usually appears between the ages of 20 and 40.

- Linear scleroderma usually occurs in children or teenagers.

- Systemic scleroderma, whether limited or diffuse, typically occurs in people from 30 to 50 years old. It affects more women of African American than European descent.

Because scleroderma can be hard to diagnose and it overlaps with or resembles other diseases, scientists can only estimate how many cases there actually are. Estimates for the number of people in the United States with systemic sclerosis range from 40,000 to 165,000. By contrast, a survey that included all scleroderma-related disorders, including Raynaud phenomenon, suggested a number between 250,000 and 992,500.

For some people, scleroderma (particularly the localized forms) is fairly mild and resolves with time. But for others, living with the disease and its effects from day to day has a significant impact on their quality of life.

How Can Scleroderma Affect My Life?

Having a chronic disease can affect almost every aspect of your life, from family relationships to holding a job. For people with scleroderma, there may be other concerns about appearance or even the ability to dress, bathe, or handle the most basic daily tasks. Here are some areas in which scleroderma could intrude.

Appearance and self-esteem: Aside from the initial concerns about health and longevity, one of the first fears people with scleroderma have is how the disease will affect their appearance. Thick, hardened skin can be difficult to accept, particularly on the face. Systemic scleroderma may result in facial changes that eventually cause the opening to the mouth to become smaller and the upper lip to virtually disappear. Linear scleroderma may leave its mark on the forehead. Although these problems can't always be prevented, their effects may be minimized with proper treatment and skin care. Special cosmetics—and in some cases, plastic surgery—can help conceal scleroderma's damage.

Caring for yourself: Tight, hard connective tissue in the hands can make it difficult to do what were once simple tasks, such as brushing your teeth and hair, pouring a cup of coffee, using a knife and fork, unlocking a door, or buttoning a jacket. If you have trouble using your hands, consult an occupational therapist, who can recommend new ways of doing things or devices to make tasks easier. Devices as simple as Velcro fasteners and built-up brush handles can help you be more independent.

Family relationships: Spouses, children, parents, and siblings may have trouble understanding why you don't have the energy to keep house, drive to soccer practice, prepare meals, and hold a job the way you used to. If your condition isn't that visible, they may even suggest you are just being lazy. On the other hand, they may be overly concerned and eager to help you, not allowing you to do the things you are able to do or giving up their own interests and activities to be with you. It's important to learn as much about your form of the disease as you can and share any information you have with your family. Involving them in counseling or a support group may also help them better understand the disease and how they can help you.

Sexual relations: Sexual relationships can be affected when systemic scleroderma enters the picture. For men, the disease's effects on the blood vessels can lead to problems achieving an erection. In women, damage to the moisture-producing glands can cause vaginal dryness that makes intercourse painful. People of either sex may find they have difficulty moving the way they once did. They may be self-conscious about their appearance or afraid that their sexual partner will no longer find them attractive. With communication between partners, good medical care, and perhaps counseling, many of these changes can be overcome or at least worked around.

Pregnancy and childbearing: In the past, women with systemic scleroderma were often advised not to have children. But thanks to better medical treatments and a better understanding of the disease itself, that advice is changing. (Pregnancy, for example, is not likely to be a problem for women with localized scleroderma.) Although blood vessel involvement in the placenta may cause babies of women with systemic scleroderma to be born early, many women with the disease can have safe pregnancies and healthy babies if they follow some precautions.

One of the most important pieces of advice is to wait a few years after the disease starts before attempting a pregnancy. During the first 3 years you are at the highest risk of developing severe problems of the heart, lungs, or kidneys that could be harmful to you and your unborn baby.

If you haven't developed organ problems within 3 years of the disease's onset, chances are you won't, and pregnancy should be safe. But it is important to have both your disease and your pregnancy monitored regularly. You'll probably need to stay in close touch with the doctor you typically see for your scleroderma as well as an obstetrician experienced in guiding high-risk pregnancies.

How Is Scleroderma Diagnosed?

Depending on your particular symptoms, a diagnosis of scleroderma may be made by a general internist, a dermatologist (a doctor who specializes in treating diseases of the skin, hair, and nails), an orthopaedist (a doctor who treats bone and joint disorders), a pulmonologist (lung specialist), or a rheumatologist (a doctor specializing in treatment of rheumatic diseases). A diagnosis of scleroderma is based largely on the medical history and findings from the physical exam. To make a diagnosis, your doctor will ask you a lot of questions about what has happened to you over time and about any symptoms you may be experiencing. Are you having a problem with heartburn or swallowing? Are you often tired or achy? Do your hands turn white in response to anxiety or cold temperatures?

Once your doctor has taken a thorough medical history, he or she will perform a physical exam. Finding one or more of the following factors can help the doctor diagnose a certain form of scleroderma:

- Changed skin appearance and texture, including swollen fingers and hands and tight skin around the hands, face, mouth, or elsewhere.
- Calcium deposits developing under the skin.
- Changes in the tiny blood vessels (capillaries) at the base of the fingernails.
- Thickened skin patches.

Finally, your doctor may order lab tests to help confirm a suspected diagnosis. At least two proteins, called antibodies, are commonly found in the blood of people with scleroderma:

- Antitopoisomerase-1 or Anti-Scl-70 antibodies appear in the blood of up to 40 percent of people with diffuse systemic sclerosis.
- Anticentromere antibodies are found in the blood of as many as 90 percent of people with limited systemic sclerosis.

A number of other scleroderma-specific antibodies can occur in people with scleroderma, although less frequently. When present, however, they are helpful in clinical diagnosis.

Because not all people with scleroderma have these antibodies and because not all people with the antibodies have scleroderma, lab test results alone cannot confirm the diagnosis.

In some cases, your doctor may order a skin biopsy (the surgical removal of a small sample of skin for microscopic examination) to aid in or help confirm a diagnosis. However, skin biopsies, too, have their limitations: biopsy results cannot distinguish between localized and systemic disease, for example.

Diagnosing scleroderma is easiest when a person has typical symptoms and rapid skin thickening. In other cases, a diagnosis may take months, or even years, as the disease unfolds and reveals itself and as the doctor is able to rule out some other potential causes of the symptoms. In some cases, a diagnosis is never made, because the symptoms that prompted the visit to the doctor go away on their own.

What Other Conditions Can Look Like Scleroderma?

Symptoms similar to those seen in scleroderma can occur with a number of other diseases. Here are some of the most common scleroderma look-alikes:

- Eosinophilic fasciitis (EF): a disease that involves the fascia, the thin connective tissue around the muscles, particularly those of the forearms, arms, legs, and trunk. EF causes the muscles to become encased in collagen, the fibrous protein that makes up tissue such as the skin and tendons. Permanent shortening of the muscles and tendons, called contractures, may develop, sometimes causing disfigurement and problems with joint motion and function. EF may begin after hard physical exertion. The disease usually fades away after several years, but people sometimes have relapses. Although the upper layers of the skin are not thickened in EF, the thickened fascia may cause the skin to look somewhat like the tight, hard skin of scleroderma. A skin biopsy easily distinguishes between the two.

- Undifferentiated connective tissue disease (UCTD): a diagnosis for patients who have some signs and symptoms of various related diseases, but not enough symptoms of any one disease to make a definite diagnosis. In other words, their condition hasn't differentiated into a particular connective tissue disease. In time, UCTD can go in one of three directions: it can change into a systemic disease such as systemic sclerosis, systemic lupus erythematosus, or rheumatoid arthritis; it can remain undifferentiated; or it can improve spontaneously.

- Overlap syndromes: a disease combination in which patients have symptoms and lab findings characteristic of two or more conditions.

At other times, symptoms resembling those of scleroderma can be the result of an unrelated disease or condition. For example:

- Skin thickening on the fingers and hands also appears with diabetes, mycosis fungoides, amyloidosis, and adult celiac disease. It can also result from hand trauma.

- Generalized skin thickening may occur with scleromyxedema, graft-versus-host disease, porphyria cutanea tarda, and human adjuvant disease.

248

- Internal organ damage, similar to that seen in systemic sclerosis, may instead be related to primary pulmonary hypertension, idiopathic pulmonary fibrosis, or collagenous colitis.

- Raynaud phenomenon also appears with atherosclerosis or systemic lupus erythematosus or in the absence of underlying disease.

An explanation of most of these other diseases is beyond the scope of this chapter. What's important to understand, however, is that scleroderma isn't always easy to diagnose; it may take time for you and your doctor to establish a diagnosis. And although having a definite diagnosis may be helpful, knowing the precise form of your disease is not needed to receive proper treatment.

How Is Scleroderma Treated?

Because scleroderma can affect many different organs and organ systems, you may have several different doctors involved in your care. Typically, care will be managed by a rheumatologist, a specialist who treats people with diseases of the joints, bones, muscles, and immune system. Your rheumatologist may refer you to other specialists, depending on the specific problems you are having: for example, a dermatologist for the treatment of skin symptoms, a nephrologist for kidney complications, a cardiologist for heart complications, a gastroenterologist for problems of the digestive tract, and a pulmonary specialist for lung involvement.

In addition to doctors, professionals like nurse practitioners, physician assistants, physical or occupational therapists, psychologists, and social workers may play a role in your care. Dentists, orthodontists, and even speech therapists can treat oral complications that arise from thickening of tissues in and around the mouth and on the face.

Currently, there is no treatment that controls or stops the underlying problem—the overproduction of collagen—in all forms of scleroderma. Thus, treatment and management focus on relieving symptoms and limiting damage. Your treatment will depend on the particular problems you are having. Some treatments will be prescribed or given by your physician. Others are things you can do on your own.

Here are some of the potential problems that can occur in systemic scleroderma and the medical and nonmedical treatments for them. These problems do not occur as a result or complication of localized scleroderma. Remember that this is not a complete listing of problems or their treatments. Different people experience different problems with scleroderma and not all treatments work equally well for all people. Work with your doctor to find the best treatment for your specific symptoms.

Raynaud phenomenon: One of the most common problems associated with scleroderma, Raynaud phenomenon can be uncomfortable and can lead to painful skin ulcers on the fingertips. Smoking makes the condition worse. The following measures may make you more comfortable and help prevent problems:

- Don't smoke! Smoking narrows the blood vessels even more and makes Raynaud phenomenon worse.

- Dress warmly, with special attention to hands and feet. Dress in layers and try to stay indoors during cold weather.

- Use biofeedback (to control various body processes that are not normally thought of as being under conscious control) and relaxation exercises.

- For severe cases, speak to your doctor about prescribing drugs called calcium channel blockers, such as nifedipine (Procardia), which can open up small blood vessels and improve circulation. Other drugs are in development and may become available in the future.

- If Raynaud leads to skin sores or ulcers, increasing your dose of calcium channel blockers (under the direction of your doctor **only**) may help. You can also protect skin ulcers from further injury or infection by applying nitroglycerin paste or antibiotic cream. Severe ulcerations on the fingertips can be treated with bioengineered skin.

Stiff, painful joints: In diffuse systemic sclerosis, hand joints can stiffen because of hardened skin around the joints or inflammation of the joints themselves. Other joints can also become stiff and swollen. The following may help:

- Exercise regularly. Ask your doctor or physical therapist about an exercise plan that will help you increase and maintain range of motion in affected joints. Swimming can help maintain muscle strength, flexibility, and joint mobility.

- Use acetaminophen or an over-the-counter or prescription non-steroidal anti-inflammatory drug, as recommended by your doctor, to help relieve joint or muscle pain. If pain is severe, speak to a rheumatologist about the possibility of prescription-strength drugs to ease pain and inflammation.

- Learn to do things in a new way. A physical or occupational therapist can help you learn to perform daily tasks, such as lifting and carrying objects or opening doors, in ways that will put less stress on tender joints.

Skin problems: When too much collagen builds up in the skin, it crowds out sweat and oil glands, causing the skin to become dry and stiff. If your skin is affected, you may need to see a dermatologist. To ease dry skin, try the following:

- Apply oil-based creams and lotions frequently and always right after bathing.

- Apply sunscreen before you venture outdoors to protect against further damage by the sun's rays.

- Use humidifiers to moisten the air in your home in colder winter climates. (Clean humidifiers often to stop bacteria from growing in the water.)

- Avoid very hot baths and showers, as hot water dries the skin.

- Avoid harsh soaps, household cleaners, and caustic chemicals, if at all possible. If that's not possible, be sure to wear rubber gloves when you use such products.

- Exercise regularly. Exercise, especially swimming, stimulates blood circulation to affected areas.

Dry mouth and dental problems: Dental problems are common in people with scleroderma for a number of reasons: tightening facial skin can make the mouth opening smaller and narrower, which makes it hard to care for teeth; dry mouth due to salivary gland damage speeds up tooth decay; and damage to connective tissues in the mouth can lead to loose teeth. You can avoid tooth and gum problems in several ways:

- Brush and floss your teeth regularly. (If hand pain and stiffness make this difficult, consult your doctor or an occupational therapist about specially made toothbrush handles and devices to make flossing easier.)

- Have regular dental checkups. Contact your dentist immediately if you experience mouth sores, mouth pain, or loose teeth.

- If decay is a problem, ask your dentist about fluoride rinses or prescription toothpastes that remineralize and harden tooth enamel.

- Consult a physical therapist about facial exercises to help keep your mouth and face more flexible.

- Keep your mouth moist by drinking plenty of water, sucking ice chips, using sugarless gum and hard candy, and avoiding mouthwashes with alcohol. If dry mouth still bothers you, ask your doctor about a saliva substitute or a prescription medication called pilocarpine hydrochloride (Salagen) that can stimulate the flow of saliva.

Gastrointestinal (GI) problems: Systemic sclerosis can affect any part of the digestive system. As a result, you may experience problems such as heartburn, difficulty swallowing, early satiety (the feeling of being full after you've barely started eating), or intestinal complaints such as diarrhea, constipation, and gas. In cases where the intestines are damaged, your body may have difficulty absorbing nutrients from food. Although GI problems are diverse, here are some things that might help at least some of the problems you have:

- Eat small, frequent meals.

- Raise the head of your bed with blocks, and stand or sit for at least an hour (preferably two or three) after eating to keep stomach contents from backing up into the esophagus.

- Avoid late-night meals, spicy or fatty foods, and alcohol and caffeine, which can aggravate GI distress.

- Chew foods well and eat moist, soft foods. If you have difficulty swallowing or if your body doesn't absorb nutrients properly, your doctor may prescribe a special diet.

- Ask your doctor about prescription medications for problems such as diarrhea, constipation, and heartburn. Some drugs called proton pump inhibitors are highly effective against heartburn. Oral antibiotics may stop bacterial overgrowth in the bowel that can be a cause of diarrhea in some people with systemic sclerosis.

Lung damage: About 10 to 15 percent of people with systemic sclerosis develop severe lung disease, which comes in two forms: pulmonary fibrosis (hardening or scarring of lung tissue because of excess collagen) and pulmonary hypertension (high blood pressure in the artery that carries blood from the heart to the lungs). Treatment for the two conditions is different.

- Pulmonary fibrosis may be treated with drugs that suppress the immune system such as cyclophosphamide (Cytoxan) or azathioprine (Imuran), along with low doses of corticosteroids.

- Pulmonary hypertension may be treated with drugs that dilate the blood vessels such as prostacyclin (Iloprost).

Regardless of the problem or its treatment, your role in the treatment process is essentially the same. To minimize lung complications, work closely with your medical team. Do the following:

- Watch for signs of lung disease, including fatigue, shortness of breath or difficulty breathing, and swollen feet. Report these symptoms to your doctor.

- Have your lungs closely checked, using standard lung-function tests, during the early stages of skin thickening. These tests, which can find problems at the earliest and most treatable stages, are needed because lung damage can occur even before you notice any symptoms.

- Get regular flu and pneumonia vaccines as recommended by your doctor. Contracting either illness could be dangerous for a person with lung disease.

Heart problems: About 15 to 20 percent of people with systemic sclerosis develop heart problems, including scarring and weakening of the heart (cardiomyopathy), inflamed heart muscle (myocarditis), and abnormal heartbeat (arrhythmia). All of these problems can be treated. Treatment ranges from drugs to surgery, and varies depending on the nature of the condition.

Kidney problems: About 15 to 20 percent of people with diffuse systemic sclerosis develop severe kidney problems, including loss of kidney function. Because uncontrolled high blood pressure can quickly lead to kidney failure, it's important that you take measures to minimize the problem. Things you can do:

- Check your blood pressure regularly and, if you find it to be high, call your doctor right away.

- If you have kidney problems, take your prescribed medications faithfully. In the past two decades, drugs known as ACE (angiotensin-converting enzyme) inhibitors, including captopril (Capoten), enalapril (Vasotec), and quinapril (Accupril), have made scleroderma-related kidney failure a less-threatening problem than it was in the past. But for these drugs to work, you must take them.

Cosmetic problems: Even if scleroderma doesn't cause any lasting physical disability, its effects on the skin's appearance—particularly on the face—can take their toll on your self-esteem. Fortunately, there are procedures to correct some of the cosmetic problems scleroderma causes.

- The appearance of telangiectasis, small red spots on the hands and face caused by swelling of tiny blood vessels beneath the skin, may be lessened or even eliminated with the use of guided lasers.

- Facial changes of localized scleroderma, such as the *en coup de sabre* that may run down the forehead in people with linear scleroderma, may be corrected through cosmetic surgery. (However, such surgery is not appropriate for areas of the skin where the disease is active.)

How Can I Play a Role in My Health Care?

Although your doctors direct your treatment, you are the one who must take your medicine regularly, follow your doctor's advice, and report any problems promptly. In other words, the relationship between you and your doctors is a partnership, and you are the most important partner. Here's what you can do to make the most of this important role:

- Get educated: Knowledge is your best defense against this disease.

- Learn as much as you can about scleroderma, both for your own benefit and to educate the people in your support network.

- Seek support: Recruit family members, friends, and coworkers to build a support network. This network will help you get through difficult times: when you are in pain; when you feel angry, sad, or afraid; and when you're depressed. Also, look for a scleroderma support group in your community by calling a national scleroderma organization. If you can't find a support group, you might want to consider organizing one.

- Assemble a health care team: You and your doctors will lead the team. Other members may include physical and occupational therapists, a psychologist or social worker, a dentist, and a pharmacist.

- Be patient: Understand that a final diagnosis can be difficult and may take a long time. Find a doctor with experience treating people with systemic and localized scleroderma. Then, even if you don't yet have a diagnosis, you will get understanding and the right treatment for your symptoms.

- Speak up: When you have problems or notice changes in your condition, don't feel too self-conscious to speak up during your appointment or even call your doctor or another member of your health care team. No problem is too small to inquire about, and early treatment for any problem can make the disease more manageable for you and your health care team.

- Don't accept depression: While it's understandable that a person with a chronic illness like scleroderma would become depressed, don't accept depression as a normal consequence of your condition. If depression makes it hard for you to function well, don't hesitate to ask your health care team for help. You may benefit from speaking with a psychologist or social worker or from using one of the effective medications on the market.

- Learn coping skills: Skills like meditation, calming exercises, and relaxation techniques may help you cope with emotional difficulties as well as help relieve pain and fatigue. Ask a member of your health care team to teach you these skills or to refer you to someone who can.

- Ask the experts: If you have problems doing daily activities, from brushing your hair and teeth to driving your car, consult an occupational or physical therapist. They have more helpful hints and devices than you can probably imagine. Social workers can often help resolve financial and insurance matters.

Is Research Close to Finding a Cure?

No one can say for sure when—or if—a cure will be found. But research is providing the next best thing: better ways to treat symptoms, prevent organ damage, and improve the quality of life for people with scleroderma. In the past two decades, multidisciplinary research has also provided new clues to understanding the disease, which is an important step toward prevention or cure.

Leading the way in funding for this research is the National Institute of Arthritis and Musculoskeletal and Skin Diseases (NIAMS), a part of the National Institutes of Health (NIH). Other sources of funding for scleroderma research include pharmaceutical companies and organizations such as the Scleroderma Foundation, the Scleroderma Research Foundation, and the Arthritis Foundation. Scientists at universities and medical centers throughout the United States conduct much of this research.

Studies of the immune system, genetics, cell biology, and molecular biology have helped reveal the causes of scleroderma, improve existing treatment, and create entirely new treatment approaches. Research advances in recent years that have led to a better understanding of and/or treatment for the diseases include:

- The use of a hormone produced in pregnancy to soften skin lesions. Early studies suggest relaxin, a hormone that helps a woman's body to stretch to meet the demands of a growing pregnancy and delivery, may soften the connective tissues of women with scleroderma. The hormone is believed to work by blocking fibrosis, or the development of fibrous tissue between the body's cells.

- Finding a gene associated with scleroderma in Oklahoma Choctaw Native Americans. Scientists believe the gene, which codes for a protein called fibrillin-1, may put people at risk for the disease.

- The use of the drug Iloprost for pulmonary hypertension. This drug has increased the quality of life and life expectancy for people with this dangerous form of lung damage.

- The use of the drug cyclophosphamide (Cytoxan) for lung fibrosis. One recent study suggested that treating lung problems early with this immunosuppressive drug may help prevent further damage and increase chances of survival.

- The increased use of ACE inhibitors for scleroderma-related kidney problems. For the past two decades, ACE inhibitors have greatly reduced the risk of kidney failure in people with sclero-derma. Now there is evidence that use of ACE inhibitors can actually heal the kidneys of people on dialysis for scleroderma-related kidney failure. As many as half of people who continue ACE inhibitors while on dialysis may be able to go off dialysis in 12 to 18 months.

Other studies are examining the following:

- Changes in the tiny blood vessels of people with scleroderma. By studying these changes, scientists hope to find the cause of cold sensitivity in Raynaud phenomenon and how to control the problem.

- Immune system changes (and particularly how those changes affect the lungs) in people with early diffuse systemic sclerosis.

- The role of blood vessel malfunction, cell death, and autoimmu-nity in scleroderma.

- Skin changes in laboratory mice in which a genetic defect prevents the breakdown of collagen, leading to thick skin and patchy hair loss. Scientists hope that by studying these mice, they can answer many questions about skin changes in scleroderma.

- The effectiveness of various treatments, including (1) meth-otrexate, a drug commonly used for rheumatoid arthritis and some other inflammatory forms of arthritis; (2) collagen pep-tides administered orally; (3) halofuginone, a drug that inhibits the synthesis of type I collagen, which is the primary compo-nent of connective tissue; (4) ultraviolet light therapy for local-ized forms of scleroderma; and (5) stem cell transfusions, a form of bone marrow transplant that uses a patient's own cells, for early diffuse systemic sclerosis.

Scleroderma research continues to advance as scientists and doc-tors learn more about how the disease develops and its underlying mechanisms. Recently, the NIAMS funded a Specialized Center of Research (SCOR) in scleroderma at the University of Texas-Houston. SCOR scientists are conducting laboratory and clinical research on the disease. The SCOR approach allows researchers to translate ba-sic science findings quickly into improved treatment and patient care.

Scleroderma poses a series of challenges for both patients and their health care teams. The good news is that scientists, doctors, and other health care professionals continue to find new answers—ways to make earlier diagnoses and manage disease better. In addition, active patient support groups share with, care for, and educate each other. The impact of all of this activity is that people with scleroderma do much better and remain active far longer than they did 20 or 30 years ago. As for tomorrow, patients and the medical community will continue to push for longer, healthier, and more active lives for people with the diseases collectively known as scleroderma.

National Resources for Scleroderma

National Institute of Arthritis and Musculoskeletal and Skin Diseases
1 AMS Circle
Bethesda, MD 20892-3675
Toll-Free: (877) 22-NIAMS (226-4267)
Phone: (301) 495-4484
TTY: (301) 565-2966
Fax: (301) 718-6366
Website: http://www.niams.nih.gov
E-mail: niamsinfo@mail.nih.gov

American Academy of Dermatology
P.O. Box 4014
Schaumburg, IL 60168-4014
Phone: (847) 330-0230
Website: http://www.aad.org

American College of Rheumatology
1800 Century Place, Suite 250
Atlanta, GA 30345-4300
Phone: (404) 633-3777
Fax: (404) 633-1870
Website: http://www.rheumatology.org

Scleroderma Foundation
12 Kent Way, Suite 101
Byfield, MA 01922
Toll-Free: 800-722-HOPE (4673)
Phone: (978) 463-5843
Fax: (978) 463-5809
Website: http://www.scleroderma.org
E-mail: sfinfo@scleroderma.org

Scleroderma Research Foundation
2320 Bath Street, Suite 315
Santa Barbara, CA 93105
Toll-Free: (800) 441-CURE
Phone: (805) 563-9133
Website: http://www.srfcure.org

Arthritis Foundation
1330 West Peachtree Street
Atlanta, GA 30309
Toll-Free: (800) 283-7800
Phone: (404) 872-7100
Website: http://www.arthritis.org

Glossary

Adult celiac disease—A chronic nutritional disorder in which the body cannot effectively digest fats and wheat gluten. The condition, which results in a distended abdomen and loose, fatty stools, is associated with several autoimmune diseases.

Amyloidosis—A disease in which excessive protein is deposited around cells in various organs and tissues of the body.

Antibodies—Special proteins produced by the body's immune system. They recognize and help fight infectious agents, such as bacteria and other foreign substances that invade the body. The presence of certain antibodies in the blood can help in making a diagnosis of some diseases, including some forms of scleroderma.

Atherosclerosis—Abnormal fatty deposits in the inner layers of large or medium-sized arteries, which can lead to hardening and narrowing of the arteries and blockages of the blood supply, especially to the heart.

Autoimmune disease—A disease in which the body's immune system turns against and damages the body's own tissues.

Calcinosis—The buildup of calcium deposits in the tissues. It may occur under the skin of the fingers, arms, feet, and knees, causing pain and infection if the calcium deposits pierce the surface of the skin.

Calcium channel blockers—Medicines that lower blood pressure, relieve chest pain, and stabilize normal heart rhythms by inhibiting calcium movement into the heart muscles and smooth muscle cells. They are used to treat a variety of conditions and to prevent circulatory and kidney problems in scleroderma.

Colitis—An inflammatory disease of the large intestine that results in diarrhea, discharge of mucus and blood, cramping, and abdominal pain. It is characterized by swelling, inflammation, and ulceration of the mucous membrane of the intestine.

Collagen—A fabric-like material of fibrous threads that is a key component of the body's connective tissues. In scleroderma, too much collagen is produced or it is produced in the wrong places, causing stiff and inflamed skin, blood vessels, and internal organs.

Connective tissue—Tissues such as skin, tendons, and cartilage that support and hold body parts together. The chief component of connective tissue is collagen.

CREST syndrome—An acronym for a collection of symptoms that occur to some degree in all people with systemic sclerosis. The symptoms are Calcinosis, Raynaud phenomenon, Esophageal dysfunction, Sclerodactyly, and Telangiectasia. Because of the predominance of CREST symptoms in people with limited systemic sclerosis, some people use the term CREST syndrome when referring to that form of the disease.

Eosinophilic fasciitis—A scleroderma-like disorder (often considered to be a localized form of scleroderma) featuring inflammation of the fascia (the thin, sheet-like connective tissues surrounding the muscles and other body structures) and an abnormally high number of a specific kind of white blood cells (eosinophils). The result of the inflammation may be fibrous buildup in the skin of arms and legs, contractures, and carpal tunnel syndrome.

Esophageal dysfunction—Improper functioning of the esophagus (the tube that attaches the throat to the stomach) that can lead to heartburn and swallowing problems.

Fibroblast—A type of cell in connective tissue that secretes proteins, including collagen.

Fibrosis—A condition marked by increased fibrous tissue that develops between the cells of various organs or tissues. It is a common feature of scleroderma and some other diseases. Fibrosis causes hardening or stiffening of tissues in the skin, joints, and internal organs.

Graft versus-host disease—A major complication of bone marrow transplantations and sometimes blood transfusions in which white blood cells, called lymphocytes, in the marrow or blood attack tissues in the body into which they were transplanted.

Human adjuvant disease—An autoimmune syndrome in which the body becomes extremely sensitive to a foreign material injected into the body.

Mycosis fungoides—A form of lymph cancer characterized by scaly skin patches. It progresses over several years to form elevated skin lesions and then tumors.

Pulmonary fibrosis—Hardening or scarring of lung tissue because of excess collagen. Pulmonary fibrosis occurs in a small percentage of people with systemic sclerosis.

Pulmonary hypertension—Abnormally high blood pressure in the arteries supplying the lungs that may be caused by a number of factors, including damage from fibrosis.

Raynaud phenomenon—A disorder of the small blood vessels of the extremities, causing coldness and reduced blood flow. In response to cold or anxiety, these vessels go into spasms, causing pain, the sensations of burning and tingling, and color changes.

Rheumatic—An adjective used to describe a group of conditions characterized by inflammation or pain in the muscles, joints, and fibrous tissue. Rheumatic diseases or disorders can be related to autoimmunity or other causes.

Sclerodactyly—The hard, shiny appearance of fingers caused by excess connective tissue buildup. This is a common feature of scleroderma, but it may also occur in other conditions.

Systemic condition—A condition involving the body as a whole, as opposed to limited conditions that affect particular parts of the body.

Systemic lupus erythematosus—A systemic rheumatic disease that occurs predominantly in women and is characterized by autoimmune activity, a facial rash across the bridge of the nose and cheeks, Raynaud's phenomenon, joint pain and swelling, fever, chest pain, hair loss, and other symptoms. Many of its symptoms overlap with those of scleroderma.

Telangiectasia—Small red dots, usually on the face and hands, resulting from tiny blood vessels showing through the skin's surface.

Chapter 22

Sjögren Syndrome

Sjögren syndrome is an autoimmune disease—that is, a disease in which the immune system turns against the body's own cells. In Sjögren syndrome, the immune system targets moisture-producing glands and causes dryness in the mouth and eyes. Other parts of the body can be affected as well, resulting in a wide range of possible symptoms.

Normally, the immune system works to protect us from disease by destroying harmful invading organisms like viruses and bacteria. In the case of Sjögren syndrome, disease-fighting cells attack the glands that produce tears and saliva (the lacrimal and salivary glands). Damage to these glands keeps them from working properly and causes dry eyes and dry mouth. In technical terms, dry eyes are called keratoconjunctivitis sicca, or KCS, and dry mouth is called xerostomia. Your doctor may use these terms when talking to you about Sjögren syndrome.

The disease can affect other glands, too, such as those in the stomach, pancreas, and intestines, and can cause dryness in other places that need moisture, such as the nose, throat, airways, and skin.

You might hear Sjögren syndrome called a rheumatic disease. A rheumatic disease causes inflammation in joints, muscles, skin, or other body tissue, and Sjögren syndrome can do that. The many forms of arthritis, which often involve inflammation in the joints, among other problems, are examples of rheumatic diseases. Sjögren syndrome is also

"Questions and Answers About Sjögren's Syndrome," National Institute of Arthritis and Musculoskeletal and Skin Diseases (NIAMS), January 2001. Available online at http://www.niams.nih.gov; accessed February 2004.

considered a disorder of connective tissue, which is the framework of the body that supports organs and tissues (joints, muscles, and skin).

Sjögren syndrome is classified as either primary or secondary disease. Primary Sjögren syndrome occurs by itself, and secondary Sjögren syndrome occurs with another disease. Both are systemic disorders, although the symptoms in primary are more restricted.

In primary Sjögren syndrome, the doctor can trace the symptoms to problems with the tear and saliva glands. People with primary disease are more likely to have certain antibodies (substances that help fight a particular disease) circulating in their blood than people with secondary disease. These antibodies are called SS-A and SS-B. People with primary Sjögren syndrome are more likely to have antinuclear antibodies (ANAs) in their blood. ANAs are autoantibodies, which are directed against the body.

In secondary Sjögren syndrome, the person had an autoimmune disease like rheumatoid arthritis or lupus before Sjögren syndrome developed. People with this type tend to have more health problems because they have two diseases, and they are also less likely to have the antibodies associated with primary Sjögren syndrome.

What Are the Symptoms of Sjögren Syndrome?

The main symptoms are:

* Dry eyes—Your eyes may be red and burn and itch. People say it feels like they have sand in their eyes. Also, your vision may be blurry, and bright light, especially fluorescent lighting, might bother you.

* Dry mouth—Dry mouth feels like a mouth full of cotton. It's difficult to swallow, speak, and taste. Your sense of smell can change, and you may develop a dry cough. Also, because you lack the protective effects of saliva, dry mouth increases your chances of developing cavities and mouth infections.

Both primary and secondary Sjögren syndrome can affect other parts of the body as well, including the skin, joints, lungs, kidneys, blood vessels, and nervous system, and cause symptoms such as:

* dry skin
* skin rashes
* thyroid problems
* joint and muscle pain

- pneumonia
- vaginal dryness
- numbness and tingling in the extremities

When Sjögren syndrome affects other parts of the body, the condition is called extraglandular involvement because the problems extend beyond the tear and salivary glands. These problems are described in more detail later.

Finally, Sjögren syndrome can cause extreme fatigue that can seriously interfere with daily life.

Who Gets Sjögren Syndrome?

Experts believe 1 to 4 million people have the disease. Most—90 percent—are women. It can occur at any age, but it usually is diagnosed after age 40 and can affect people of all races and ethnic backgrounds. It's rare in children, but it can occur.

What Causes Sjögren Syndrome?

Researchers think Sjögren syndrome is caused by a combination of genetic and environmental factors. Several different genes appear to be involved, but scientists are not certain exactly which ones are linked to the disease because different genes seem to play a role in different people. For example, there is one gene that predisposes Caucasians to the disease. Other genes are linked to Sjögren syndrome in people of Japanese, Chinese, and African-American descent. Simply having one of these genes will not cause a person to develop the disease, however. Some sort of trigger must activate the immune system.

Scientists think that the trigger may be a viral or bacterial infection. It might work like this: A person who has a Sjögren syndrome-associated gene gets a viral infection. The virus stimulates the immune system to act, but the gene alters the attack, sending fighter cells (lymphocytes) to the eye and mouth glands. Once there, the lymphocytes attack healthy cells, causing the inflammation that damages the glands and keeps them from working properly. These fighter cells are supposed to die after their attack in a natural process called apoptosis, but in people with Sjögren syndrome, they continue to attack, causing further damage.

Scientists think that resistance to apoptosis may be genetic. The possibility that the endocrine and nervous systems play a role is also under investigation.

How Is Sjögren Syndrome Diagnosed?

The doctor will first take a detailed medical history, which includes asking questions about general health, symptoms, family medical history, alcohol consumption, smoking, or use of drugs or medications. The doctor will also do a complete physical exam to check for other signs of Sjögren syndrome.

You may have some tests, too. First, the doctor will want to check your eyes and mouth to see whether Sjögren syndrome is causing your symptoms and how severe the problem is. Then, the doctor may do other tests to see whether the disease is elsewhere in the body as well.

Common eye and mouth tests are:

- Schirmer test—This test measures tears to see how the lacrimal gland is working. It can be done in two ways: In Schirmer I, the doctor puts thin paper strips under the lower eyelids and measures the amount of wetness on the paper after 5 minutes. People with Sjögren syndrome usually produce less than 8 millimeters of tears. The Schirmer II test is similar, but the doctor uses a cotton swab to stimulate a tear reflex inside the nose.

- Staining with vital dyes (rose bengal or lissamine green)—The tests show how much damage dryness has done to the surface of the eye. The doctor puts a drop of a liquid containing a dye into the lower eye lid. These drops stain on the surface of the eye, highlighting any areas of injury.

- Slit lamp examination—This test shows how severe the dryness is and whether the outside of the eye is inflamed. An ophthalmologist (eye specialist) uses equipment that magnifies to carefully examine the eye.

- Mouth exam—The doctor will look in the mouth for signs of dryness and to see whether any of the major salivary glands are swollen. Signs of dryness include a dry, sticky mouth; cavities; thick saliva, or none at all; a smooth look to the tongue; redness in the mouth; dry, cracked lips; and sores at the corners of the mouth. The doctor might also try to get a sample of saliva to see how much the glands are producing and to check its quality.

- Salivary gland biopsy of the lip—This test is the best way to find out whether dry mouth is caused by Sjögren syndrome. The doctor removes tiny minor salivary glands from the inside of the lower lip and examines them under the microscope. If the glands contain lymphocytes in a particular pattern, the test is positive for Sjögren syndrome.

Because there are many causes of dry eyes and dry mouth, the doctor will take other possible causes into account. Generally, you are considered to have definite Sjögren syndrome if you have dry eyes, dry mouth, and a positive lip biopsy. But the doctor may decide to do additional tests to see whether other parts of the body are affected. These tests may include:

- Routine blood tests—The doctor will take blood samples to check blood count and blood sugar level, and to see how the liver and kidneys are working.

- Immunological tests—These blood tests check for antibodies commonly found in the blood of people with Sjögren syndrome. For example, antithyroid antibodies are created when antibodies migrate out of the salivary glands into the thyroid gland. Antithyroid antibodies cause thyroiditis (inflammation of the thyroid), a common problem in people with Sjögren syndrome. Immunoglobulins and gamma globulins are antibodies that everyone has in their blood, but people with Sjögren syndrome usually have too many of them. Rheumatoid factors (RFs) are found in the blood of people with rheumatoid arthritis, as well as in people with Sjögren syndrome. Substances known as cryoglobulins may be detected; these indicate risk of lymphoma. Similarly, the presence of antinuclear antibodies (ANAs) can indicate an autoimmune disorder, including Sjögren syndrome. Sjögren syndrome antibodies, called SS-A (or SS-Ro) and SS-B (or SS-La), are specific antinuclear antibodies common in people with Sjögren syndrome. However, you can have Sjögren syndrome without having these ANAs.

- Chest x-ray—Sjögren syndrome can cause inflammation in the lungs, so the doctor may want to take an x-ray to check them.

- Urinalysis—The doctor will probably test a sample of your urine to see how well the kidneys are working.

What Type of Doctor Diagnoses and Treats Sjögren Syndrome?

Because the symptoms of Sjögren syndrome are similar to those of many other diseases, getting a diagnosis can take time—in fact, the average time from first symptom to diagnosis ranges from 2 to 8 years. During those years, depending on the symptoms, a person might see a number of doctors, any of whom may diagnose the disease and be involved in treatment. Usually, a rheumatologist (a doctor who specializes in diseases of the joints, muscles, and bones) will coordinate treatment among a number of specialists. Other doctors who may be involved include:

- allergist
- dentist
- dermatologist (skin specialist)
- gastroenterologist (digestive disease specialist)
- gynecologist (women's reproductive health specialist)
- neurologist (nerve and brain specialist)
- ophthalmologist (eye specialist)
- otolaryngologist (ear, nose, and throat specialist)
- pulmonologist (lung specialist)
- urologist

How Is Sjögren Syndrome Treated?

Treatment is different for each person, depending on what parts of the body are affected. But in all cases, the doctor will help relieve your symptoms, especially dryness. For example, you can use artificial tears to help with dry eyes and saliva stimulants and mouth lubricants for dry mouth. Treatment for dryness is described in more detail below.

If you have extraglandular involvement, your doctor—or the appropriate specialist—will also treat those problems. Treatment may include nonsteroidal anti-inflammatory drugs for joint or muscle pain, saliva- and mucus-stimulating drugs for nose and throat dryness, and corticosteroids or drugs that suppress the immune system for lung, kidney, blood vessel, or nervous system problems. Hydroxychloroquine, methotrexate, and cyclophosphamide are examples of such immunosuppressants (drugs that suppress the immune system).

What Can I Do about Dry Eyes?

Artificial tears can help. They come in different thicknesses, so you may have to experiment to find the right one. Some drops contain preservatives that might irritate your eyes. Drops without preservatives don't usually bother the eyes. Nonpreserved tears typically come in single-dose packages to prevent contamination with bacteria.

At night, an eye ointment might provide more relief. Ointments are thicker than artificial tears and moisturize and protect the eye for several hours. They may blur your vision, which is why some people prefer to use them while they sleep.

Hydroxypropyl methylcellulose (Lacrisert) is a chemical that lubricates the surface of the eye and slows the evaporation of natural tears. It comes in a small pellet that you put in your lower eyelid. When you add artificial tears, the pellet dissolves and forms a film over your own tears that traps the moisture.

Another alternative is surgery to close the tear ducts that drain tears from the eye. The surgery is called punctal occlusion. For a temporary closure, the doctor inserts collagen or silicone plugs into the ducts. Collagen plugs eventually dissolve, and silicone plugs are permanent until they are removed or fall out. For a longer lasting effect, the doctor can use a laser or cautery to seal the ducts.

General Tips for Eye Care

- Don't use artificial tears that irritate your eyes—try another brand or preparation.

- Nonpreserved drops may be more comfortable.

- Blink several times a minute while reading or working on the computer.

- Protect your eyes from drafts, breezes, and wind.

- Put a humidifier in the rooms where you spend the most time, including the bedroom, or install a humidifier in your heating and air conditioning unit.

- Don't smoke and stay out of smoky rooms.

- Apply mascara only to the tips of your lashes so it doesn't get in your eyes. If you use eyeliner or eye shadow, put it only on the skin above your lashes, not on the sensitive skin under your lashes, close to your eyes.

- Ask your doctor whether any of your medications contribute to dryness and, if so, how to reduce that effect.

What Can I Do about Dry Mouth?

If your salivary glands still produce some saliva, you can stimulate them to make more by chewing gum or sucking on hard candy. However, gum and candy must be sugar free because dry mouth makes you extremely prone to cavities. Take sips of water or another sugar-free drink often throughout the day to wet your mouth, especially when you are eating or talking. Note that you should take sips of water—drinking large amounts of liquid throughout the day will not make your mouth any less dry. It will only make you urinate more often and may strip your mouth of mucus, causing even more dryness. You can soothe dry, cracked lips by using oil- or petroleum-based lip balm or lipstick. If your mouth hurts, the doctor may give you medicine in a mouth rinse, ointment, or gel to apply to the sore areas to control pain and inflammation.

If you produce very little saliva or none at all, your doctor might recommend a saliva substitute. These products mimic some of the properties of saliva, which means they make the mouth feel wet, and if they contain fluoride, they can help prevent cavities. Gel-based saliva substitutes tend to give the longest relief, but all saliva products are limited since you eventually swallow them.

At least two drugs that stimulate the salivary glands to produce saliva are available. These are pilocarpine and cevimeline. The effects last for a few hours, and you can take them three or four times a day. However, they are not suitable for everyone, so talk to your doctor about whether they might help you.

People with dry mouth can easily get mouth infections. Candidiasis, a fungal mouth infection, is one of the most commonly seen infections in people with Sjögren syndrome. It most often shows up as white patches inside the mouth that you can scrape off, or as red, burning areas in the mouth. Candidiasis is treated with antifungal drugs. Various viruses and bacteria can also cause infections; they're treated with the appropriate antiviral or antibiotic medicines.

The Importance of Oral Hygiene

Natural saliva contains substances that rid the mouth of the bacteria that cause cavities and mouth infections, so good oral hygiene is extremely important when you have dry mouth. Here's what you can do to prevent cavities and infections:

- Visit a dentist at least three times a year to have your teeth examined and cleaned.

- Rinse your mouth with water several times a day. Don't use mouthwash that contains alcohol because alcohol is drying.

- Use fluoride toothpaste to gently brush your teeth, gums, and tongue after each meal and before bedtime. Nonfoaming toothpaste is less drying.

270

- Floss your teeth every day.

- Avoid sugar. That means choosing sugar-free gum, candy, and soda. If you do eat or drink sugary foods, brush your teeth immediately afterward.

- Look at your mouth every day to check for redness or sores. See a dentist right away if you notice anything unusual or have any mouth pain or bleeding.

- Ask your dentist whether you need to take fluoride supplements, use a fluoride gel at night, or have a protective varnish put on your teeth to protect the enamel.

What Other Parts of the Body Are Involved in Sjögren Syndrome?

The autoimmune response that causes dry eyes and mouth can cause inflammation throughout the body. People with Sjögren syndrome often have skin, lung, kidney, and nerve problems, as well as disorders of the digestive system and connective tissue. Following are examples of extraglandular problems.

Skin Problems

About half of the people who have Sjögren syndrome have dry skin. Some experience only itching, but it can be severe. Others develop cracked, split skin that can easily become infected. Infection is a risk for people with itchy skin, too, particularly if they scratch vigorously. The skin may darken in infected areas, but it returns to normal when the infection clears up and the scratching stops.

To treat dry skin, apply heavy moisturizing creams and ointments three or four times a day to trap moisture in the skin. Lotions, which are lighter than creams and ointments, aren't recommended because they evaporate quickly and can contribute to dry skin. Also, doctors suggest that you take only a short shower (less than 5 minutes), use a moisturizing soap, pat your skin almost dry, and then cover it with a cream or ointment. If you take baths, it's a good idea to soak for 10 to 15 minutes to give your skin time to absorb moisture. Having a humidifier in the bedroom can help hydrate your skin, too. If these steps don't help the itching, your doctor might recommend that you use a skin cream or ointment containing steroids.

Some patients who have Sjögren syndrome, particularly those who have lupus, are sensitive to sunlight and can get painful burns from even

271

a little sun exposure, such as through a window. So, if you're sensitive to sunlight, you need to wear sunscreen (at least SPF 15) whenever you go outdoors and try to avoid being in the sun for long periods of time.

Vaginal Dryness

Vaginal dryness is common in women with Sjögren syndrome. Painful intercourse is the most common complaint. A vaginal moisturizer helps retain moisture, and a vaginal lubricant can make intercourse more comfortable. Vaginal moisturizers attract liquid to the dry tissues and are designed for regular use. Vaginal lubricants should be used only for intercourse—they don't moisturize. Oil-based lubricants, such as petroleum jelly, trap moisture and can cause sores and hinder the vagina's natural cleaning process. A water-soluble lubricant is better. Regular skin creams and ointments relieve dry skin on the outer surface of the vagina (the vulva).

Lung Problems

Dry mouth can cause lung problems. For example, aspiration pneumonia can happen when a person breathes in food instead of swallowing it (dry mouth can keep you from swallowing food properly), and the food gets stuck in the lungs. Pneumonia can also develop when bacteria in the mouth migrate into the lungs and cause infection, or when bacteria get into the lungs and coughing doesn't remove them. (Some people with Sjögren syndrome don't produce enough mucus in the lungs to remove bacteria, and others are too weak to be able to cough.) Pneumonia is treated with various antibiotics, depending on the person and the type of infection. It is important to get treatment for pneumonia to prevent lung abscess (a hole in the lung caused by severe infection).

People with Sjögren syndrome also tend to have lung problems caused by inflammation, such as bronchitis (affecting the bronchial tubes), tracheobronchitis (affecting the windpipe and bronchial tubes), and laryngotracheobronchitis (affecting the voice box, windpipe, and bronchial tubes). Depending on your condition, the doctor may recommend using a humidifier, taking medicines to open the bronchial tubes, or taking corticosteroids to relieve inflammation. Pleurisy is inflammation of the lining of the lungs and is treated with corticosteroids and nonsteroidal antiinflammatory drugs.

Kidney Problems

The kidneys filter waste products from the blood and remove them from the body through urine. The most common kidney problem in people

272

with Sjögren syndrome is interstitial nephritis, or inflammation of the tissue around the kidney's filters, which can occur even before dry eyes and dry mouth. Inflammation of the filters themselves, called glomerulonephritis, is less common. Some people develop renal tubular acidosis, which means they can't get rid of certain acids through urine. The amount of potassium in their blood drops, causing an imbalance in blood chemicals that can affect the heart, muscles, and nerves.

Often, doctors do not treat these problems unless they start to affect kidney function or cause other health problems. However, they keep a close eye on the problem through regular exams, and will prescribe medicines called alkaline agents to balance blood chemicals when necessary. Corticosteroids or immunosuppressants are used to treat more severe cases.

Nerve Problems

People with Sjögren syndrome can have nerve problems. When they do, the problem usually involves the peripheral nervous system (PNS), which contains the nerves that control sensation and movement. Involvement of the PNS is increasingly being recognized. Carpal tunnel syndrome, peripheral neuropathy, and cranial neuropathy are examples of peripheral nervous system disorders that occur in people with Sjögren syndrome. In carpal tunnel syndrome, inflamed tissue in the forearm presses against the median nerve, causing pain, numbness, tingling, and sometimes muscle weakness in the thumb and index and middle fingers. In peripheral neuropathy, an immune attack damages nerves in the legs or arms, causing the same symptoms there. (Sometimes nerves are damaged because inflamed blood vessels cut off their blood supply.) In cranial neuropathy, nerve damage causes face pain; loss of feeling in the face, tongue, eyes, ears, or throat; and loss of taste and smell.

Nerve problems are treated with medicines to control pain and, if necessary, with steroids or other drugs to control inflammation.

Digestive Problems

Inflammation in the esophagus, stomach, pancreas, and liver can cause problems like painful swallowing, heartburn, abdominal pain and swelling, loss of appetite, diarrhea, and weight loss. It can also cause hepatitis (inflammation of the liver) and cirrhosis (hardening of the liver). Sjögren syndrome is closely linked to a liver disease called primary biliary cirrhosis (PBC), which causes itching, fatigue, and, eventually, cirrhosis. Many patients with PBC have Sjögren syndrome.

Treatment varies, depending on the problem, but may include pain medicine, anti-inflammatory drugs, steroids, and immunosuppressants.

Connective Tissue Disorders

Connective tissue is the framework of the body that supports organs and tissues. Examples are joints, muscles, bones, skin, blood vessel walls, and the lining of internal organs. Many connective tissue disorders are autoimmune diseases, and several are common among people with Sjögren syndrome:

- Polymyositis is an inflammation of the muscles that causes weakness and pain, difficulty moving, and, in some cases, problems breathing and swallowing. If the skin is inflamed too, it's called dermatomyositis. The disease is treated with corticosteroids and immunosuppressants.

- In Raynaud phenomenon, blood vessels in the hands, arms, feet, and legs constrict (narrow) when exposed to cold. The result is pain, tingling, and numbness. When vessels constrict, fingers turn white. Shortly after that, they turn blue because of blood that remained in the tissue pools. When new blood rushes in, the fingers turn red. The problem is treated with medicines that dilate blood vessels. Raynaud's phenomenon usually occurs before dryness of the eyes or mouth.

- Rheumatoid arthritis (RA) is severe inflammation of the joints that can eventually deform the surrounding bones (fingers, hands, knees, etc.). RA can also damage muscles, blood vessels, and major organs. Treatment depends on the severity of the pain and swelling and which body parts are involved. It may include physical therapy, aspirin, rest, nonsteroidal anti-inflammatory agents, steroids, or immunosuppressants.

- Scleroderma causes the body to accumulate too much collagen, a protein commonly found in the skin. The result is thick, tight skin and damage to muscles, joints, and internal organs such as the esophagus, intestines, lungs, heart, kidneys, and blood vessels. Treatment is aimed at relieving pain and includes drugs, skin softeners, and physical therapy.

- Systemic lupus erythematosus (SLE) causes joint and muscle pain, weakness, skin rashes, and, in more severe cases, heart, lung, kidney, and nervous system problems. As with RA, treatment for SLE depends on the symptoms and may include aspirin, rest, steroids, and anti-inflammatory and other drugs, as well as dialysis and high blood pressure medicine.

- Vasculitis is an inflammation of the blood vessels, which then become scarred and too narrow for blood to get through to reach the organs. In people with Sjögren syndrome, vasculitis tends to occur in those who also have Raynaud phenomenon and lung and liver problems.

- Autoimmune thyroid disorders are common with Sjögren syndrome. They can appear as either the overactive thyroid of Graves disease or the underactive thyroid of Hashimoto disease. Nearly half of the people with autoimmune thyroid disorder also have Sjögren syndrome, and many people with Sjögren syndrome show evidence of thyroid disease.

Does Sjögren Syndrome Cause Lymphoma?

About 5 percent of people with Sjögren syndrome develop cancer of the lymph nodes, or lymphoma. The most common symptom of lymphoma is a painless swelling of the lymph nodes in the neck, underarm, or groin. In Sjögren syndrome, when lymphoma develops it often involves the salivary glands. Persistent enlargement of the salivary glands should be investigated further. Other symptoms may include the following:

- unexplained fever
- night sweats
- constant fatigue
- unexplained weight loss
- itchy skin
- reddened patches on the skin

These symptoms are not sure signs of lymphoma. They may be caused by other, less serious conditions, such as the flu or an infection. If you have these symptoms, see a doctor so that any illness can be diagnosed and treated as early as possible.

If you're worried that you might develop lymphoma, talk to your doctor to learn more about the disease, symptoms to watch for, any special medical care you might need, and what you can do to relieve your worry.

Medicines and Dryness

Certain drugs can contribute to eye and mouth dryness. If you take any of the drugs listed below, ask your doctor whether they could be causing symptoms. However, don't stop taking them without asking your doctor—he or she may already have adjusted the dose to help protect you against drying side effects or chosen a drug that's least likely to cause dryness.

Drugs that can cause dryness include:

- antihistamines
- decongestants
- diuretics
- some antidiarrhea drugs
- some antipsychotic drugs
- tranquilizers
- some blood pressure medicines
- antidepressants

What Research Is Being Done on Sjögren Syndrome?

Through basic research on the immune system, autoimmunity, genetics, and connective tissue diseases, researchers continue to learn more about Sjögren syndrome. As they get a better understanding of the genes involved and which environmental factors trigger disease and how, they'll be able to develop more effective treatments. For example, gene therapy studies suggest that we may someday be able to insert molecules into salivary glands that will control inflammation and prevent their destruction. Other research focuses on how the immune and hormonal systems work in people who have Sjögren syndrome and on the natural history of the disease (learning how it affects people by following those who have it).

Researchers are also looking into the use of the salivary stimulant pilocarpine for dry eyes. Other researchers are testing immune modulating drugs to treat the glandular inflammation. A drug called cevimeline has recently been approved for treating dry mouth. Work on developing an artificial salivary gland is in progress.

The National Institute of Dental and Craniofacial Research is conducting several studies on Sjögren syndrome designed to help scientists better understand, manage, and treat the disease. Some focus on the disease's natural history, while others test potential new treatments.

Talk to your doctor if you'd like more information about these clinical trials.

Where Can People Find More Information about Sjögren Syndrome?

The following organizations have information relevant to Sjögren syndrome:

American Academy of Dermatology
P.O. Box 4014
Schaumburg, IL 60168-4014
Toll-Free: (888) 462-3376
Phone: (847) 330-0230
Website: http://www.aad.org

American Academy of Ophthalmology
P.O. Box 7424
San Francisco, CA 94120
Phone: (415) 561-8500; Fax: (415) 561-8567
Website: http://www.eyenet.org

American Association for Dental Research
1619 Duke Street
Alexandria, VA 22314
Phone: (703) 548-0066
Fax: (703)548-1883
Website: http://www.iadr.com

American College of Rheumatology
1800 Century Place, Suite 250
Atlanta, GA 30345-4300
Phone: (404) 633-3777; Fax: (404) 633-1870
Website: http://www.rheumatology.org

American Dental Association
Department of Public Information and Education
211 East Chicago Avenue
Chicago, IL 60611
Phone: (312) 440-2500; Fax: (312) 440-2800
Website: http://www.ada.org
E-mail: publicinfo@ada.org

National Eye Institute
National Institutes of Health
2020 Vision Place
Bethesda, MD 20892-3655
Phone: (301) 496-5248
Website: http://www.nei.nih.gov

National Institute of Allergy and Infectious Disease
6610 Rockledge Drive
MSC 6612
Bethesda, MD 20892-6612
Phone: (301) 402-1663
Fax: (301) 402-0120
Website: http://www.niaid.nih.gov

National Institute of Arthritis and Musculoskeletal and Skin Diseases
1 AMS Circle
Bethesda, MD 20892-3675
Toll-Free: (877) 22-NIAMS (226-4267)
Phone: (301) 495-4484
TTY: (301) 565-2966
Fax: (301) 718-6366
Website: http://www.niams.nih.gov
E-mail: niamsinfo@mail.nih.gov

National Institute of Dental and Craniofacial Research
National Institutes of Health
45 Center Drive, MSC 6400
Building 45, Room 4AS-25
Bethesda, MD 20892-6400
Phone: (301) 496-4261
Website: http://www.nidcr.nih.gov
E-mail: nidrinfo@od31.nidr.nih.gov

National Institute of Neurological Disorders and Stroke
National Institutes of Health
Office of Communications and Public Liaison
P.O. Box 5801
Bethesda, MD 20824
Toll-Free: (800) 352-9424
Website: http://www.ninds.nih.gov

American Autoimmune Related Diseases Association
22100 Gratiot Avenue
Eastpointe
E. Detroit, MI 48021-2227
Toll-Free: (800) 598-4668
Phone: (586) 776-3900
Fax: (586) 776-3903
Website: http://www.aarda.org
E-mail: aarda@aarda.org

Arthritis Foundation
1330 West Peachtree Street
Atlanta, GA 30309
Toll-Free: (800) 283-7800
Phone: (404) 872-7100
Website: http://www.arthritis.org

Lupus Foundation of America, Inc.
2000 L Street, N.W.
Suite 710
Washington, DC 20036
Toll-Free: (800) 558-0121
Phone: (202) 349-1155
Fax: (202)349-1156
Website: http://www.lupus.org
E-mail: lupusinfo@lupus.org

Myositis Foundation of America
755 Cantrell Avenue, Suite C
Harrisonburg, VA 22801
Phone: (540) 433-7686
Fax: (540) 432-0206
Website: http://www.myositis.org
E-mail: maa@myositis.org

National Organization for Rare Disorders, Inc.
P.O. Box 1968
Danbury, CT 06813-1968
Phone: (203) 744-0100
Toll-Free: (800) 999-6673
Website: http://www.rarediseases.org
E-mail: orphan@rarediseases.org

Scleroderma Foundation
12 Kent Way, Suite 101
Byfield, MA 01922
Toll-Free: 800-722-HOPE (4673)
Phone: (978) 463-5843
Fax: (978) 463-5809
Website: http://www.scleroderma.org
E-mail: sfinfo@scleroderma.org

Scleroderma Research Foundation
2320 Bath Street, Suite 315
Santa Barbara, CA 93105
Toll-Free: (800) 441-CURE
Phone: (805) 563-9133
Website: http://www.srfcure.org

Sjögren's Syndrome Foundation
8120 Woodmont Avenue, Suite 530
Bethesda, MD 20814
Toll-Free: (800) 475-6473
Fax: (301) 718-0322
Website: http://sjogrens.com

Chapter 23

Systemic Lupus
Erythematosus

This chapter is for people who have systemic lupus erythemato-sus, commonly called SLE or lupus, as well as for their family and friends and others who want to better understand the disease. The chapter describes the disease and its symptoms and contains information about diagnosis and treatment as well as current research efforts supported by the National Institute of Arthritis and Musculoskeletal and Skin Diseases (NIAMS) and other components of the Department of Health and Human Services' National Institutes of Health (NIH). It also discusses issues such as health care, pregnancy, and quality of life for people with lupus. If you have further questions after reading this chapter, you may wish to discuss them with your doctor.

Defining Lupus

Lupus is one of many disorders of the immune system known as autoimmune diseases. In autoimmune diseases, the immune system turns against parts of the body it is designed to protect. This leads to inflammation and damage to various body tissues. Lupus can affect many parts of the body, including the joints, skin, kidneys, heart, lungs, blood vessels, and brain. Although people with the disease may have many different symptoms, some of the most common ones include

"Handout on Health: Systemic Lupus Erythematosus," National Institute of Arthritis and Musculoskeletal and Skin Diseases (NIAMS), August 2003. Available online at http://www.niams.nih.gov; accessed March 2004.

extreme fatigue, painful or swollen joints (arthritis), unexplained fever, skin rashes, and kidney problems.

At present, there is no cure for lupus. However, lupus can be effectively treated with drugs, and most people with the disease can lead active, healthy lives. Lupus is characterized by periods of illness, called flares, and periods of wellness, or remission.

Understanding how to prevent flares and how to treat them when they do occur helps people with lupus maintain better health. Intense research is underway, and scientists funded by the National Institutes of Health are continuing to make great strides in understanding the disease, which may ultimately lead to a cure.

Two of the major questions researchers are studying are who gets lupus and why. We know that many more women than men have lupus. Lupus is three times more common in African American women than in Caucasian women and is also more common in women of Hispanic, Asian, and Native American descent. In addition, lupus can run in families, but the risk that a child or a brother or sister of a patient will also have lupus is still quite low. It is difficult to estimate how many people in the United States have the disease because its symptoms vary widely and its onset is often hard to pinpoint.

There are several kinds of lupus:

- **Systemic lupus erythematosus (SLE)** is the form of the disease that most people are referring to when they say lupus. The word systemic means the disease can affect many parts of the body. The symptoms of SLE may be mild or serious. Although SLE usually first affects people between the ages of 15 and 45 years, it can occur in childhood or later in life as well. This chapter focuses on SLE.

- **Discoid lupus erythematosus** is a chronic skin disorder in which a red, raised rash appears on the face, scalp, or elsewhere. The raised areas may become thick and scaly and may cause scarring. The rash may last for days or years and may recur. A small percentage of people with discoid lupus have or develop SLE later.

- **Subacute cutaneous lupus erythematosus** refers to skin lesions that appear on parts of the body exposed to sun. The lesions do not cause scarring.

- **Drug-induced lupus** is a form of lupus caused by medications. Many different drugs can cause drug-induced lupus. Symptoms are similar to those of SLE (arthritis, rash, fever, and chest pain) and they typically go away completely when the drug is stopped. The kidneys and brain are rarely involved.

- **Neonatal lupus** is a rare disease that can occur in newborn babies of women with SLE, Sjögren syndrome, or no disease at all. Scientists suspect that neonatal lupus is caused by autoantibodies in the mother's blood called anti-Ro (SSA) and anti-La (SSB). Autoantibodies (*auto* means self) are blood proteins that act against the body's own parts. At birth, the babies have a skin rash, liver problems, and low blood counts. These symptoms gradually go away over several months. In rare instances, babies with neonatal lupus may have a serious heart problem that slows down the natural rhythm of the heart. Neonatal lupus is rare, and most infants of mothers with SLE are entirely healthy. All women who are pregnant and known to have anti-Ro (SSA) or anti-La (SSB) antibodies should be monitored by echocardiograms (a test that monitors the heart and surrounding blood vessels) during the 16th and 30th weeks of pregnancy.

It is important for women with SLE or other related autoimmune disorders to be under a doctor's care during pregnancy. Physicians can now identify mothers at highest risk for complications, allowing for prompt treatment of the infant at or before birth. SLE can also flare during pregnancy, and prompt treatment can keep the mother healthier longer.

Understanding What Causes Lupus

Lupus is a complex disease, and its cause is unknown. It is likely that a combination of genetic, environmental, and possibly hormonal factors work together to cause the disease. Scientists are making progress in understanding lupus, as described here and in the "Current Research" section of this chapter. The fact that lupus can run in families indicates that its development has a genetic basis. Recent research suggests that genetics plays an important role; however, no specific lupus gene has been identified yet. Studies suggest that several different genes may be involved in determining a person's likelihood of developing the disease, which tissues and organs are affected, and the severity of disease. However, scientists believe that genes alone do not determine who gets lupus and that other factors also play a role. Some of the factors scientists are studying include sunlight, stress, certain drugs, and infectious agents such as viruses.

In lupus, the body's immune system does not work as it should. A healthy immune system produces proteins called antibodies and specific cells called lymphocytes that help fight and destroy viruses, bacteria, and other foreign substances that invade the body. In lupus, the immune system produces antibodies against the body's healthy cells and tissues. These antibodies, called autoantibodies, contribute to the inflammation of various parts of the body and can cause damage to organs and tissues. The most common type of autoantibody that develops in people with lupus is called an antinuclear antibody (ANA) because it reacts with parts of the cell's nucleus (command center). Doctors and scientists do not yet understand all of the factors that cause inflammation and tissue damage in lupus, and researchers are actively exploring them.

Symptoms of Lupus

Each person with lupus has slightly different symptoms that can range from mild to severe and may come and go over time. However, some of the most common symptoms of lupus include painful or swollen joints (arthritis), unexplained fever, and extreme fatigue. A characteristic red skin rash—the so-called butterfly or malar rash—may appear across the nose and cheeks. Rashes may also occur on the face and ears, upper arms, shoulders, chest, and hands. Because many people with lupus are sensitive to sunlight (called photosensitivity), skin rashes often first develop or worsen after sun exposure.

Common symptoms of lupus include:

- Painful or swollen joints and muscle pain
- Unexplained fever
- Red rashes, most commonly on the face
- Chest pain upon deep breathing
- Unusual loss of hair
- Pale or purple fingers or toes from cold or stress (Raynaud phenomenon)
- Sensitivity to the sun
- Swelling (edema) in legs or around eyes
- Mouth ulcers
- Swollen glands
- Extreme fatigue

Other symptoms of lupus include chest pain, hair loss, anemia (a decrease in red blood cells), mouth ulcers, and pale or purple fingers and toes from cold and stress. Some people also experience headaches, dizziness, depression, confusion, or seizures. New symptoms may continue to appear years after the initial diagnosis, and different symptoms can occur at different times. In some people with lupus, only one system of the body, such as the skin or joints, is affected. Other people experience symptoms in many parts of their body. Just how seriously a body system is affected varies from person to person. The following systems in the body also can be affected by lupus.

- **Kidneys:** Inflammation of the kidneys (nephritis) can impair their ability to get rid of waste products and other toxins from the body effectively. There is usually no pain associated with kidney involvement, although some patients may notice swelling in their ankles. Most often, the only indication of kidney disease is an abnormal urine or blood test. Because the kidneys are so important to overall health, lupus affecting the kidneys generally requires intensive drug treatment to prevent permanent damage.

- **Lungs:** Some people with lupus develop pleuritis, an inflammation of the lining of the chest cavity that causes chest pain, particularly with breathing. Patients with lupus also may get pneumonia.

- **Central nervous system:** In some patients, lupus affects the brain or central nervous system. This can cause headaches, dizziness, memory disturbances, vision problems, seizures, stroke, or changes in behavior.

- **Blood vessels:** Blood vessels may become inflamed (vasculitis), affecting the way blood circulates through the body. The inflammation may be mild and may not require treatment or may be severe and require immediate attention.

- **Blood:** People with lupus may develop anemia, leukopenia (a decreased number of white blood cells), or thrombocytopenia (a decrease in the number of platelets in the blood, which assist in clotting). Some people with lupus may have an increased risk for blood clots.

- **Heart:** In some people with lupus, inflammation can occur in the heart itself (myocarditis and endocarditis) or the membrane that surrounds it (pericarditis), causing chest pains or other symptoms. Lupus can also increase the risk of atherosclerosis (hardening of the arteries).

Diagnosing Lupus

Diagnosing lupus can be difficult. It may take months or even years for doctors to piece together the symptoms to diagnose this complex disease accurately. Making a correct diagnosis of lupus requires knowledge and awareness on the part of the doctor and good communication on the part of the patient. Giving the doctor a complete, accurate medical history (for example, what health problems you have had and for how long) is critical to the process of diagnosis. This information, along with a physical examination and the results of laboratory tests, helps the doctor consider other diseases that may mimic lupus, or determine if the patient truly has the disease. Reaching a diagnosis may take time as new symptoms appear.

No single test can determine whether a person has lupus, but several laboratory tests may help the doctor to make a diagnosis. The most useful tests identify certain autoantibodies often present in the blood of people with lupus. For example, the antinuclear antibody (ANA) test is commonly used to look for autoantibodies that react against components of the nucleus, or command center, of the body's cells. Most people with lupus test positive for ANA; however, there are a number of other causes of a positive ANA besides lupus, including infections, other autoimmune diseases, and occasionally as a finding in healthy people. The ANA test simply provides another clue for the doctor to consider in making a diagnosis. In addition, there are blood tests for individual types of autoantibodies that are more specific to people with lupus, although not all people with lupus test positive for these and not all people with these antibodies have lupus. These antibodies include anti-DNA, anti-Sm, anti-RNP, anti-Ro (SSA), and anti-La (SSB). The doctor may use these antibody tests to help make a diagnosis of lupus.

Some tests are used less frequently but may be helpful if the cause of a person's symptoms remains unclear. The doctor may order a biopsy of the skin or kidneys if those body systems are affected. Some doctors may order a test for anticardiolipin (or antiphospholipid) antibody. The presence of this antibody may indicate increased risk for blood clotting and increased risk for miscarriage in pregnant women with lupus. Again, all these tests merely serve as tools to give the doctor clues and information in making a diagnosis. The doctor will look at the entire picture-medical history, symptoms, and test results to determine if a person has lupus.

Other laboratory tests are used to monitor the progress of the disease once it has been diagnosed. A complete blood count, urinalysis, blood chemistries, and the erythrocyte sedimentation rate (ESR) test can provide valuable information. Another common test measures the blood level of a group of substances called complement. People with lupus often have increased ESRs and low complement levels, especially during flares of the disease. X-rays and other imaging tests can help doctors see the organs affected by SLE.

Treating Lupus

Diagnosing and treating lupus are often a team effort between the patient and several types of health care professionals. A person with lupus can go to his or her family doctor or internist or can visit a rheumatologist. A rheumatologist is a doctor who specializes in rheumatic diseases (arthritis and other inflammatory disorders, often involving the immune system). Clinical immunologists (doctors specializing in immune system disorders) may also treat people with lupus. As treatment progresses, other professionals often help. These may include nurses, psychologists, social workers, nephrologists (doctors who treat kidney disease), hematologists (doctors specializing in blood disorders), dermatologists (doctors who treat skin disease), and neurologists (doctors specializing in disorders of the nervous system).

The range and effectiveness of treatments for lupus have increased dramatically, giving doctors more choices in how to manage the disease. It is important for the patient to work closely with the doctor and take an active role in managing the disease. Once lupus has been diagnosed, the doctor will develop a treatment plan based on the patient's age, sex, health, symptoms, and lifestyle. Treatment plans are tailored to the individual's needs and may change over time. In developing a treatment plan, the doctor has several goals: to prevent flares, to treat them when they do occur, and to minimize organ damage and complications. The doctor and patient should reevaluate the plan regularly to ensure it is as effective as possible.

NSAIDs: For people with joint or chest pain or fever, drugs that decrease inflammation, called nonsteroidal anti-inflammatory drugs (NSAIDs), are often used. While some NSAIDs, such as ibuprofen and naproxen, are available over the counter, a doctor's prescription is necessary for others. NSAIDs may be used alone or in combination with other types of drugs to control pain, swelling, and fever. Even though some NSAIDs may be purchased without a prescription, it is

287

important that they be taken under a doctor's direction. Common side effects of NSAIDs can include stomach upset, heartburn, diarrhea, and fluid retention. Some people with lupus also develop liver, kidney, or even neurological complications, making it especially important to stay in close contact with the doctor while taking these medications.

Antimalarials: Antimalarials are another type of drug commonly used to treat lupus. These drugs were originally used to treat malaria, but doctors have found that they also are useful for lupus. A common antimalarial used to treat lupus is hydroxychloroquine (Plaquenil). It may be used alone or in combination with other drugs and generally is used to treat fatigue, joint pain, skin rashes, and inflammation of the lungs. Clinical studies have found that continuous treatment with antimalarials may prevent flares from recurring. Side effects of antimalarials can include stomach upset and, extremely rarely, damage to the retina of the eye.

Corticosteroids: The mainstay of lupus treatment involves the use of corticosteroid hormones, such as prednisone (Deltasone), hydrocortisone, methylprednisolone (Medrol), and dexamethasone (Decadron, Hexadrol). Corticosteroids are related to cortisol, which is a natural anti-inflammatory hormone. They work by rapidly suppressing inflammation. Corticosteroids can be given by mouth, in creams applied to the skin, or by injection. Because they are potent drugs, the doctor will seek the lowest dose with the greatest benefit. Short-term side effects of corticosteroids include swelling, increased appetite, and weight gain. These side effects generally stop when the drug is stopped. It is dangerous to stop taking corticosteroids suddenly, so it is very important that the doctor and patient work together in changing the corticosteroid dose. Sometimes doctors give very large amounts of corticosteroid by vein over a brief period of time (days) (called bolus or pulse therapy). With this treatment, the typical side effects are less likely and slow withdrawal is unnecessary.

Long-term side effects of corticosteroids can include stretch marks on the skin, weakened or damaged bones (osteoporosis and osteonecrosis), high blood pressure, damage to the arteries, high blood sugar (diabetes), infections, and cataracts. Typically, the higher the dose and the longer they are taken, the greater the risk and severity of side effects. Researchers are working to develop ways to limit or offset the use of corticosteroids. For example, corticosteroids may be used in combination with other, less potent drugs, or the doctor may try to slowly decrease the dose once the disease is under control. People with lupus who are using corticosteroids should talk to their doctors about taking supplemental calcium and vitamin D or other drugs to reduce the risk of osteoporosis (weakened, fragile bones).

Immunosuppressives: For some patients whose kidneys or central nervous systems are affected by lupus, a type of drug called an immunosuppressive may be used. Immunosuppressives, such as cyclophosphamide (Cytoxan) and mycophenolate mofetil (CellCept), restrain the overactive immune system by blocking the production of immune cells. These drugs may be given by mouth or by infusion (dripping the drug into the vein through a small tube). Side effects may include nausea, vomiting, hair loss, bladder problems, decreased fertility, and increased risk of cancer and infection. The risk for side effects increases with the length of treatment. As with other treatments for lupus, there is a risk of relapse after the immunosuppressives have been stopped.

Other Therapies: In some patients, methotrexate (Folex, Mexate, Rheumatrex), a disease-modifying antirheumatic drug, may be used to help control the disease. Working closely with the doctor helps ensure that treatments for lupus are as successful as possible. Because some treatments may cause harmful side effects, it is important to report any new symptoms to the doctor promptly. It is also important not to stop or change treatments without talking to the doctor first.

Alternative and Complementary Therapies: Because of the nature and cost of the medications used to treat lupus and the potential for serious side effects, many patients seek other ways of treating the disease. Some alternative approaches people have tried include special diets, nutritional supplements, fish oils, ointments and creams, chiropractic treatment, and homeopathy. Although these methods may not be harmful in and of themselves, and may be associated with symptomatic or psychosocial benefit, no research to date shows that they affect the disease process or prevent organ damage. Some alternative or complementary approaches may help the patient cope or reduce some of the stress associated with living with a chronic illness. If the doctor feels the approach has value and will not be harmful, it can be incorporated into the patient's treatment plan. However, it is important not to neglect regular health care or treatment of serious symptoms. An open dialogue between the patient and physician about the relative values of complementary and alternative therapies allows the patient to make an informed choice about treatment options.

Lupus and Quality of Life

Despite the symptoms of lupus and the potential side effects of treatment, people with lupus can maintain a high quality of life overall. One key to managing lupus is to understand the disease and its impact. Learning to recognize the warning signs of a flare can help the patient take steps to ward it off or reduce its intensity. Many people with lupus experience increased fatigue, pain, a rash, fever, abdominal discomfort, headache, or dizziness just before a flare. Developing strategies to prevent flares can also be helpful, such as learning to recognize your warning signals and maintaining good communication with your doctor.

It is also important for people with lupus to receive regular health care, instead of seeking help only when symptoms worsen. Results from a medical exam and laboratory work on a regular basis allow the doctor to note any changes and to identify and treat flares early. The treatment plan, which is tailored to the individual's specific needs and circumstances, can be adjusted accordingly. If new symptoms are identified early, treatments may be more effective. Other concerns also can be addressed at regular checkups. The doctor can provide guidance about such issues as the use of sunscreens, stress reduction, and the importance of structured exercise and rest, as well as birth control and family planning. Because people with lupus can be more susceptible to infections, the doctor may recommend yearly influenza vaccinations or pneumococcal vaccinations for some patients.

Women with lupus should receive regular preventive health care, such as gynecological and breast examinations. Men with lupus should have the prostate-specific antigen (PSA) test. Both men and women need to have their blood pressure and cholesterol checked on a regular basis. If a person is taking corticosteroids or antimalarial medications, an eye exam should be done at least yearly to screen for and treat eye problems.

Staying healthy requires extra effort and care for people with lupus, so it becomes especially important to develop strategies for maintaining wellness. Wellness involves close attention to the body, mind, and spirit. One of the primary goals of wellness for people with lupus is coping with the stress of having a chronic disorder. Effective stress management varies from person to person. Some approaches that may help include exercise, relaxation techniques such as meditation, and setting priorities for spending time and energy.

Developing and maintaining a good support system is also important. A support system may include family, friends, medical professionals, community organizations, and support groups. Participating in a support group can provide emotional help, boost self-esteem and morale, and help develop or improve coping skills.

Learning more about lupus may also help. Studies have shown that patients who are well-informed and participate actively in their own care experience less pain, make fewer visits to the doctor, build self-confidence, and remain more active.

Tips for Working with Your Doctor

- Seek a health care provider who is familiar with SLE and who will listen to and address your concerns.
- Provide complete, accurate medical information.
- Make a list of your questions and concerns in advance.
- Be honest and share your point of view with the health care provider.
- Ask for clarification or further explanation if you need it.
- Talk to other members of the health care team, such as nurses, therapists, or pharmacists.
- Do not hesitate to discuss sensitive subjects (for example, birth control or intimacy) with your doctor.
- Discuss any treatment changes with your doctor before making them.

Pregnancy for Women with Lupus

Although a lupus pregnancy is considered high risk, most women with lupus carry their babies safely to the end of their pregnancy. Women with lupus have a higher rate of miscarriage and premature births compared with the general population. In addition, women who have antiphospholipid antibodies are at a greater risk of miscarriage in the second trimester because of their increased risk of blood clotting in the placenta. Lupus patients with a history of kidney disease have a higher risk of preeclampsia (hypertension with a buildup of excess watery fluid in cells or tissues of the body). Pregnancy counseling and planning before pregnancy are important. Ideally, a woman should have no signs or symptoms of lupus and be taking no medications for at least 6 months before she becomes pregnant.

Pregnancy counseling and planning before pregnancy are important. Some women may experience a mild to moderate flare during or after their pregnancy; others do not. Pregnant women with lupus, especially those taking corticosteroids, also are more likely to develop high blood pressure, diabetes, hyperglycemia (high blood sugar), and kidney complications, so regular care and good nutrition during pregnancy are essential. It is also advisable to have access to a neonatal (newborn) intensive care unit at the time of delivery in case the baby requires special medical attention.

Current Research

Lupus is the focus of intense research as scientists try to determine what causes the disease and how it can best be treated. Some of the questions they are working to answer include: Why are women more likely than men to have the disease? Why are there more cases of lupus in some racial and ethnic groups? What goes wrong in the immune system, and why? How can we correct the way the immune system functions once something goes wrong? What treatment approaches will work best to lessen lupus symptoms? How do we cure lupus?

To help answer these questions, scientists are developing new and better ways to study the disease. They are doing laboratory studies that compare various aspects of the immune systems of people with lupus with those of other people both with and without lupus. They also use mice with disorders resembling lupus to better understand the abnormalities of the immune system that occur in lupus and to identify possible new therapies.

The National Institute of Arthritis and Musculoskeletal and Skin Diseases (NIAMS), a component of the Department of Health and Human Services' National Institutes of Health (NIH), has a major focus on lupus research in its on campus program in Bethesda, Maryland. By evaluating patients with lupus and their relatives, researchers on campus are learning more about how lupus develops and changes over time. The NIAMS also funds many lupus researchers across the United States. Some of these researchers are studying the genetic factors that increase a person's risk for developing lupus. To help scientists gain new knowledge, the NIAMS also has established Specialized Centers of Research devoted specifically to lupus research. In addition, the NIAMS is funding lupus registries that gather medical information as well as blood and tissue samples from patients and their relatives. This gives researchers across the country access to information and materials they can use to help identify genes that determine susceptibility to the disease.

Identifying genes that play a role in the development of lupus is an active area of research. For example, researchers suspect that a genetic defect in a cellular process called apoptosis, or programmed cell death, exists in people with lupus. Apoptosis is similar to the process that causes leaves to turn color in autumn and fall from trees; it allows the body to eliminate cells that have fulfilled their function and typically need to be replaced. If there is a problem in the apoptosis process, harmful cells may stay around and do damage to the body's own tissues. For example, in a mutant mouse strain that develops a lupus-like illness, one of the genes that controls apoptosis is defective. When it is replaced by a normal gene, the mice no longer develop signs of the disease. Scientists are studying what role genes involved in apoptosis may play in human disease development.

Studying genes for complement, a series of proteins in the blood that play an important part in the immune system, is another active area of lupus research. Complement acts as a backup for antibodies, helping them destroy foreign substances that invade the body. If there is a decrease in complement, the body is less able to fight or destroy foreign substances. If these substances are not removed from the body, the immune system may become overactive and begin to make autoantibodies.

Recent large studies of families with lupus have identified a number of genetic regions that appear to be associated with risk of SLE. Although the specific genes and their function remain unknown, intensive work in mapping the entire human genome offers promise that these genes will be identified in the near future. This should provide knowledge of the complex factors that contribute to lupus susceptibility.

NIAMS-funded researchers are uncovering the impact of genetic, socioeconomic, and cultural factors on the course and outcome of lupus in Hispanics, African Americans, and Caucasians. Preliminary data show that African American and Hispanic lupus patients typically have more kidney damage compared with Caucasians. In addition, NIAMS-funded researchers found that African American lupus patients have more skin damage compared with Hispanics and Caucasians, and that the death rate from lupus is higher in African Americans and Hispanics compared with Caucasians.

It is thought that autoimmune diseases, such as lupus, occur when a genetically susceptible individual encounters an unknown environmental agent or trigger. In this circumstance, an abnormal immune response can be initiated that leads to the signs and symptoms of lupus. Research has focused on both the genetic susceptibility and the environmental trigger. Although the environmental trigger remains unknown, microbial agents such as Epstein-Barr virus and others have been considered.

Researchers also are studying other factors that may affect a person's susceptibility to lupus. For example, because lupus is more common in women than in men, some researchers are investigating the role of hormones and other male-female differences in the development and course of the disease. A current study funded by the NIH is focusing on the safety and effectiveness of oral contraceptives (birth control pills) and hormone replacement therapy in women with lupus. Doctors have worried about the wisdom of prescribing oral contraceptives or estrogen replacement therapy for women with lupus because of a widely held view that estrogens can make the disease worse. Oral contraceptives and estrogen replacement therapy do not, as once feared, appear to intensify lupus symptoms. Scientists do not know the effects of oral contraceptives on women with antiphospholipid antibody syndrome.

Patients with lupus are at risk of developing atherosclerotic vascular disease (hardening of the blood vessels that can cause heart attack, angina, or stroke). The increased risk is due partly to having lupus and partly to steroid therapy. Preventing atherosclerotic vascular disease in lupus patients is a new area of study. NIAMS-funded researchers are studying the most effective ways to manage cardiovascular risk factors and prevent cardiovascular disease in adult lupus patients.

In childhood lupus, researchers are evaluating the safety and effectiveness of drugs called statins that lower LDL (or bad) cholesterol levels as a method of preventing fat buildup in the blood vessels.

One out of five lupus patients experiences symptoms such as headaches, dizziness, memory disturbances, stroke, or changes in behavior that result from changes in the brain or other parts of the central nervous system. Such lupus patients have what is called neuropsychiatric lupus. NIAMS-funded scientists are applying new tools such as brain imaging techniques to discover cellular activity and specific genes that may cause neuropsychiatric lupus. By uncovering the mechanisms responsible for central nervous system damage in lupus patients, researchers hope to move closer to improved diagnosis and treatment for patients with neuropsychiatric lupus.

Researchers are focusing on finding better treatments for lupus. A primary goal of this research is to develop treatments that can effectively minimize the use of corticosteroids. Scientists are trying to identify combination therapies that may be more effective than single treatment approaches. Another goal is to improve the treatment and management of lupus in the kidneys and central nervous system. For example, a 20-year study supported by the NIAMS and the NIH found that combining cyclophosphamide with prednisone helped delay or prevent kidney failure, a serious complication of lupus.

On the basis of new information about the disease process, scientists are using novel biologic agents to selectively block parts of the immune system. Development and testing of these new drugs, which are based on compounds that occur naturally in the body, comprise an exciting and promising new area of lupus research. The hope is that these treatments not only will be effective, but also will have fewer side effects. Preliminary research suggests that white blood cells known as B cells may play a key role in the development of lupus. Biologics that interfere with B cell function or block the interactions of immune cells are active areas of research. These targeted treatments hold promise because they have the advantage of reduced side effects and adverse reactions compared with conventional therapies. Clinical trials are testing the safety and effectiveness of rituximab (also called anti-CD20) in treating people with lupus. Rituximab is a genetically engineered antibody that blocks the production of B cells. Other treatment options currently being explored include reconstructing the immune system by bone marrow transplantation. In the future, gene therapy also may play an important role in lupus treatment.

Hope for the Future

With research advances and a better understanding of lupus, the prognosis for people with lupus today is far brighter than it was even 20 years ago. It is possible to have lupus and remain active and involved with life, family, and work. As current research efforts unfold, there is continued hope for new treatments, improvements in quality of life, and, ultimately, a way to prevent or cure the disease. The research efforts of today may yield the answers of tomorrow, as scientists continue to unravel the mysteries of lupus.

Additional Resources

National Institute of Arthritis and Musculoskeletal and Skin Diseases
1 AMS Circle
Bethesda, MD 20892-3675
Toll-Free: (877) 22-NIAMS (226-4267); Phone: (301) 495-4484
TTY: (301) 565-2966; Fax: (301) 718-6366
Website: http://www.niams.nih.gov
E-mail: niamsinfo@mail.nih.gov

American College of Rheumatology
1800 Century Place, Suite 250
Atlanta, GA 30345-4300
Phone: (404) 633-3777
Fax: (404) 633-1870
Website: http://
www.rheumatology.org

Alliance for Lupus Research, Inc.
28 West 44th Street, Suite 1217
New York, NY 10036
Toll-Free: (800) 867-1743
Phone: (212) 218-2840
Website: http://
www.lupusresearch.org

American Autoimmune Related Diseases Association
22100 Gratiot Avenue
Eastpointe
East Detroit, MI 48021-2227
Toll-Free: (800) 598-4668
Phone: (586) 776-3900
Website: http://www.aarda.org
E-mail: aarda@aarda.org

Arthritis Foundation
1330 West Peachtree Street
Atlanta, GA 30309
Toll-Free: (800) 283-7800
Phone: (404) 872-7100
Website: http://www.arthritis.org
E-mail:
arthritis@finelinesolutions.com

Lupus Clinical Trials Consortium Inc. (LCTC)
47 Hulfish Street, Suite 442
Princeton, NJ 08540
Phone: (609) 921-1532

Lupus Foundation of America (LFA), Inc.
2000 L Street, N.W., Suite 710
Washington, DC 20036
Toll-Free: (800) 558-0121
Phone: (202) 349-1155
Website: http://www.lupus.org

Rheuminations, Inc.
221 East 48th Street,
Ground Floor
New York, NY 10017
Phone: (212) 593-5180
Fax: (212) 593-5181
Website: http://www.dxlupus.org

SLE Foundation, Inc.
149 Madison Avenue, Suite 205
New York, NY 10016
Phone: (212) 685-4118
Website: http://www.lupusny.org

Part Four

Management of Arthritis and Arthritis-Related Pain

Chapter 24

Arthritis: A Major Public Health Problem

What Is Arthritis?

Arthritis comprises over 100 different diseases and conditions. The most common are osteoarthritis, rheumatoid arthritis, fibromyalgia, and gout. Common symptoms include pain, aching, stiffness, and swelling in or around the joints. Some forms of arthritis, such as rheumatoid arthritis and lupus, can affect multiple organs and cause widespread symptoms.

Why Is Arthritis a Public Health Problem?

In 2001, 49 million American adults reported doctor-diagnosed arthritis and another 21 million reported chronic joint symptoms, making arthritis one of the nation's most common health problems. As the U.S. population ages, this number is likely to increase dramatically. For example, the number of people aged 65 or older who have arthritis or chronic joint symptoms is projected to nearly double from 2001 (21.4 million) to 2030 (41.4 million).

Arthritis limits everyday activities for 8 million Americans. Arthritis and the disability it causes create huge burdens for individuals, their families, and the nation. Each year, arthritis results in 750,000

"Targeting Arthritis: The Nation's Leading Cause of Disability," Centers for Disease Control and Prevention (CDC), 2004. Available online at http://www.cdc.gov; accessed March 2004.

hospitalizations and 36 million outpatient visits. In 1997, medical care for arthritis cost over $51 billion.

Arthritis is not just an old person's disease. Nearly two thirds of people with arthritis are younger than 65 years. Arthritis affects children and people of all racial and ethnic groups; however, it is more common among women and older Americans.

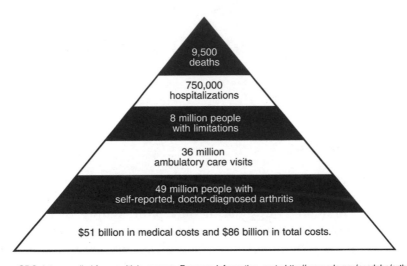

Source: CDC data compiled from multiple sources. For more information, go to http://www.cdc.gov/nccdphp/arthritis.

Figure 24.1. Arthritis in the United States

What Can Be Done to Target Arthritis?

Fortunately, there are effective ways not only to prevent arthritis, but also to reduce the symptoms, lessen the disability, and improve the quality of life for people with arthritis.

- Weight control and injury prevention measures can lower the risk for osteoarthritis.

- The pain and disability that accompany arthritis can be decreased through early diagnosis and appropriate management, including self-management activities such as weight control and physical activity.

- Self-management education programs are also effective in reducing both pain and costs. One successful program, the Arthritis Self-Help Course, disseminated by the Arthritis Foundation, teaches people how to manage their arthritis and lessen its effects. This 6-week course reduces arthritis pain by 20% and physician visits by 40%. Unfortunately, less than 1% of Americans with doctor-diagnosed arthritis participate in such programs, and courses are not offered in all areas of the country. More widespread use of the Arthritis Self-Help Course and similar programs could save money and reduce the burden of arthritis.

What Are CDC and Its Partners Doing about Arthritis?

The *National Arthritis Action Plan: A Public Health Strategy* was developed by CDC, the Arthritis Foundation, the Association of State and Territorial Health Officials, and 90 other organizations to address

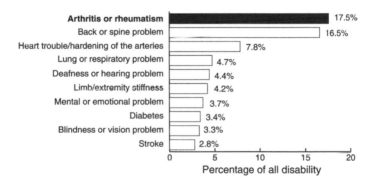

Figure 24.2. *Most Common Causes of Disability* among U.S. Adults, 1999. *In this analysis, people were considered to have a disability if they had difficulty with any one of a wide range of activities, such as lifting or carrying 10 pounds, climbing a flight of stairs without resting, walking three city blocks, getting in and out of bed, bathing, dressing, preparing meals, or doing light housework. In addition, people were considered to have a disability if they used a wheelchair, crutches, cane, or walker for more than 6 months; were limited in their ability to work at a job; or had any one of a number of other limitations. For the full definition of disability, see: CDC. Prevalence of disabilities and associated health conditions among adults—United States, 1999. MMWR 2001;50:120-5.*

the growing problem of arthritis. This landmark plan recommends a national coordinated effort to reduce pain and disability and improve the quality of life for people with arthritis. This plan forms the foundation of CDC's work in arthritis.

With nearly $15 million in fiscal year 2004 funding, CDC is working with the Arthritis Foundation and other partners to implement the *National Arthritis Action Plan* and is supporting activities in 36 states. By carrying out the goals of the action plan, CDC and its partners are also moving toward achieving the arthritis-related objectives in *Healthy People 2010,* a comprehensive, national agenda for promoting health and preventing disease.

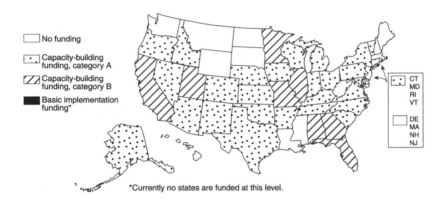

Figure 24.3. *CDC Funding for 36 State Arthritis Programs, Fiscal Year 2003*

What Activities Does CDC's Arthritis Program Support?

The primary goal of CDC's arthritis program is to increase the quality of life for people affected by arthritis. The program achieves this goal by supporting five key activities:

#1: Building state arthritis programs.

States use CDC funding to strengthen partnerships with state Arthritis Foundation chapters and others, increase public awareness, improve their ability to monitor the burden of arthritis, coordinate activities, and conduct interventions. The central aim is to let people know that something can be done to lessen the effects of arthritis and to increase the number of people who participate in arthritis self-help programs. CDC has the following levels of program funding:

- **Capacity building funding** (formerly known as establishment or core funding; up to $600,000). *Category A funding* (average level $140,000) allows states to begin building an arthritis program. States funded at this level have developed state arthritis action plans and are building programs and partnerships to reduce the burden of arthritis. In 2003, 28 states were funded at this level. *Category B funding* (average level $300,000) carries this process further and also allows states to conduct pilot projects to improve the quality of life for people with arthritis. Many states funded at this level have been able to make the Arthritis Self-Help Course and physical activity programs available to more people, especially in underserved areas. In 2003, eight states were funded at this level.

- **Basic implementation funding** (formerly known as comprehensive funding; $600,000 to $1,000,000) would allow states to further reduce the burden of arthritis by more broadly implementing evidence-based interventions. States could also work with additional partners to enhance arthritis activities. No states are funded at this level.

#2: *Reaching the public.*

CDC, working with state health departments and Arthritis Foundation chapters, has developed a campaign that promotes physical activity to relieve arthritis pain among people aged 45 to 64 in lower socioeconomic levels. Radio spots, brochures, and print pieces carry the theme "Physical Activity. The Arthritis Pain Reliever." Of the 36 CDC-funded states, 35 will implement the campaign as part of their efforts to reach populations with arthritis.

#3: *Improving the science base.*

CDC supports research to learn more about why arthritis occurs and progresses and how to deal with it, as these examples show:

- Hip and knee osteoarthritis, the primary causes of expensive joint replacement surgery, are becoming more common as the

303

population ages. CDC collaborated with the University of North Carolina and the National Institutes of Health to study these conditions among 3,200 residents of rural Johnson County, North Carolina. This study found that the prevalence and rate of progression of hip and knee osteoarthritis was higher among blacks than among whites.

- Self-management programs are integral to reducing pain and disability. To learn which approaches are most effective and how these programs can be improved, CDC is working with the Arthritis Foundation and several universities to evaluate programs. PACE® (People with Arthritis Can Exercise) is being evaluated at the University of Missouri and the University of North Carolina. The University of North Carolina is also evaluating the effectiveness of Active Living Every Day—a program designed to help people overcome barriers to physical activity—for increasing physical activity among people with arthritis.

#4: Measuring the burden of arthritis.

CDC's Behavioral Risk Factor Surveillance System, which all 50 states use to collect health information from adults, is the main source of state arthritis data. These data are used to monitor trends, define the burden of arthritis, and assess how arthritis affects quality of life. CDC is also developing a survey to collect national data on the effects of arthritis on the daily activities and mental health of people with arthritis and on their knowledge, attitudes, and behaviors related to arthritis self-management.

#5: Making policy and systems changes.

CDC and its partners are making the policy and systems changes recommended in the *National Arthritis Action Plan*. For example, CDC is working with the Group Health Cooperative of Puget Sound to pilot test strategies to integrate self-management support into routine medical care.

Future Directions

With funded states and other partners, CDC hopes to:

- Create a nationwide program to improve the quality of life for people affected by arthritis.

- Help state arthritis programs reach more people.

- Develop and evaluate culturally appropriate programs to better serve diverse communities.

- Fund evaluation efforts to deliver effective arthritis programs.

- Develop health communications programs to increase physical activity among minority communities, the elderly, and people of low socioeconomic status.

Chapter 25

Arthritis Health Care Providers

Chapter Contents

Section 25.1

Introducing Your Arthritis Health Care Team

Excerpted from *Managing Your Health Care*. ©2001. Reprinted with permission of the Arthritis Foundation, 1330 W. Peachtree St., Suite 100, Atlanta, GA 30309. To order a free copy of this brochure or other titles from the Arthritis Foundation, call 800-283-7800 or visit www.arthritis.org.

Introduction

Arthritis causes pain, stiffness and sometimes swelling in or around joints. Its symptoms can make it difficult to move and do daily tasks, but that doesn't mean nothing can be done about it. In fact, much can be done to help treat arthritis, both by your health-care team and you. You play the most important role in the management of your condition. By learning all you can about the various medications, treatments and Arthritis Foundation-related services, you can learn to become a self-manager and take steps to reduce pain and keep moving.

Who Makes up Your Health Care Team?

Many health professionals may be involved in your care, depending on your condition and their availability in your area. The following health-care professionals may play a role in your treatment.

Doctors

Family physicians, general practitioners and primary-care physicians provide medical care for adults and children with different types of arthritis. These doctors also can help you find a specialist, if necessary.

Internists specialize in internal medicine and in treating adult diseases. They provide general care to adults and often help select specialists. Internists should not be confused with interns, who are doctors doing a year's training in a hospital after graduating from medical school.

Pediatricians provide medical care for children from birth to adolescence.

308

Rheumatologists specialize in treating people with arthritis or related diseases that affect the joints, muscles, bones, skin and other tissues. You may be referred to a rheumatologist if you need special care or treatment. Most rheumatologists are internists who have had further training in the care of people with arthritis and related diseases. Some rheumatologists also have pediatrics training.

Pediatric rheumatologists specialize in treating children through adolescence with arthritis or related diseases that affect the joints, muscles, bones, skin and other tissues.

Orthopaedic surgeons specialize in the treatment of musculoskeletal conditions and may be consulted to perform certain surgical procedures if your joints are damaged.

Ophthalmologists (opf-THAL-mall-o-gists) provide eye care and treatment.

Physiatrists (fiz-ee-AT-rists) may direct your physical therapy and rehabilitation.

Podiatrists are experts in foot care. If arthritis affects your feet, a podiatrist can prescribe special supports and shoes for you. Podiatrists may also perform surgery to correct foot deformities.

Psychiatrists give you the tools necessary for managing emotional and mental distress related to your disease. They are physicians and can prescribe medication.

Forming a Partnership with Your Health-Care Team

Some people see their family physician only once or twice a year—perhaps for an annual checkup or to receive treatment for an acute (sudden, but usually short-lived) condition. Most people with acute conditions carefully follow their doctor's recommendations for treatment. Their condition clears up and there is no need to make a follow-up appointment.

Other people must see their family physician more often because they have a chronic (long-lasting) medical condition such as arthritis. People who are newly diagnosed with arthritis often must see their doctor several times and try different medications and treatments before they find one that suits them.

Unlike someone seeking treatment for an acute condition, you probably will need to see members of your health-care team on an ongoing basis. It's to your advantage to have a good relationship with them, because by helping them, you help yourself. By working as partners, you and your health-care team can increase your chances of getting the maximum benefits from your treatment program.

Section 25.2

What Is a Rheumatologist?

A rheumatologist is an internist or pediatrician who is qualified by additional training and experience in the diagnosis and treatment of arthritis and other diseases of the joints, muscles, and bones. Many rheumatologists conduct research to determine the cause and better treatments for these disabling and sometimes fatal diseases.

What Kind of Training Do Rheumatologists Have?

After four years of medical school and three years of training in either internal medicine or pediatrics, rheumatologists devote an additional two to three years in specialized rheumatology training. Most rheumatologists who plan to treat patients choose to become board certified. Upon completion of their training, they must pass a rigorous exam conducted by the American Board of Internal Medicine to become certified.

What Do Rheumatologists Treat?

Rheumatologists treat arthritis, certain autoimmune diseases, musculoskeletal pain disorders, and osteoporosis. There are more than 100 types of these diseases, including rheumatoid arthritis, osteoarthritis, gout, lupus, back pain, osteoporosis, fibromyalgia, and tendonitis. Some of these are very serious diseases that can be difficult to diagnose and treat.

When Should You See a Rheumatologist?

If musculoskeletal pains are not severe or disabling and last just a few days, it makes sense to give the problem a reasonable chance to be resolved. But sometimes, pain in the joints, muscles, or bones is severe or persists for more than a few days. At that point, you should see your physician.

Many types of rheumatic diseases are not easily identified in the early stages. Rheumatologists are specially trained to do the detective work necessary to discover the cause of swelling and pain. It's important to determine a correct diagnosis early so that appropriate treatment can begin early. Some musculoskeletal disorders respond best to treatment in the early stages of the disease.

Because some rheumatic diseases are complex, one visit to a rheumatologist may not be enough to determine a diagnosis and course of treatment. These diseases often change or evolve over time. Rheumatologists work closely with patients to identify the problem and design an individualized treatment program.

How Does the Rheumatologist Work with Other Health Care Professionals?

The role the rheumatologist plays in health care depends on several factors and needs. Typically the rheumatologist works with other physicians, sometimes acting as a consultant to advise another physician about a specific diagnosis and treatment plan. In other situations, the rheumatologist acts as a manager, relying upon the help of many skilled professionals including nurses, physical and occupational therapists, psychologists, and social workers. Team work is important, since musculoskeletal disorders are chronic. Health care professionals can help people with musculoskeletal diseases and their families cope with the changes the diseases cause in their lives.

Is Specialty Care More Expensive?

You may be surprised to learn that specialized care may save time and money and reduce the severity of disease. A rheumatologist is specially trained to spot clues in the medical history and physical examination. The proper tests done early may save money in the long run. Prompt diagnosis and specially tailored treatment often save money and buy time in treating the disease.

For More Information

To find a rheumatologist in your area, check the American College of Rheumatology's directory at http://www.rheumatology.org/directory/geo.asp. For more information on this or any other form of arthritis, contact the Arthritis Foundation at (800) 283-7800 or visit the Arthritis Foundation website at www.arthritis.org.

Chapter 26

Medical Tests That Aid in Arthritis Diagnosis

Chapter Contents

Section 26.1

Blood Tests for Arthritis

"Blood Tests," ©2003 The Cleveland Clinic Foundation, 9500 Euclid Avenue, Cleveland, OH 44195, 800-223-2273 ext. 48950, www.clevelandclinic .org. Additional information is available from the Cleveland Clinic Health Information Center, 216-444-3771, or www.clevelandclinic.org/health.

Patients with arthritis will probably have blood tests as part of their initial evaluation and follow-up care. This is because blood is the most easily and safely sampled body tissue and contains traces of material from every other part of the body. The most common blood tests used to assist in the diagnosis and management of arthritis include:

Complete Blood Count (CBC)

The complete blood count is a series of blood tests that provides information about the components of blood including red blood cells, white blood cells, and platelets. Automated machines rapidly count the cell types. The CBC test results can help diagnose diseases and determine their severity.

Under normal conditions, the white blood cell count is between 5,000 to 10,000. A high white blood cell count could suggest inflammation, which can be due to rheumatoid arthritis (RA). However, infections, stress, exercise and cold will temporarily elevate the white blood cell count, too.

A CBC also measures hemoglobin, the iron-containing component of red cells that carries oxygen. The hematocrit is the percent of total blood volume that is made up of red cells. Normal value for males is 40–55 percent, and 36–48 percent for females. A lower hematocrit can be caused by a number of factors or conditions including rheumatoid arthritis or anemia.

Erythrocyte Sedimentation Rate (ESR)

The erythrocyte sedimentation rate is a test that involves placing a blood sample in a tube and determining how far the red blood cells settle in one hour. When there is inflammation in the body, it produces proteins in the blood which make the red cells clump together, causing them to fall faster than the healthy blood cells. Since inflammation can be caused by conditions other than arthritis, the ESR test alone is not diagnostic of arthritis.

Rheumatoid Factor (RF)

Rheumatoid factor is an antibody found in many patients with rheumatoid arthritis. It is one of several criteria used in diagnosing RA, as 80 percent of RA patients have RF in their blood. RF can take many months to show up in a patient's blood, and if tested for too early in the course of the disease the test could be negative. This may lead to the need for retesting at a later date. An RF test can be positive in response to other inflammatory or infectious diseases other than RA.

Antinuclear Antibody (ANA)

Patients with certain rheumatic diseases, such as lupus and RA, make antibodies that are directed at the nucleus of the body's cells. These antibodies, known as antinuclear antibodies, are detected by viewing the patient's blood serum (clear liquid separated from the blood) under a microscope. A substance containing fluorescent dye that causes the antibodies to bind is then added to the serum. This allows the abnormal antibodies to be seen binding to the nuclei. Over 95 percent of patients with lupus have a positive ANA test. Fifty percent of RA patients are positive for ANA. However, patients with other diseases also can have positive ANA test results, and even perfectly healthy people can have positive ANA test results, so other tests must be completed before a definitive diagnosis can be given.

Section 26.2

Other Tests Used to Diagnose Arthritis

Excerpted from "Questions and Answers about Arthritis and Rheumatic Diseases," National Institute of Arthritis and Musculoskeletal and Skin Diseases (NIAMS), February 2002. Available online at http://www.niams .nih.gov; accessed December 2003.

How Are Rheumatic Diseases Diagnosed?

Diagnosing rheumatic diseases can be difficult because some symptoms and signs are common to many different diseases. A general practitioner or family doctor may be able to evaluate a patient or refer him or her to a rheumatologist (a doctor who specializes in treating arthritis and other rheumatic diseases).

The doctor will review the patient's medical history, conduct a physical examination, and obtain laboratory tests and x-rays or other imaging tests. The doctor may need to see the patient more than once to make an accurate diagnosis.

Medical History

It is vital for people with joint pain to give the doctor a complete medical history. Answers to the following questions will help the doctor make an accurate diagnosis:

- Is the pain in one or more joints?
- When does the pain occur?
- How long does the pain last?
- When did you first notice the pain?
- What were you doing when you first noticed the pain?
- Does activity make the pain better or worse?
- Have you had any illnesses or accidents that may account for the pain?
- Is there a family history of any arthritis or other rheumatic disease?

- What medicine(s) are you taking?

Because rheumatic diseases are so diverse and sometimes involve several parts of the body, the doctor may ask many other questions. It may be helpful for people to keep a daily journal that describes the pain. Patients should write down what the affected joint looks like, how it feels, how long the pain lasts, and what they were doing when the pain started.

Physical Examination and Laboratory Tests

The doctor will examine the patient's joints for redness, warmth, damage, ease of movement, and tenderness. Because some forms of arthritis, such as lupus, may affect other organs, a complete physical examination that includes the heart, lungs, abdomen, nervous system, eyes, ears, and throat may be necessary. The doctor may order some laboratory tests to help confirm a diagnosis. Samples of blood, urine, or synovial fluid (lubricating fluid found in the joint) may be needed for the tests.

Common laboratory tests and procedures include the following:

Antinuclear antibody (ANA)—This test checks blood levels of antibodies that are often present in people who have connective tissue diseases or other autoimmune disorders, such as lupus. Since the antibodies react with material in the cell's nucleus (control center), they are referred to as antinuclear antibodies. There are also tests for individual types of ANAs that may be more specific to people with certain autoimmune disorders. ANAs are also sometimes found in people who do not have an autoimmune disorder. Therefore, having ANAs in the blood does not necessarily mean that a person has a disease.

C-reactive protein test—This is a nonspecific test used to detect generalized inflammation. Levels of the protein are often increased in patients with active disease such as rheumatoid arthritis, and may decline when corticosteroids or nonsteroidal anti-inflammatory drugs (NSAIDs) are used to reduce inflammation.

Complement—This test measures the level of complement, a group of proteins in the blood. Complement helps destroy foreign substances, such as germs, that enter the body. A low blood level of complement is common in people who have active lupus.

Complete blood count (CBC)—This test determines the number of white blood cells, red blood cells, and platelets present in a

317

sample of blood. Some rheumatic conditions or drugs used to treat arthritis are associated with a low white blood count (leukopenia), low red blood count (anemia), or low platelet count (thrombocytopenia). When doctors prescribe medications that affect the CBC, they periodically test the patient's blood.

Creatinine—This blood test is commonly ordered in patients who have a rheumatic disease, such as lupus, to monitor for underlying kidney disease. Creatinine is a breakdown product of creatine, which is an important component of muscle. It is excreted from the body entirely by the kidneys, and the level remains constant and normal when kidney function is normal.

Erythrocyte sedimentation rate (sed rate)—This blood test is used to detect inflammation in the body. Higher sed rates indicate the presence of inflammation and are typical of many forms of arthritis, such as rheumatoid arthritis and ankylosing spondylitis, and many of the connective tissue diseases.

Hematocrit (PCV, packed cell volume)—This test and the test for hemoglobin (a substance in the red blood cells that carries oxygen throughout the body) measure the number of red blood cells present in a sample of blood. A decrease in the number of red blood cells (anemia) is common in people who have inflammatory arthritis or another rheumatic disease.

Rheumatoid factor—This test detects the presence of rheumatoid factor, an antibody found in the blood of most (but not all) people who have rheumatoid arthritis. Rheumatoid factor may be found in many diseases besides rheumatoid arthritis, and sometimes in people without health problems.

Synovial fluid examination—Synovial fluid may be examined for white blood cells (found in patients with rheumatoid arthritis and infections), bacteria or viruses (found in patients with infectious arthritis), or crystals in the joint (found in patients with gout or other types of crystal-induced arthritis). To obtain a specimen, the doctor injects a local anesthetic, then inserts a needle into the joint to withdraw the synovial fluid into a syringe. The procedure is called arthrocentesis or joint aspiration.

Urinalysis—In this test, a urine sample is studied for protein, red blood cells, white blood cells, and bacteria. These abnormalities may indicate kidney disease, which may be seen in several rheumatic diseases, including lupus. Some medications used to treat arthritis can also cause abnormal findings on urinalysis.

White blood cell count (WBC)—This test determines the number of white blood cells present in a sample of blood. The number may increase as a result of infection or decrease in response to certain medications or in certain diseases, such as lupus. Low numbers of white blood cells increase a person's risk of infections.

X-Rays and Other Imaging Procedures

To see what the joint looks like inside, the doctor may order x-rays or other imaging procedures. X-rays provide an image of the bones, but they do not show cartilage, muscles, and ligaments. Other noninvasive imaging methods such as computed tomography (CT or CAT scan), magnetic resonance imaging (MRI), and arthrography show the whole joint. The doctor may look for damage to a joint by using an arthroscope, a small, flexible tube which is inserted through a small incision at the joint and which transmits the image of the inside of a joint to a video screen.

Chapter 27

Understanding the Diagnosis of Arthritis

Chapter Contents

Section 27.1

Now You Have a Diagnosis: What Is Next?

"Now You Have a Diagnosis: What's Next? Using Healthcare Information to Help Make Treatment Decisions." Agency for Healthcare Research and Quality and the Kanter Family Foundation, Rockville, MD. December 1999. Reviewed by David A. Cooke, M.D., on November 27, 2003.

If you were recently diagnosed with a serious illness or chronic condition, what would you do?

This resource will help you to use research and other information to make the best treatment decisions for you.

Using Healthcare Information to Help Make Treatment Decisions

It may have taken you only a visit or two to your doctor or other healthcare provider to find out what's causing your health problem. It may have taken longer. But now you have a diagnosis, and it's time to make some decisions about your treatment.

For many conditions, there is no one right treatment. You may have several options—each with its up sides and down sides. Some of your options may have been proven by healthcare research to be effective, whereas others may not.

In the future, your doctor or other healthcare provider may be able to tap into a nationwide database containing the results of treatments for thousands of people like you with your condition. This would help you and your doctor make a good decision about the treatment that would be right for you.

Initial efforts to develop this national database are under way, but until that database is available, there are still things you can do to make sure you get the best health care possible—right now.

Finding out more about your condition is a good place to start. By contacting groups that support your condition, visiting your local library, and searching on the Internet, you can find good information to help guide your treatment decisions. Some information may be hard to find—especially if you don't know where to look. This information has been created to point you in the right direction.

Healthcare Quality Can Vary

Many things can affect the quality of your healthcare, depending on your doctor or other healthcare provider, your health plan, your hospital, and where you live.

Online Resource: Healthcare Quality is an Internet site sponsored by the Federal Government's Quality Interagency Coordination Task Force. This site explains what quality healthcare is, why it matters, and how you can get it.
Go to: http://www.consumer.gov/qualityhealth.

Finding Reliable Information

Books, newspapers, magazines, television and radio programs, and the Internet offer access to a lot of health-related information. However, not all information is good information.

You can begin your search and figure out what's good information and what's not by following these three steps:

- Contact a group that advocates for your condition
- Visit your local library
- Get on the Internet

Contact a Group That Advocates for Your Condition

Groups such as the American Heart Association, the American Cancer Society, and the American Diabetes Association will probably have a local chapter in your community. These organizations can be a valuable source of information and support.

How to find them: If you can't find them in the phone book, most libraries have directories that provide phone numbers and Internet addresses for their national headquarters.

The National Health Information Center (NHIC) offers a toll-free telephone referral service to help people get in touch with organizations and resources that can provide information about specific conditions and illnesses. Visit their website at http://www.health.gov/nhic.

Visit Your Local Library

At the library you can find:

- Medical texts and reference books
- Consumer health books
- Newspapers and magazines
- Medical and healthcare journals

You can ask reference librarians for help with your search. They may know about resources that would be unfamiliar to you.

Get on the Internet

Another way is to search for information on the Internet. If you don't have your own computer, many libraries provide access to the Internet through their computers. Ask your librarian if this is available to you and don't hesitate to ask for help if how to get online isn't clear.

Here are some ways to get good information on the Internet:

- Start at a site that focuses on health
- Look for a name you can trust
- Look at the latest and best studies
- Exercise caution

Start at a Site That Focuses on Health. There are many sites that focus on health information on the Internet. Some are commercial sites; others are sponsored by universities or the Federal Government. Using a site that is devoted to health information is an easy way to get going.

Online Resource: The healthfinder® site is a good place to start. Sponsored by the U.S. Department of Health and Human Services, it offers links to hundreds of sites that contain reliable healthcare information.

Go to: http://www.healthfinder.gov.

Look for a Name You Can Trust. Besides government-sponsored sites, many medical schools and university medical centers have consumer health education sites that contain a wide range of information. The information in these sites is most likely to be science-based and reputable.

Look at the Latest and Best Studies. You might find clues or pieces of information in articles from medical journals. Although these articles are written in medical language, sites that direct you to summaries of the articles can be helpful.

Online Resource: The National Library of Medicine offers a free online catalog of medical journal articles and article abstracts called MEDLINEplus® that provides current information on specific diseases and conditions.

Go to: http://www.nlm.nih.gov/medlineplus.

Exercise Caution. Genuine medical miracles are few and far between. Beware of any drugs or treatments that make big claims. Not all information is objective and honest. If you are not sure about any treatment you find discussed on the Internet, ask your doctor or other healthcare provider about it.

Online Resource: Virtual Treatments Can Be Real-World Deceptions, from the Federal Trade Commission (FTC), offers a list of words and key phrases to be on the lookout for. These words and phrases could indicate phony, exaggerated, or unproven claims on Internet health sites.

Go to: http://www.ftc.gov/bcp/conline/pubs/alerts/mrclalrt.htm.

Understanding Different Types of Healthcare Research

Healthcare research plays a critical role in providing up-to-date information on what works, and what doesn't work, in treating many different kinds of diseases and conditions. This information helps improve healthcare quality by making sure that:

- You receive the right treatment, at the right time, and in the right way.

- You don't receive treatments that are unnecessary, costly, or even harmful to your health.

- You may hear about the results of healthcare research—perhaps even studies about your condition—on the news, or read about it in a newspaper or magazine. That's because scientists are constantly involved in a variety of research projects supported by the federal government, charitable foundations, and other public- and private-sector groups.

Main Types of Research Studies

There are four main types of studies that researchers conduct about health conditions:

- Laboratory experiments
- Clinical trials
- Epidemiological research
- Outcomes research

Laboratory Experiments. Laboratory experiments are done to find out the cause of a disease, or how a drug or treatment works. They are usually carried out on cells or tissue, or on laboratory animals.

Clinical Trials. Clinical trials use different study methods to make sure the results they get are true and not due to outside influences. People are randomly assigned to different treatment groups—some get the research treatment, others get a standard treatment or may be given a placebo or no treatment. The groups are monitored, and results are compared to evaluate whether the treatment works.

Epidemiological Research. Epidemiological research looks at:

- The natural course of diseases in a particular group of people.
- Relationships between people and their health habits, lifestyles, and environment.
- Risk factors for certain diseases.

Example: Data shows that people who smoke have a higher risk of developing lung cancer.

Outcomes Research. Outcomes research uses a wide variety of information about how well treatments work in the real world. Outcomes research can tell whether treatments work better for certain types of patients or in specific situations. Then, recommendations can be made about treatments based on whether they work or not, and which ones are most likely to give the best results with the fewest risks. This is known as evidence-based medicine.

Sometimes these recommendations are gathered together in clinical practice guidelines. Doctors and other healthcare providers can use this kind of information to help you weigh the risks and benefits of your treatment options.

Making Your Decision

Once you have found out as much as you can about your diagnosis—and perhaps, sought out a second opinion—it's time to talk to your doctor or other healthcare provider about the information you have gathered. You may want to create a list of questions to ask.

Online Resource: Your Guide to Choosing Quality Healthcare: Choosing Treatments, from the Agency for Health Care Policy and Research, offers some sample questions to get you going.
Go to: http://www.ahrq.gov/consumer/qntool.htm.

Now is the time to start making decisions with your doctor or other healthcare provider about how to treat or manage your condition. Find out how you can make the right decision:

- Check out your options
- Look at the benefits and risks of each treatment
- Develop a treatment plan with your doctor

Check out Your Options

Evidence-based medicine, in the form of clinical practice guidelines, can help you and your doctor or other healthcare provider decide what would be the best treatment for you. Selecting the best treatment is a decision that depends on the following:

- What research shows has worked or hasn't worked for your particular condition.
- How you feel about the different treatments.

Online Resource: The National Guideline Clearinghouse offers hundreds of evidence-based clinical practice guidelines for treating the most common medical conditions.
Go to: http://www.guideline.gov.

Look at the Benefits and Risks of Each Treatment

Every treatment has benefits and risks. There are tradeoffs to be made—and they all depend on what you determine is best for you, both medically and psychologically. How do you decide which treatment is best for you? What matters is what matters most to you.

Example: If you are an older man with a prostate problem that makes it hard to urinate, there are a number of treatments a doctor or other healthcare provider can recommend. Surgery is one option; medicine is another.

Online Resource: Your Guide to Choosing Quality Health Care: Choosing Treatments, from the Agency for Health Care Policy and Research, gives good advice on how to make a treatment decision.

Go to: http://www.ahrq.gov/consumer/qntool.htm.

Develop a Treatment Plan with Your Doctor

Once you and your doctor or other healthcare provider have decided on a treatment, you can work together to develop a treatment plan—one you know you can stick to. Studies have shown that people who take an active role in developing their treatment plan have a better chance of staying on course and feel more satisfied with their care.

How to Make the Visit Work: You may want to prepare a list of questions before your visit, and then write down the answers you receive during your visit. Or, you might consider bringing along a friend or a family member with you. That way, if you have difficulty remembering everything that your doctor or other healthcare provider tells you, you can refer to your notes or ask your companion. If you have information that you have found on the Internet, bring it with you and ask your doctor or other healthcare provider to discuss it with you.

Getting Support

Sometimes the emotional side of illness is just as hard to deal with as the physical side. You may have fears and concerns or feel overwhelmed by your situation. Everyone has different ways of dealing with these feelings. Your attitude about your condition, your expectations, and how well you cope with your condition can play a big part in the success of your treatment.

Find out about the resources for support that are available to you:

- Ask family and friends for help
- Talk to a counselor
- Join a support group
- Use online support services

Ask Family and Friends for Help

In general, having close and supportive ties with friends and family seems to have a positive impact on health. The people you're closest to are the most likely to give you the support you need. Even so, you may have trouble asking for help.

How to ask for help: If you do have trouble asking for help, think about specific ways in which people can help, and start by asking one person to assist you with the easiest thing on the list. You may be surprised at how glad people are to help.

Talk to a Counselor

A good counselor can help you cope with sadness, depression, and feelings of being overwhelmed. If you think counseling might be right for you, ask your doctor or other healthcare provider to recommend someone in your area.

Join a Support Group

Healthcare research has shown that support groups—groups of people with the same condition who get together on a regular basis to discuss their illness—often help people cope better with their condition.

Example: A study looking at women breast cancer survivors revealed that the women who participated in a support group lived longer and had a better quality of life than similar women who did not participate in the group. The women in the support group learned coping skills and they shared their feelings with other women who were in the same situation.

If you are interested in a support group, ask your doctor or other healthcare provider about available groups for your condition. If there is a fee for your group, you might want to check with your health plan to see if the cost will be covered.

Churches and synagogues, and other houses of worship, as well as senior centers, might also have groups that could offer you the social support you need. Ask your friends or family members if they know of any.

Use Online Support Services

Commercial Internet service providers offer forums and chat rooms for people with different illnesses and conditions. Other Internet sites may also offer similar types of online groups. These online self-help communities can help you connect with a network of people whose concerns are similar to yours.

Caution: Online support groups are places where people talk informally. All the treatments or discoveries you hear about may not be scientifically proven to be safe and effective. If you read about something interesting and new, check it out with your doctor or other healthcare provider. The more you know, the better you will be able to cope with your condition on a day-to-day basis.

Online Resource: The National Health Council has a list of Internet links to patient-based groups, or voluntary agencies, for more than 40 different chronic diseases and/or disabilities.

Go to: http://www.nationalhealthcouncil.org/aboutus/membership .htm.

Section 27.2

How to Find Medical Info

National Institute of Arthritis and Musculoskeletal and Skin Diseases (NIAMS), April 2001. Available online at http://www.niams.nih.gov; accessed March 2004.

Searching for medical information can be confusing, especially for first-timers. However, if you are patient and stick to it, you can find a wealth of information. Today's computer technology is making it easier than ever for people to track down medical and health information. There are also many other sources of medical information available in textbooks, journal articles, and reference books and from health care organizations. This chapter explains how to locate these important sources of information.

Where to find medical information:

- Community library
- Federal Government clearinghouses
- Associations and voluntary organizations

- Medical, hospital, or university libraries
- Personal physician
- Nurse, pharmacist, dietitian, or other health professional
- Telephone or fax services
- Computer databases
- Internet

Start with Your Community Library

Most people have a library in or near their community, and it's a good place to start to look for medical information. Before going to the library, you may find it helpful to make a list of topics you want information about and questions you have. Also, if you've received a National Institute of Arthritis and Musculoskeletal and Skin Diseases (NIAMS) information package, you'll notice the list of additional references at the end of most articles. You may want to get a copy of some of these articles. Your topic list and the information package will make it easier for the librarian to direct you to the best resources.

Basic Medical References

Many community libraries have a collection of basic medical references. These references may include medical dictionaries or encyclopedias, drug information handbooks, basic medical and nursing textbooks, and directories of physicians and medical specialists (listings of doctors). You may also wish to find magazine articles on a certain topic. Look in the *Reader's Guide to Periodical Literature* for articles on health and medicine that were published in consumer magazines.

Other Resources

Infotrac, a CD-ROM computer database available at libraries or on the Web, indexes hundreds of popular magazines and newspapers, as well as some medical journals such as the *Journal of the American Medical Association* and *New England Journal of Medicine.* Your library may also carry MEDLINE® (http://www.ncbi.nlm.nih.gov/entrez/query.fcgi), *Index Medicus,* or the *Cumulative Index to Nursing and Allied Health Literature* in print format or on a computer database. The *Consumer Health and Nutrition Index* may be available in print form as well. These resources will help you find journal articles written for health professionals. Many of the indexes have abstracts that provide a summary of each journal article. Articles published in medical journals can be technical, but they may be the most current source of information on medical topics.

Interlibrary Loans

Although most community libraries don't have a large collection of medical and nursing journals, your librarian may be able to get copies of the articles you want. Interlibrary loans allow your librarian to request a copy of an article from a library that carries that particular medical journal. Your library may charge a fee for this service.

Medical and Health Directories

You may find many useful medical and health information directories at your library. Ask your librarian about the following resources:

- *Directory of Physicians in the United States.* Chicago, IL: American Medical Association (AMA) updated yearly—provides information such as address, medical school attended, year of license, specialty, and certifications for physicians who are members of the AMA.

- *Health Hotlines*—a booklet of toll-free numbers of health information hotlines available from the National Library of Medicine (NLM) or on the Internet at sis.nlm.nih.gov/hotlines.

- *Medical and Health Information Directory.* 13th edition. Detroit, MI: Gale Research, 2001—includes publications, organizations, libraries, and health services (three volumes).

- *The Official ABMS Directory of Board Certified Medical Specialists.* New Providence, NJ: Marquis Who's Who, updated yearly—provides information on physicians certified in various specialties by the American Board of Medical Specialists.

- Rees, A., editor. *The Consumer Health Information Sourcebook.* 6th edition. Phoenix, AZ: Oryx Press, 2000—lists information clearinghouses, books, and other resources.

- White, B.J., & Madone, E., editors. *The Self-Help Sourcebook: The Comprehensive Reference of Self-Help Group Resources.* 5th edition. Denville, NJ: Northwest Covenant Medical Center, 1997—lists over 700 organizations that offer support groups.

If you find a particularly useful book at the library, you can buy a copy at your local bookstore. If the book isn't in stock, your bookstore can probably order a copy for you.

Some medical references have been converted from book form to a CD-ROM or disk for use on a personal computer. If you have a computer with a CD-ROM drive, color monitor, and sound card, you can use compact disks to locate medical information. Check with your local bookstore or computer store for software programs that contain health information.

Some Popular References for the Home Library

- *American Medical Association Complete Guide to Women's Health.* 1996; and American Medical Association Family Medical Guide. 3rd edition. 1994. New York, NY: Random House (available in book and CD-ROM format).

- *The Columbia University College of Physicians and Surgeons Complete Home Medical Guide.* 3rd edition. New York, NY: Crown Publishers, 1995.

- *Everything You Need to Know About Medical Tests.* Springhouse, PA: Springhouse Corporation, 1997.

- *Johns Hopkins Symptoms and Remedies: The Complete Home Medical Reference.* New York: Rebus Publishing, 1999.

- *Mayo Clinic Family Health.* 2nd edition. New York, NY: William Morrow, Inc., 1996 (available as a book, CD-ROM, or computer disk).

- *The Merck Manual of Medical Information (Home Edition).* Rahway, NJ: The Merck Publishing Group, 1997.

- *Professional Guide to Disease.* 7th edition. Springhouse, PA: Springhouse Corporation, 2001.

Take Advantage of Services Provided by the Federal Government and Other Organizations

Federal Government

The Federal Government operates a number of clearinghouses and information centers—the NIAMS Information Clearinghouse is one of them. Services vary but may include publications, referrals, and answers to consumer inquiries. To obtain a free list of Federal information clearinghouses, visit the National Health Information Center's home page (www.health.gov/nhic), write to P.O. Box 1133, Washington, DC 20013-1133, or call (800) 336-4797.

Associations and Voluntary Organizations

Many associations and voluntary organizations are excellent sources of information. Some are devoted to specific diseases or conditions, such as the Scleroderma Foundation, National Alopecia Areata Foundation, National Psoriasis Foundation, and numerous others. Other organizations, such as the American Association of Retired Persons, serve a particular population group and provide a variety of information, including health-related topics. Your librarian or a NIAMS Information Clearinghouse information specialist can help you locate appropriate organizations and support networks. Many of these organizations offer referrals, publications, newsletters, educational programs, and local support groups. Your doctor may be able to tell you about support groups in your community as well.

Examples of health-related associations and organizations:

- American Academy of Dermatology
- American Academy of Orthopaedic Surgeons
- American College of Rheumatology
- American Skin Association
- Arthritis Foundation
- Lupus Foundation of America
- American Physical Therapy Association

There are many more organizations; call the NIAMS Information Clearinghouse for additional information.

Look for a Medical Library

Medical libraries can usually be found at medical, nursing, and dental schools; large medical centers; and community hospitals. Not all hospital or academic libraries are open to the public, but a librarian at your community library may be able to give you information about the closest medical library open to the public. Medical libraries may also be listed in your telephone book under "hospitals," "schools," or "universities." In addition, you can call the National Network of Libraries of Medicine of the NLM, National Institutes of Health, at (800) 338-7657 to find the location of the nearest medical library open to the public.

A medical library has a large collection of resources, including many medical and nursing textbooks and a comprehensive collection of medical and health-related journals. Although you may not be allowed to check out materials, most libraries have photocopiers you can use to copy material you want to take home.

Library resources include:

- Computer databases
- Directories of board-certified medical specialists
- Drug reference books
- Medical and diagnostic laboratory testing manuals
- Medical and health information directories
- Medical dictionaries
- Medical encyclopedias
- Medical, nursing, and allied health textbooks

Investigate Other Options for Finding Information

People who are unable to get to a community or medical library have several options for finding additional medical information. Some community libraries provide access to online databases that can be searched from a home computer via a modem. In addition, your doctor, nurse, pharmacist, dietitian, or the patient education department at your local hospital may be able to provide you with pamphlets, brochures, and journal articles or direct you to classes, seminars, and health screenings.

Use Telephone and Fax Services

Some communities have a telephone medical service that allows callers to listen to audiotapes on certain disease topics. Also, your health insurance company or health maintenance organization may have a nurse available to answer health-related questions over the telephone.

If you have access to a fax machine, you can get health information from some organizations in just a few minutes. If a faxback system is available, use the telephone on your fax machine to call the faxback number of the organization and listen to the instructions. In most cases, you can request a list or menu of information to be sent to you first.

The Centers for Disease Control and Prevention at (888) 232-3299 (toll free) is an example of an organization that has information available by fax. Your librarian can help you locate other fax services.

Explore Computer Databases

The computer has become an important tool for helping people locate medical and health information quickly and easily. Most software and information services are user friendly and allow people with no formal training in computer searching to use databases to obtain information. Using a computer at home or in the library, you can find health information by searching CD-ROM databases, searching on-line on the Internet, or using a health-related software program.

As mentioned earlier, many public libraries have Infotrac, a database that includes consumer health information. It indexes popular magazines and newspapers and 2 to 4 years' worth of medical publications. Medical libraries have more extensive medical databases. Start with the following list and ask your librarian to help you find the most appropriate CD-ROM or online (Internet) databases for your needs:

- **MEDLINE®.** MEDLINE® contains citations and often abstracts for over 11 million articles in 4,300 biomedical journals on all aspects of biomedicine and allied health fields. MEDLINE® now covers the literature from the mid-1950s to the present and is available free of charge through the NLM Web site at www.nlm.nih.gov.

- **DIRLINE®.** This database contains location and description information about a wide variety of resources, including organizations, research resources, projects, databases, and electronic bulletin boards concerned with health and biomedicine. The database is available online through the NLM at no fee at dirline.nlm.nih.gov.

- **CHID (Combined Health Information Database).** Developed and managed by health-related agencies of the Federal Government, this database can help people find information and educational resources such as brochures, books, and audiovisuals on selected topics. CHID contains 16 subfiles, including the Arthritis and Musculoskeletal and Skin Diseases subfile. It is available on the Internet at no fee at chid.nih.gov.

Search the Internet

The Internet is a worldwide network of computers that can exchange information almost instantaneously. The World Wide Web (abbreviated www in computer addresses), or more simply, the Web, is a system of electronic documents linked together and available on the Internet for anyone with a computer, a modem, and an Internet provider account. While the terms "Internet" and "World Wide Web" are often used interchangeably, the Web is actually the part of the Internet that supports the use of graphics, pictures, sound, and even video.

If you have access to the Web, you can find information on everything from the latest medical research to facts on particular conditions. You may have access at home or at work to Internet databases through a commercial service such as America Online or through a local Internet provider. Many public libraries have computer stations that provide Internet access.

You'll find extensive health and medical information on the Internet. America Online and other Internet providers and sites offer MEDLINE®; some sites may charge a search fee. The Internet also offers other resources such as bulletin boards, online publications, forums for discussion of current medical issues, and on-line support groups. For example, the American Self-Help Clearinghouse offers an on-line version of its *Self-Help Sourcebook* at www.mentalhelp.net/selfhelp that provides information on support groups and networks available in your community and throughout the world. The site also provides a link to the Self-Help Resource Room that contains information about on-line support groups and other health resources.

Some health resources to check out on the WWW:

- National Institute of Arthritis and Musculoskeletal and Skin Diseases (www.niams.nih.gov)
- National Institutes of Health (www.nih.gov)
- CHID (chid.nih.gov)
- healthfinder® (www.healthfinder.gov)
- National Library of Medicine (www.nlm.nih.gov)
- Agency for Healthcare Research and Quality (www.ahrq.gov)
- Arthritis Foundation (www.arthritis.org)

- American Academy of Dermatology (www.aad.org)

Help with Searching on the Internet

Searching for health information on the Internet can be confusing and difficult. The sheer volume of information can be overwhelming, and people often find it difficult to narrow down search topics or find specific Web sites. Although an Internet search engine such as Yahoo!® or Netscape® is meant to help you find information, search results on specific topics often reveal thousands of websites, many of which may be unrelated to the information you want. You may want to get a copy of a reference book that provides tips on how to find health information on the Internet. *Health Online,* by Tom Ferguson, M.D. (Addison-Wesley Publishing Company, 1996), is an example of one reference that can help you use the Internet to find health information and support groups.

National Library of Medicine

You can search the NLM's MEDLINE® database, free of charge, on the Web. The link to this database can be found on the NLM home page at www.nlm.nih.gov. You can conduct a search in the Web-based product, PubMed. It provides you with free access to MEDLINE® and, for a fee, allows you to use Loansome Doc Delivery Service to order copies of articles. PubMed links you to publishers' sites for approximately 1,200 full-text journals; some are by subscription only. You can access NLM through its gateway, gateway.nlm.nih.gov/gw/Cmd, which searches many NLM databases simultaneously.

MEDLINEplus

MEDLINEplus from the NLM is designed to assist consumers in locating authoritative health information on the Internet. This service provides access to extensive information about specific diseases and conditions and has links to consumer health information from the National Institutes of Health, dictionaries, lists of hospitals and physicians, health information in Spanish and other languages, and clinical trials. Links to preformulated searches of the MEDLINE® database allow you to find references to the latest health professional articles on each topic. The adam.com medical encyclopedia included in MEDLINEplus brings health consumers an extensive library of medical images, as well as over 4,000 articles about diseases, tests, symptoms, injuries, and surgeries. Drug information is also available on the site.

ClinicalTrials.gov

ClinicalTrials.gov is an information service of the National Institutes of Health (NIH) developed by the NLM that provides patients, family members, health care professionals, and the public with easy access to information on clinical trials for a wide range of diseases and conditions. This database provides opportunities to participate in the evaluation of new treatments. The NLM is developing the database in collaboration with all NIH institutes, other Federal agencies, the pharmaceutical industry, and academic and other nonprofit organizations. You can access this database on the Web at www.clinicaltrials.gov.

healthfinder®

To help people find health information on the Internet, the Federal Government's Department of Health and Human Services has developed a website—healthfinder® (www.healthfinder.gov). This site serves as a gateway or point of entry to the broad range of consumer health information resources produced by the Federal Government and many of its partners. healthfinder® includes a searchable index and locator aids for news, publications, on-line journals, support and self-help groups, online discussions, and toll-free numbers

Don't Believe Everything You Read

As you make purchases for your home library or search the Internet, keep in mind that not all information is written by qualified medical experts. Your doctor or a health organization may be able to recommend some good books or helpful Internet sites. When looking for health information on the Internet, don't believe everything you see. Articles published in peer-reviewed medical journals are checked for accuracy, but anyone can put information on the Internet, so there's no guarantee that the information you find is accurate or up-to-date. In addition, many companies set up websites primarily to sell their products. It may be helpful to ask a health professional about the information you find on the Internet, particularly before you buy any products. If you search and shop with care, you can add some medically sound reference materials to your home library and find accurate information on the Internet.

Use Information Wisely

It can be hard to judge the accuracy and credibility of medical information you read in books or magazines, see on television, or find on the Internet. Even people with medical backgrounds sometimes find this task challenging. Following are some important tips to help you decide what information is believable and accurate.

Books, Articles, and Television Reports

* Compare several different resources on the same topic. Check two or three other articles or books to see whether the information or advice is similar.

* Check the author's credentials by looking up his or her affiliations, such as university and medical school attended, associations, and lists of other publications. For doctors, this information can be found in one of the physician directories at your library or on the AMA's website at www.ama-assn.org (click on AMA Physician Select). You can also call the American Board of Medical Specialists at (866) ASK-ABMS (275-2267) to see whether a physician is board certified in his or her specialty. Your librarian can help you find other resources to check the credentials of nonphysicians.

* Ask yourself if the information or advice "rings true." That is, is it feasible, plausible, and common sense, or is it wishful thinking or sensationalism?

* Look for a list of references at the end of the article or book. Information that is backed up by other medical professionals and researchers is more likely to be accurate.

* Check out your information source. Was the article published in a peer-reviewed journal? Look for a list of editorial or review board members at the beginning of a journal. In a peer-reviewed journal, articles are reviewed by other qualified members of the profession for accuracy and reliability.

* Look very carefully at information published in newspapers and magazines or reported on television. Most reporters are journalists rather than medical experts. In addition, newspapers and television reporters may use sensationalism to attract more readers or viewers. Medical facts and statistics can be misrepresented or incomplete. Check to see whether the newspaper or

magazine cites a source for its information and includes the credentials of the persons cited.

- Examine a magazine's list of editors. Do medical experts serve as editors and review articles? Be especially wary of personal testimonials of miracle cures. There's often no way of judging whether the story is true. Furthermore, don't trust medical product advertisements claiming miracle cures or spectacular results.

The Internet

- Compare the information you find on the Internet with other resources. Check two or three articles in the medical literature or medical textbooks to see whether the information or advice is similar.

- Check the author's or organization's credentials. They should be clearly displayed on the Web site. If the credentials are missing, consider this a red flag. Unfortunately, there are many phony doctors and other health professionals making false claims on the Internet.

- Find out if the Web site is maintained by a reputable health organization. Remember that no one regulates information on the Internet. Anyone can set up a home page and claim anything. Some reliable websites providing health information include those of government agencies, health foundations and associations, and medical colleges.

- Be wary of websites advertising and selling products that claim to improve your health. More important, be very careful about giving out credit-card information on the Internet. Further, even if nothing is being sold on a website, ask yourself if the site host has an interest in promoting a particular product or service.

- Ask yourself whether the information or advice seems to contradict what you've learned from your doctor. If so, talk to your doctor to clarify the differences in the information.

- Be cautious when using information found on bulletin boards or during "chat" sessions with others. Testimonials and personal stories are based on one person's experience rather than on objective facts or proven medical research.

To Make Informed Decisions about Your Health Care, You Need to Understand Your Health Problem

Medical information, especially material written for health care providers, can be hard to understand, confusing, and sometimes frightening. As you read through your materials, write down any words or information you don't understand or find confusing. Make a list of your questions and concerns. During your next office visit, ask your doctor, nurse, or other health professional to review the information with you so that you understand clearly how it might be helpful to you.

If the medical information you gathered is for a personal health problem, you may want to share what you found with your spouse, other family members, or a close friend. Family members and friends who understand your health problem are better able to provide needed support and care. Finally, you might want to consider joining a support group in your community. You may find it helpful to be able to talk with others who have the same health problem and share your feelings or concerns.

Ultimately, the information you gather from print and electronic resources can help you make decisions about your health care—how to prevent illness, maintain optimal health, and address your specific health problems. Armed with this knowledge, you can more actively work in partnership with your doctor and other health care professionals to explore treatment options and make health care decisions. Health care experts predict that today's computer and telecommunication systems will result in a new era—the health care system information age—built around health-savvy, health-responsible consumers who are the primary managers of their own health and medical care.

For More Information

National Institute of Arthritis and Musculoskeletal and Skin Diseases (NIAMS)
1 AMS Circle
Bethesda, MD 20892-3675
Toll-Free: (877) 22-NIAMS (226-4267)
Phone: (301) 495-4484
TTY: (301) 565-2966
Fax: (301) 718-6366
Website: http://www.niams.nih.gov
E-mail: niamsinfo@mail.nih.gov

Chapter 28

Arthritis: Timely Treatments for an Ageless Disease

Myth: Arthritis affects only older people.

Fact: Arthritis affects any age, including children. There's no question that the incidence of arthritis increases with age, but nearly three of every five sufferers are under age 65.

Myth: Arthritis is just minor aches and pains.

Fact: Arthritis can be permanently debilitating.

Myth: Arthritis cannot be treated.

Fact: The FDA recently approved several new treatments for osteoarthritis and rheumatoid arthritis.

The fact is, these myths keep people from seeking a doctor's help against the number-one cause of disability in the United States, according to the national Centers for Disease Control and Prevention (CDC). Arthritis disables more Americans than heart disease and stroke, and the CDC says it's what Americans don't know about the disease that can hurt them.

"People ignore arthritis both as public and personal health problems because it doesn't kill you," says Chad Helmick, a medical epidemiologist at the CDC. "But what they don't realize is that as Americans

U.S. Food and Drug Administration, *FDA Consumer,* May/June 2000. Written by Carol Lewis. Available online at http://www.fda.gov/fdac; accessed March 2004.

work and live longer, arthritis can affect their quality of life and eventually lead to disability." Current costs to the U.S. economy total nearly $65 billion annually—an impact equal to a moderate recession.

And the extent of the suffering is going to get worse. Arthritis already affects more than 42 million Americans in its chronic form, including 300,000 children. By 2020, CDC estimates that 60 million people will be affected, and that more than 12 million will be disabled.

The Arthritis Foundation and the American College of Rheumatology agree that awareness, early diagnosis, and an aggressive treatment plan developed by a doctor are key to stopping arthritis from taking over your life.

What Is Arthritis?

Although the term literally means joint inflammation, arthritis really refers to a group of more than 100 rheumatic diseases and conditions that can cause pain, stiffness, and swelling in the joints. Certain conditions may affect other parts of the body—such as the muscles, bones, and some internal organs—and can result in debilitating, and sometimes life-threatening, complications. If left undiagnosed and untreated, arthritis can cause irreversible damage to the joints.

The two most common forms of the disease, osteoarthritis and rheumatoid arthritis, have the greatest public health implications, according to the Arthritis Foundation.

Osteoarthritis, previously known as degenerative joint disease, results from the wear and tear of life. The pressure of gravity—the load of living—causes physical damage to the joints and surrounding tissues, leading to pain, tenderness, swelling, and decreased function. Initially, osteoarthritis is noninflammatory and its onset is subtle and gradual, usually involving one or only a few joints. The joints most often affected are the knee, hip, and hand. Pain is the earliest symptom, usually made worse by repetitive use. Osteoarthritis affects 21 million people, and the risk of getting it increases with age. Other risk factors include joint trauma, obesity, and repetitive joint use.

Rheumatoid arthritis is an autoimmune disease that occurs when the body's own immune system mistakenly attacks the synovium (cell lining inside the joint). This chronic, potentially disabling disease causes pain, stiffness, swelling, and loss of function in the joints.

While the cause remains elusive, doctors suspect that genetic factors are important in rheumatoid arthritis. Recent studies have begun to tease out the genetic characteristics that can be passed from generation to generation. However, the inherited trait alone does not cause the illness. Researchers think this trait, along with some other unknown factor—probably in the environment—triggers the disease.

But rheumatoid arthritis can be difficult to diagnose early because it may begin gradually with subtle symptoms. According to the CDC, this form of arthritis affects more than 2 million people in the United States, and two to three times more women are affected than men.

Finding Effective Treatments

For years, the pain and inflammation of arthritis have been treated with varying success, using medications, local steroid injections, and joint replacement. Seldom did the therapies make the pain go away completely or for very long, nor did they affect the underlying joint damage. Just ask Jo Ellen Gluscevich, who has tried more drugs and treatments than she can remember, to no avail.

"It seems I've tried them all," says the 50-year-old from Frederick, Md., who was diagnosed with rheumatoid arthritis 10 years ago. "Every year continues to be a challenge for me medically."

But now there are some new treatments available, and patients should consult with their doctors to determine which are the most appropriate for their conditions.

Osteoarthritis

When taken regularly and at high doses, traditional nonsteroidal anti-inflammatory drugs (NSAIDs) used for pain relief can cause gastrointestinal (GI) bleeding or ulcers. But a new type of NSAID, cyclooxygenase-2 inhibitors, better known as COX-2 inhibitors, has joined the old standbys. These drugs help suppress arthritis with less stomach irritation.

Cyclooxygenases are enzymes needed for the synthesis of hormone-like substances called prostaglandins. There are two types of cyclooxygenases: the COX-2 enzyme that mediates inflammation and pain, and the COX-1 enzyme that helps maintain other physiological functions in the body. Traditional NSAIDs inhibit both enzymes. The new NSAIDs, however, block mostly the COX-2 enzyme, offering a new treatment option for people who have had difficulty tolerating the old NSAIDs.

"COX-2 inhibitors are just as effective in treating osteoarthritis as other NSAIDs," says Maria Villalba, M.D., a medical officer with the Food and Drug Administration's Center for Drug Evaluation and Research.

The FDA approved the first COX-2 inhibitor, Celebrex (celecoxib), in 1998 to treat rheumatoid arthritis and osteoarthritis. Vioxx (rofecoxib) became the second COX-2 inhibitor to receive approval, in 1999, for the treatment of osteoarthritis, dysmenorrhea (pain with menstrual periods), and the relief of acute pain in adults, such as that caused by dental surgery.

Both drugs, taken orally, were found to substantially lower the risk of stomach and upper intestinal ulcers detected by endoscopy in clinical trials, compared with some of the other NSAIDs tested. However, two recently completed large clinical studies of approximately one-year duration did not support removal of the standard NSAID warning of the risk of serious gastrointestinal events from the Celebrex and Vioxx labels. These large studies did not show an advantage in overall safety (as measured by the total number of deaths, serious adverse events, discontinuations, and hospitalizations due to adverse events) favoring the selective COX-2 inhibitors compared to the other NSAIDs tested.

Two non-drug alternatives for the treatment of pain in osteoarthritis of the knee were approved by the FDA's Center for Devices and Radiological Health in 1997 for patients who have failed to respond adequately to simple analgesics, such as acetaminophen, and to conservative nonpharmacologic therapy. Hyalgan and Synvisc are viscous solutions composed of hyaluronan (hyaluronic acid, a lubricant found naturally in the joints), and are injected directly into the knee joint. Both are believed to increase the quality of synovial fluid, although the mechanism of action for these products is not well understood. The most common side effects reported from these treatments—injection site pain and knee pain and/or swelling—were found to be temporary. For patients who cannot tolerate oral medications and who are not candidates for surgical knee replacement, these treatments may be an ideal option.

Rheumatoid Arthritis

Typical treatments for rheumatoid arthritis have relied on a combination of NSAIDs, such as ibuprofen or aspirin (which reduce swelling and alleviate pain but do not change the course of the disease) and disease-modifying anti-rheumatic drugs (DMARDs) such as methotrexate and sulfasalazine, also called slow-acting drugs. DMARDs work to slow inflammation and can, in many cases, alter the course of the disease. Until recently, most doctors reserved the use of DMARDs for patients who failed to respond to other therapies. Now, most physicians use DMARDs early and aggressively in the hope of slowing disease progression and damage to joints and internal organs.

The most recently approved treatment regimen for rheumatoid arthritis is one that combines the genetically engineered biological drug Remicade (infliximab) with the drug methotrexate. (Not all patients with rheumatoid arthritis can tolerate or respond to methotrexate alone, a standard treatment for the disease.) Remicade is the second in a new class of drugs known as biologic response modifiers, which bind to and block the action of a naturally occurring protein called tumor necrosis factor (TNF), believed to play a role in joint inflammation and damage. Elevated levels of TNF are found in the synovial fluid of rheumatoid arthritis patients.

Remicade, which is administered intravenously by a health-care professional in a two-hour outpatient procedure, was approved by the FDA in 1999 to reduce the signs and symptoms in patients who have not experienced significant relief from methotrexate alone.

Approved in 1996, Enbrel (etanercept) is the first biologic response modifier to receive FDA approval for patients with moderate to severe rheumatoid arthritis.

Taken twice weekly by injection, Enbrel was shown to decrease pain and morning stiffness and improve joint swelling and tenderness. In 2000, the drug's uses were expanded to include delaying structural damage. Jeffrey N. Siegel, M.D., a medical officer with FDA's Center for Biologics Evaluation and Research, says that Enbrel is an exciting breakthrough because it helps a majority of patients who have not responded to any of the other commonly used therapies. Although it is injected, the treatment can be administered at home. In addition, Enbrel has been shown to be effective for children with the juvenile form of rheumatoid arthritis. In clinical trials, Enbrel was generally well tolerated, and one of the most common side effects was an injection site reaction.

Both Remicade and Enbrel show promise in treating rheumatoid arthritis, although the long-term risks and benefits of these agents are unknown. In post-marketing reports, serious infections, including fatalities, have been reported with these agents. Caution should be used in patients with a history of recurring infections or with underlying conditions that may predispose patients to infections.

Arava (leflunomide) is the first oral treatment approved for slowing the progression of rheumatoid arthritis. Although its effects are similar to those of methotrexate, this drug works by a different chemical mechanism that blocks at least one enzyme in certain immune cells called lymphocytes (a type of white blood cell that is part of the immune system), and thereby retards the progression of the disease.

However, Arava is not a cure for rheumatoid arthritis. It may cause birth defects, and the label carries a special warning for pregnant women and those planning to become pregnant. Liver damage, including deaths, also has been reported. The drug is not recommended for patients with severe immunodeficiency, bone marrow dysplasia, or severe, uncontrolled infections.

The first non-drug alternative for adult patients with moderate to severe rheumatoid arthritis and longstanding disease was approved by the FDA in 1999. The Prosorba column, which was initially approved in 1987 to treat an immune blood disorder, is a single-use medical device, about the size of a coffee mug, containing a material that binds antibodies and antigen-antibody complexes.

In a two-hour process performed in a hospital or specialized treatment center, a patient's blood is removed and passed through a machine that separates the blood cells from the plasma (the liquid portion of the blood). The plasma is then passed through the Prosorba column, recombined with the blood cells, and returned to the patient. Although this filtering process is believed to remove proteins that may inadvertently attack the joint cells, the mechanism of action of the Prosorba column is not well understood. The treatment is given once a week for 12 weeks. The most common side effects include joint pain and/or swelling, fatigue, hypotension (low blood pressure), and anemia.

"For those patients who have failed or are intolerant to DMARDs, including Arava and the anti-TNF agents," says Sahar M. Dawisha, M.D., a medical officer in the FDA's Center for Devices and Radiological Health, "the Prosorba column may be an additional treatment option."

Exercise and Arthritis

Proper exercises performed on a regular basis are an important part of arthritis treatment, according to the Arthritis Foundation. Twenty years ago, doctors advised exactly the opposite, fearing that activity would cause more damage and inflammation. Not exercising causes weak muscles, stiff joints, reduced mobility, and lost vitality, say rheumatologists, who now routinely advise a balance of physical activity and rest.

According to the 1996 Surgeon General's Report on Physical Activity and Health, regular, moderate physical activity is beneficial in decreasing fatigue, strengthening muscles and bones, increasing flexibility and stamina, and improving the general sense of well-being. The National Institutes of Health (NIH) advises that the amount and form of exercise should depend on which joints are involved, the amount of inflammation, how stable the joints are, and whether a joint replacement procedure has been done. A skilled physician who is knowledgeable about the medical and rehabilitation needs of people with arthritis, working with a physical therapist, can design an exercise plan for each patient.

Three main types of exercises are recommended:

- Range-of-motion—moving a joint as far as it will comfortably go and then stretching it a little further to increase and maintain joint mobility, decrease pain, and improve joint function. These can be done daily, or at least every other day.

- Strengthening—using muscles without moving joints to help increase muscle strength and stabilize weak joints. These can be done daily, or at least every other day, unless there is severe pain or swelling.

- Endurance—aerobic exercises such as walking, swimming, and bicycling to strengthen the heart and lungs and increase stamina. These should be done for 20 to 30 minutes, three times a week, unless there is severe pain or swelling.

Unproven Remedies

Many people with arthritis become discouraged with typical treatments because the disease progresses over time and the symptoms worsen. Consequently, they search for alternative therapies aimed at arthritis. But arthritis patients need to be careful because treatments not shown to be safe and effective through controlled scientific studies may be dangerous. According to the Arthritis Foundation, the benefits of a treatment in controlling arthritis should be greater than the risk of unwanted or harmful effects. Since arthritis symptoms may come and go, a person using an unproven remedy may mistakenly think the remedy worked simply because he or she tried it when symptoms were going into a natural remission.

Two controversial nutritional supplements, not approved by the FDA, have catapulted into the spotlight because of claims that they rebuild joint tissues damaged by osteoarthritis—or halt the disease entirely. But at this time, the use of glucosamine and chondroitin sulfate supplements warrant further in-depth studies on their safety and effectiveness, according to the Arthritis Foundation. The NIH plans to study the effectiveness of these supplements.

Both glucosamine and chondroitin sulfate occur in the body naturally and are vital to normal cartilage formation, but the Arthritis Foundation says there's no evidence that swallowed chondroitin is absorbed into the body and deposited into the joints. Moreover, no one knows how much glucosamine and chondroitin sulfate are in the bottles since current law does not require dietary supplements to be manufactured under the same good manufacturing practice standards as pharmaceuticals. As reported in the December 1999 *UC Berkeley Wellness Letter,* "It's a hit-or-miss proposition because there's no standardization and no guarantee that you're getting what the label says."

The Arthritis Foundation urges anyone considering using these supplements to become "fully educated about potential positive and negative effects." In addition, people are encouraged to consult their physicians about how the supplements fit within their existing treatment regimens. Above all, do not stop proven treatments and disease-management techniques in favor of the supplements.

The Arthritis Foundation also says that copper bracelets, mineral springs, vibrators, magnets, vinegar and honey, dimethyl sulfoxide, large doses of vitamins, drugs with hidden ingredients (such as steroids), and snake venom are all unproven remedies. And any unproven remedy, no matter how harmless, can become harmful if it stops or delays someone from seeking a prescribed treatment program from a knowledgeable physician.

Prevention Measures

There are ways to help prevent arthritis. Both CDC and the American College of Rheumatology recommend maintaining ideal weight, taking precautions to reduce repetitive joint use and injury on the job, avoiding sports injuries by performing warm-ups and strengthening exercises using weights, and by choosing appropriate sports equipment.

Lyme arthritis may develop after a bacterial infection is transmitted to humans through tick bites. To prevent this type of arthritis, health experts advise people to use insect repellents, wear long-sleeved shirts and pants while walking near wooded areas, and check for and remove ticks to help reduce the risk of getting the disease. CDC also recommends the prompt use of antibiotics for Lyme disease symptoms. In December 1998, FDA approved the first vaccine, LYMErix, to help prevent Lyme disease.

In an efficacy and safety trial, the vaccine's effectiveness in preventing Lyme disease was 49 percent after two injections and 76 percent after three. Vaccination should be considered by people 15 to 70 years old who live in or visit high-risk areas and have frequent or prolonged exposure to ticks. The vaccine has not yet been approved for use in children.

Hope for the Future

Recently approved drugs offer patients new options. For Jo Ellen Gluscevich, the results have not been so dramatic. She remains mostly housebound and must avoid crowds because her immune system is compromised and susceptible to infection.

But as the population ages and arthritis becomes a growing problem, the Arthritis Foundation believes that "more physicians are recognizing the severity of the disease and the need for a broader approach toward treatment."

Other Forms of Arthritis and Related Conditions

In addition to rheumatoid and osteoarthritis, there are a number of diseases and conditions that can cause joint pain and stiffness.

Juvenile arthritis is a general term for all types of arthritis that occur in children. Juvenile rheumatoid arthritis is the most prevalent form in children, and there are three major types: polyarticular (affecting many joints), pauciarticular (pertaining to only a few joints), and systemic (affecting the entire body). The signs and symptoms of juvenile rheumatoid arthritis vary from child to child. There is no single test that establishes conclusively a diagnosis of juvenile arthritis, and the condition must be present consistently for six or more consecutive weeks before a correct diagnosis can be made. Heredity is thought to play some part in the development of juvenile arthritis. However, the inherited trait alone does not cause the illness. Researchers think this trait, along with some other unknown factor (probably in the environment), triggers the disease. The Arthritis Foundation says that juvenile arthritis is even more prevalent than juvenile diabetes and cerebral palsy.

Gout is a disease that causes sudden, severe attacks of pain, tenderness, redness, warmth, and swelling in some joints. It usually affects one joint at a time, especially the joint of the big toe. The pain and swelling associated with gout are caused by uric acid crystals that precipitate out of the blood and are deposited in the joint. Factors leading to increased levels of uric acid and then gout include excessive alcohol intake, hypertension, kidney disease, and certain drugs.

Ankylosing spondylitis is a chronic inflammatory disease of the spine that can fuse the vertebrae to produce a rigid spine. Spondylitis is a result of inflammation that usually starts in tissue outside the joint. The most common early symptoms of spondylitis are low back pain and stiffness that continues for months. Although the cause of spondylitis is unknown, scientists have discovered a strong genetic or family link, according to the Arthritis Foundation. Most people with spondylitis have a genetic marker known as HLA-B27. Genetic markers are protein molecules located on the surface of white blood cells that act as a type of name tag. Having this genetic marker does not mean a person will develop spondylitis, but people with the marker are more likely to develop the disease than those without it. Ankylosing spondylitis usually affects men between the ages of 16 and 35, but it also affects women. Other joints besides the spine may be involved.

Systemic lupus erythematosus is an autoimmune disease that can involve the skin, kidneys, blood vessels, joints, nervous system, heart, and other internal organs. Symptoms vary among those affected, but may include a skin rash, arthritis, fever, anemia, hair loss, ulcers in the mouth, and kidney damage. In most cases, the symptoms first appear in women of childbearing age; however, lupus can occur in young children or older people. Studies suggest that there is an inherited tendency to get lupus. Lupus affects women about 9 to 10 times as often as men. It is also more common in African American women.

Related Arthritis Conditions

Bursitis, tendinitis, and myofascial pain are localized, non-systemic (not affecting the whole body) painful conditions. Bursitis is inflammation of the sac surrounding any joint that contains a lubricating fluid. Tendinitis is inflammation of a tendon, and myofascial pain is a problem that results from the strain or improper use of a muscle. These conditions may start suddenly, and usually stop within a matter of days or weeks.

Carpal tunnel syndrome is a condition in which pressure on the median nerve at the wrist causes tingling and numbness in the fingers. It can begin suddenly or gradually, and can be associated with another disease, such as rheumatoid arthritis, or it may be unrelated to other conditions. If untreated, it can result in permanent nerve and muscle damage. With early diagnosis and treatment, there is an excellent chance of complete recovery.

Fibromyalgia syndrome is a condition with generalized muscular pain, fatigue, and poor sleep that is believed to affect nearly 4 million people. The name fibromyalgia means pain in the muscles, ligaments, and tendons. The condition mainly affects muscles and their attachments to bones. Although it may feel like a joint disease, the Arthritis Foundation says it is not a true form of arthritis and does not cause deformities of the joints. Fibromyalgia is instead a form of soft tissue or muscular rheumatism.

Infectious arthritis is a form of joint inflammation that is caused by bacteria, viruses, or fungi. The diagnosis is made by culturing the organism from the joint. Most infectious arthritis can be cured by antibiotic medications.

Psoriatic arthritis is similar to rheumatoid arthritis. About 5 percent of people with psoriasis, a chronic skin disease, also develop psoriatic arthritis. In psoriatic arthritis, there is inflammation of the joints and sometimes the spine. Fewer joints may be involved than in rheumatoid arthritis, and there is no rheumatoid factor in the blood.

Reiter syndrome (also called reactive arthritis) involves inflammation in the joints, and sometimes where ligaments and tendons attach to bones. This form of arthritis usually develops following an intestinal or a genital/urinary tract infection. People with Reiter syndrome have arthritis and one or more of the following conditions: urethritis, prostatitis, cervicitis, cystitis, eye problems, or skin sores.

Scleroderma is a disease of the body's connective tissue that causes thickening and hardening of the skin. It can also affect joints, blood vessels, and internal organs. There are two types of scleroderma: localized and generalized.

—Carol Lewis is a staff writer for *FDA Consumer.*

Chapter 29

Help Your Arthritis Treatment Work

Ease the Pain, Help Prevent More Damage

Arthritis can strike at any age. It hurts the joints, where two bones meet. It damages the joints and makes them stiff and painful. Sometimes it's so bad it can cripple a person.

Correct treatment can ease the pain and help prevent more damage. You can help your treatment work. This information tells how.

If Your Joints Have Signs of Arthritis, Talk to Your Doctor

If you have arthritis, the doctor may prescribe a medicine for you or tell you to use a medicine you buy without a prescription, like aspirin.

You may need to take more than one medicine.

Joints with arthritis may have:

- swelling
- warmth
- redness
- pain

Before Taking New Medicine, Ask Your Doctor about It

Ask:

- How should I take this medicine?
- Are there any special instructions?

U.S. Food and Drug Administration, May 2000. Available online at http://www.fda.gov; accessed March 2004.

355

- What side effects could there be?
- If I have any side effects, what should I do?
- What should I do if I forget to take a dose?

If you took the medicine before and it caused problems, tell the doctor.

Tell the doctor if you are taking other medicines. And ask if you should keep taking them.

Read the Label of Medicine You Buy without a Prescription

Like arthritis medicine, many medicines for headaches or colds or flu have painkillers in them. Some common painkillers are aspirin, acetaminophen, ibuprofen, ketoprofen, and naproxen.

So before you buy any medicine, read the label to see what's in it.

Does it have a painkiller? If it does, ask your doctor or pharmacist if it's OK for you to take it.

Be Careful with Medicine

- Never take any medicine for arthritis without your doctor's advice.
- Never take someone else's medicine.
- Keep all medicine away from children.
- Throw out medicine that reaches its "Discard" or "Exp" (expiration) date.

Remember: There can be problems with any medicine, even those you can buy without a prescription.

Rest and Exercise

You may need extra rest when your arthritis gets worse, or flares up. But even then, it's good to gently exercise the joints that hurt.

Gentle exercise can ease the pain and help you sleep better. Ask your doctor how to exercise your joints.

Learn about Your Arthritis

It helps to learn about your arthritis. Many people do this by joining a group with other people who have the disease.

To find a group, look in the newspaper. Or ask your doctor or the hospital. The local Arthritis Foundation office has information, too.

Remember: Never take someone else's medicine.

Watch out for Cures That Don't Work

Some people with arthritis can't find any treatment that helps very much. That's why there are so many ads for gadgets, health foods, and supplements to treat arthritis.

Many of these have never been tested. They're just a waste of money.

Protect Yourself with the Facts

Pain and stiffness often come and go by themselves, for no known reason. You may use an untested product and then feel better. But you may have felt better even without the product.

There is no cure for arthritis. But correct treatment can ease pain and stiffness.

If you use worthless products, you delay real help. So the damage gets worse.

Remember: If it sounds too good to be true, it probably isn't true

What If Correct Treatment Doesn't Help?

If all else fails, an operation might help. Talk about this with your doctor

Do You Have More Questions about an Arthritis Treatment?

Ask your doctor or other health-care worker.

Chapter 30

Understanding Arthritis Medications

First Line Drugs: NSAIDs and Other Painkillers

Nonsteroidal Anti-Inflammatory Drugs (NSAIDs)

Two thirds of people with rheumatoid arthritis (RA) ranked pain as their primary reason for seeking professional help. The most common pain relievers for RA are the nonsteroidal anti-inflammatory drugs (NSAIDs). These agents block prostaglandins, the substances that dilate blood vessels and cause inflammation and pain. There are dozens of NSAIDs. The most common pain relievers are the following:

- Over-the-counter NSAIDs include aspirin, ibuprofen (Motrin IB, Advil, Nuprin, Rufen), naproxen (Aleve), ketoprofen (Actron, Orudis KT). One study suggested that ibuprofen or naproxen is more effective than aspirin or acetaminophen for acute tension-type headache.

- Prescription NSAIDs include ibuprofen (Motrin), naproxen (Naprosyn, Anaprox), flurbiprofen (Ansaid), diclofenac (Voltaren), tolmetin (Tolectin), ketoprofen (Orudis, Oruvail), and dexibuprofen (Seractil).

Studies have indicated that the optimal times for taking an NSAID might be after the evening meal and then again on awakening. The reason for this is RA symptoms increase gradually during the night, reaching their greatest severity at the time of awakening. Taking NSAIDs with food can reduce stomach discomfort, although it may slow down the pain-relieving effect.

Regular use of even over-the-counter NSAIDs may be hazardous for anyone and has been associated with the following side effects:

- Ulcers and gastrointestinal bleeding. This is the major danger with long-term use of NSAIDs.

- Increased blood pressure. Most NSAIDs appear to pose this risk, with higher risks observed with piroxicam (Feldene), naproxen (Aleve), and indomethacin (Indocin). (Sulindac has the smallest effect and aspirin as no risk.) People with hypertension, severe vascular disease, kidney, or liver problems and those taking diuretics must be closely monitored if they need to take NSAIDs.

- May delay the emptying of the stomach, which could interfere with the actions of other drugs. The elderly are at special risk.

- Dizziness

- Tinnitus (ringing in the ear)

- Headache

- Skin rash

- Depression

- Confusion or bizarre sensation (in some higher-potency NSAIDs, such as indomethacin)

- As with acetaminophen, high daily doses of aspirin have been associated with an increased risk of kidney failure, although the risk remains low in those with healthy kidney function. Kidney abnormalities have been reported in people taking other NSAIDs as well, which resolve when the drugs are withdrawn. Any sudden weight gain or swelling should be reported to a physician. Anyone with kidney disease should avoid these drugs.

- Diabetics taking oral hypoglycemics may need to adjust the dosage if they also need to take NSAIDs because of possible harmful interactions between the drugs.

Some studies have reported that ibuprofen (but not other NSAIDs) may blunt the heart-protective effects of low-dose aspirin. Additional research is needed to confirm these findings.

NSAID-Induced Ulcers and Gastrointestinal Bleeding

Long-term use of nonsteroidal anti-inflammatory drugs (NSAIDs) is the second most common cause of ulcers and the rate of NSAID-caused ulcers in increasing. Ulcers caused by nonsteroidal anti-inflammatory drugs (NSAIDs) are more likely to bleed than those caused by the bacteria *H. pylori*. NSAID-related bleeding and stomach problems may be responsible for 107,000 hospital admissions and 16,500 deaths each year. Because there are usually no gastrointestinal symptoms from NSAIDs until bleeding begins, physicians cannot predict which patients taking these drugs will develop bleeding. Among the groups at high risk for bleeding are elderly people, anyone with a history of ulcers of GI bleeding, patients with serious heart conditions, alcohol abusers, and those on certain medications, such anticoagulants (blood thinners), corticosteroids, or bisphosphonates (drugs used for osteoporosis).

One study ranked the sixteen most commonly used NSAIDs according to risk for ulcers and bleeding.

- Lowest Risk: nabumetone (Relafen), etodolac (Lodine), salsalate, and sulindac (Clinoril).

- Medium Risk: diclofenac (Voltaren), ibuprofen (Motrin, Advil, Nuprin, Rufen), aspirin, naproxen (Aleve, Naprosyn, Naprelan, Anaprox), and tolmetin (Tolectin). (Drugs within this group vary in risk. Studies show, for example, that short-term use of naproxen is twice as likely as ibuprofen to be associated with hospitalization from GI bleeding. Although ketoprofen (Actron, Orudis KT) was considered a medium-risk drug, another study reported that even one week of taking the drug at low doses causes significant GI injury.

- Highest Risk: flurbiprofen (Ansaid), piroxicam (Feldene), fenoprofen, indomethacin (Indocin), meclofenamate (Meclomen), and oxaprozin.

If NSAID-induced ulcers are identified, the following steps have been suggested:

- Switching to alternative pain relievers is the first step in preventing or healing ulcers caused by NSAIDs. If people cannot change drugs, then they should use the lowest NSAID dose possible. For example, Arthrotec is a combination of an ulcer protective agent called misoprostol and the NSAID diclofenac that may reduce the risk for gastrointestinal bleeding. One

361

study found that patients taking Arthrotec had 65% to 80% fewer ulcers than those who took NSAIDs alone.

- In addition, agents are available that may help prevent ulcers in people who need to take NSAIDs. For example, proton-pump inhibitors (PPIs) are the first choice for preventing ulcers in high-risk individuals and have been demonstrated to reduce NSAID-ulcer rates by as much as 80% compared with no treatment. Brands include omeprazole (Prilosec), esomeprazole (Nexium), lansoprazole (Prevacid), rabeprazole (Aciphex), and pantoprazole (Protonix). Prevacid is the first proton-pump inhibitor to be specifically indicated for protecting against ulcers in chronic NSAID users.

COX-2 Inhibitors (Coxibs)

Celecoxib (Celebrex), rofecoxib (Vioxx), and valdecoxib (Bextra) are known as COX-2 (cyclooxygenase-2) inhibitors, or coxibs. They inhibit an inflammation-promoting enzyme called COX-2. Meloxicam (Mobicox) is a related drug known as a COX-2 preferential.

Most studies have found coxibs to be about equally effective to each other (and to NSAIDs) for allaying arthritic pain of osteoarthritis. Furthermore, evidence is increasing that the coxibs are somewhat less harmful to the GI tract than the common NSAID naproxen. Celebrex may be superior to Vioxx in this regard, although more studies are needed to confirm this. Some early evidence also suggests that, like NSAIDs, they may be partially protective against colon cancer and possibly even Alzheimer's disease.

In spite of their potential promise, some researchers theorize that inhibiting COX-2 may have some negative side effects over the long term. The effects of these drugs on the heart particularly require clarification. The following are possible adverse effects or complications:

- Some studies have reported twice the incidence of heart attacks in patients taking Vioxx compared to those taking standard NSAIDs. There were limitations to these studies, however, and 2003 study found no higher risk. Some (but not all evidence) suggests that the COX-2 inhibitors may increase the risk for blood clots. On the other hand, some studies have suggested that the anti-inflammatory effects, at least in Celebrex and meloxicam (Mobicox) may have beneficial effects on blood vessels, which would be heart protective.

- In one study, people who took Celebrex or Vioxx experienced an increase in blood pressure, with Vioxx having the greater effect.

- A few cases of psychiatric side effects (hallucinations) have been observed with higher doses of Celebrex or Vioxx.

- Coxibs may have some adverse effects on kidney function, particularly in elderly people, which is similar to the effects of standard NSAIDs. Liver abnormalities, which are side effects of many drugs, have also been reported with coxibs and need further follow-up. They may have negative effects on pregnancy and fertility.

- No one who has allergic reactions, hives, or asthma from sulfa drugs, aspirin, or other NSAIDs should take a coxib. For example, life-threatening and widespread reactions have been reported in patients taking valdecoxib (Bextra). Anyone who develops a rash after taking these agents should stop taking them immediately.

- Coxibs can interfere with other drugs taken concurrently. Patients taking anticoagulant drugs such as warfarin may experience a higher risk for bleeding with the use of these agents. The use of coxibs can interfere with many other drugs taken concurrently, including lithium, methotrexate, and many others taken for heart disease, high blood pressure, or epilepsy. Patients should discuss all other medications with their physician.

COX-2 inhibitors are also currently more expensive than traditional NSAIDs, however, costing about $80 per month, compared to about $15 for an NSAID like naproxen, and some insurers do not pay for them. More research is needed to confirm or refute any possible hazards from taking coxibs and also to determine whether their benefits are worth the higher cost.

Second-Line Agents: Disease-Modifying Anti-Rheumatic Drugs (DMARDs)

Disease-modifying anti-rheumatic drugs (DMARDs) are the standard second line drugs. Early treatment with DMARDs improves patients' long-term outcome and quality of life and may also help slow down progression of the disease. Evidence supporting early use was reflected in a five-year 2001 study published in 2001 that compared RA progression rates in patients from different countries. The slowest disease progression rates were observed in patients from Finland, who were given the most effective DMARDs immediately upon diagnosis.

The worst and most rapid progression occurred in patients from Sweden, who tended to be given less potent DMARDs and whose treatment was delayed by three months. This group also tended to stay on treatment for shorter duration (two years) compared to the Finnish group (the majority was treated for five years).

There is also some evidence that early use of DMARDs may help protect against heart problems, which are major complications of RA.

DMARDs do not have any common properties other than their ability to slow down the progression of rheumatoid arthritis. Many were used for other diseases and were found accidentally to help RA. They include the following:

- Methotrexate (considered to be the current second-line standard of care. Newer agents called biologic modifiers, however, may prove to be as effective with fewer side effects.)
- Hydroxychloroquine
- Sulfasalazine
- Gold
- D-penicillamine
- Cyclosporine
- Leflunomide

Unfortunately, they all tend to lose effectiveness over time, even methotrexate. Patients rarely use one for more than two years. It is now apparent that combining DMARDs with each other or with drugs in other categories offers the best approach for many patients. The addition of a corticosteroid to any combination may be important.

All DMARDs may produce stomach and intestinal side effects, and, over the long term, each poses some risk for rare but serious reactions. (In some cases, however, they may be less harmful than long-term NSAID treatment.)

Methotrexate

Methotrexate (Rheumatrex) acts as an anti-inflammatory agent and is now the most frequently used DMARD, particularly for severe disease. It has the following advantages over other DMARDs:

- A faster mode of action than other DMARDs (starts working within a few weeks).
- The best record to date for long-term use.

- A 2002 study suggested that it reduced mortality rates from heart disease by 70%, compared to other DMARDs. (Death rates from other causes were also lower, although less significantly.)

Even this drug loses effectiveness, however, when used alone. It is more effective when used in combination with other DMARDs or agents. Studies indicating effective combinations are as follows:

- Using it with cyclosporine and a corticosteroid may be effective and allow lower doses of methotrexate, thereby minimizing side effects. (Methotrexate has a wide range of actions against the immune system, while cyclosporine is fairly specific; it prevents T-cells from proliferating.)
- The combination of methotrexate and leflunomide (which has different effects on the immune system) is very effective compared to methotrexate alone. (This combination poses a risk for liver toxicity and requires monitoring.)
- Combinations with the newer agents, the tumor-necrosis factor (TNF) modifiers and the interleukin-1 antagonist anakinra, are very promising.

About 20% of patients withdraw because of side effects. They include nausea and vomiting, rash, mild hair loss, headache, mouth sores, and muscle aches.

Methotrexate has fewer serious toxic effects than many DMARDs, although rare, they can include the following:

- Kidney and liver damage. People at particular risk for liver damage from methotrexate include diabetics with existing liver or kidney problems, alcoholics, those who are obese, the elderly, and (at very high risk) those with psoriasis. (Taking folate supplements may be very helpful in reducing liver toxicity as well as relieving less serious side effects, although folate may interfere slightly with the effectiveness of methotrexate.)
- Possibly osteoporosis at high doses. (A 2001 study reported no higher risk for bone loss at low doses.)
- Increased risk for infections, particularly herpes zoster and pneumonia.
- Lung disease occurs in up to 5% of people who take methotrexate and deserves special mention. There are five key risk factors for methotrexate-induced lung diseases: age, diabetes, existing

rheumatoid involvement in the lung, protein in the urine, and previous use of other DMARDs, particularly sulfasalazine, oral gold and d-penicillamine. Patients with multiple risk factors should report any symptoms, such as coughing, that might indicate lung injury.

- The drug increases the risk for birth defects when taken by pregnant women.

- There have been a few reports of lymphomas in some patients taking methotrexate. In such cases, the disease appears to go into remission when the drug is stopped. Most studies have found no significant risk for cancer in patients taking this agent.

Leflunomide

Leflunomide (Arava) blocks autoimmune antibodies and reduces inflammation. It also may inhibit metalloproteinases (MMP), which are involved in cartilage destruction. It has the following benefits:

- It is the first oral treatment approved for RA.

- It slows disease progression as early as six months into treatment.

- Comparison studies with methotrexate report a better quality of life with leflunomide, including more energy, greater vitality, and fewer emotional side effects. (Studies comparing their risk for serious adverse effects are mixed. One, for example, showed fewer problems with leflunomide, while another reported identical rates.)

The combination of methotrexate and leflunomide (which has different effects on the immune system) is very effective compared to either agent alone. (This combination poses a risk for liver toxicity and requires monitoring.)

Reports of adverse effects are comparable to those with methotrexate. Common problems include nausea, diarrhea, hair loss, and rash. Potentially serious side effects infections and liver injury. Everyone taking leflunomide should be monitored regularly, and anyone with liver problems should avoid this drug until further research has determined its full effects.

Sulfasalazine

Sulfasalazine (Azulfidine) was developed in the 1930s for treating rheumatoid arthritis, but fell into disfavor when gold treatment emerged.

It has regained popularity, however, and is now beneficial for both adult and juvenile RA. (It is most effective when the disease is confined to the joints.)

Symptomatic relief can occur in four weeks. A 1999 study suggested that sulfasalazine was more effective than hydroxychloroquine and had fewer side effects than gold therapy (although also possibly fewer benefits).

Side effects are common, particularly stomach and intestinal distress. A coated-tablet form may help reduce them. Other side effects include skin rash, sensitivity to sunlight, and, in rare cases, lung problems. People with intestinal or urinary obstructions or who have allergies to sulfa drugs or salicylates should not take sulfasalazine.

Hydroxychloroquine

Hydroxychloroquine (Plaquenil) was originally used for preventing malaria and is now also used for mild, slowly progressive arthritis. It has the following benefits:

- Relieves pain

- Improve mobility

- Has one of least toxic profiles of the DMARDs

The downside is that it takes three to six months to achieve full benefit. It also does not appear to slow disease progression. One study concluded that joint erosion after two years was worse than with no DMARD at all.

As with all DMARDs, gastrointestinal complaints are fairly common. Mild headaches and eye problems may be more common with this drug than with others. The most serious side effect is damage to the retina, although this is very uncommon when low doses are used and can be reversed if treated in time. Some experts recommend eye examinations every six months in people over 60 who take hydroxychloroquine. It may aggravate psoriasis, and it poses a slight risk for birth defects.

Gold

Gold has been a long-standing DMARD for rheumatoid arthritis. Rather than suppressing immune factors that cause inflammation, research in 2002 suggests that it may stimulate specific protective factors.

It can be administered in one of two ways:

- Orally as auranofin (Ridaura). The oral form has fewer side effects but is less effective than the injected form.

- Injected (known as chrysotherapy). This form uses either gold sodium thiomalate (Myochrysine) or aurothioglucose (Solganal). Although injected gold used to be the favorite second-line drug, it is generally used for mild, slowly progressive cases.

Side effects differ according to the method of administration:

- Oral gold can cause skin rash and mouth sores as well as stomach irritation. About 50% of people taking oral gold experience diarrhea, which can be offset by reducing the dosage or taking bulk formers, such as Metamucil.

- Injected gold is the most toxic of all the DMARDs during early stages of treatment, and in one study 43% of the patients stopped taking it. (Nevertheless, over the long term, it may be among the least toxic.) The injected form can cause skin problems and sores in the mucous membranes in about 20% of people. The most serious side effects of gold injections are kidney damage and decreased white blood cell count. Women who are pregnant or people with major medical conditions of the heart, kidney, liver, skin, and blood should be very cautious about using this therapy.

Penicillamine

It may take up to a year for penicillamine (Cuprimine, Depen) to be effective in reducing the effects of RA, and its use is declining. More than half the patients who take it withdraw because of side effects. It causes stomach and intestinal side effects similar to those of gold. In addition, it may leave the patient with a metallic taste in the mouth or, even, no taste at all. Other side effects include inflamed muscles, skin blisters, and fever. Serious side effects include liver and kidney damage and problems in the lungs.

Cyclosporine

Cyclosporine (Sandimmune, Neoral) is actually an immunosuppressant that started out as a third-line drug. It has proven to be an effective and safe agent when used in combinations or as a sole agent for RA, however, so it is now often listed as one of the DMARDs. It is particularly effective when used in combination with methotrexate.

Side effects include gum disease, hair growth, and flare-ups in the joints, but they are usually manageable. There has been some concern over reports associating cyclosporine with an increased risk for cancer, but one controlled study found no such danger.

Third-Line Immunosuppressants

For treatment of very severe active rheumatoid arthritis, physicians are now prescribing third-line drugs that suppress the body's immune system. These agents include the following:

- Azathioprine (Imuran). Azathioprine is the most commonly used of these drugs, with the most usual side effects being stomach and intestinal distress, skin rash, mouth sores, and anemia.

- Cyclophosphamide (Cytoxan)

- Chlorambucil (Leukeran)

All are potentially very toxic and should not be used unless other drugs are ineffective. Grapefruit juice has an enzyme that may enhance the effects of some immunosuppressants. Blood counts should be taken frequently to check for anemia and more serious blood problems. Some increase in certain cancers has been associated with the use of some of these agents, such as lymphoma with azathioprine and bladder cancer with cyclophosphamide, although the benefits of these therapies in patients with severe disease may outweigh any risk.

Corticosteroids (Steroids)

Corticosteroids work rapidly to control inflammation and pain and are about as effective as aspirin for RA. Long-time use, however, can have severe adverse effects. Still, they are often used under the following conditions:

- Oral corticosteroids, such as prednisolone and prednisone (Deltasone, Orasone), are most often used in combination with DMARDs, which significantly enhances the benefits of DMARDs.

- Oral corticosteroids are sometimes used in early stage-RA for patients who cannot tolerate NSAIDs. Studies, in fact, suggest

369

that low-dose corticosteroids may significantly slow joint when it is the first drug administered and then used for two years. (Even low-dose oral steroids have adverse effects on bone density, blood sugar, and weight.)

- Corticosteroids are sometimes injected directly into joints for relief of flare-ups when only one or a few joints are affected. Experts suggest no more than three or four injections a year. Steroid injections in the joints may be a safe and effective treatment for juvenile rheumatoid arthritis and reduce the need for oral medications.

- Corticosteroid pulse therapy (intravenous administration) may be as beneficial as DMARDs.

Side Effects of Oral Corticosteroids

Serious side effects are associated with long-term use of oral steroids. (Low doses may reduce these risks but they do not eliminate them.) Osteoporosis is a common and particularly severe long-term side effect of prolonged steroid use. Medications that can prevent osteoporosis include calcium supplements, parathyroid hormone, or bisphosphonates (alendronate etidronate, risedronate). Other adverse effects include cataracts, glaucoma, diabetes, fluid retention, susceptibility to infections, weight gain, hypertension, capillary fragility, acne, excess hair growth, wasting of the muscles, menstrual irregularities, irritability, insomnia, and, rarely, psychosis.

Withdrawal from Long-Term Use of Oral Corticosteroids

Long-term use of oral steroid medications suppresses secretion of natural steroid hormones by the adrenal glands. After withdrawal from these drugs, this so-called adrenal suppression persists and it can take the body a while (sometimes up to a year) to regain its ability to produce natural steroids again. There have been a few cases of severe adrenal insufficiency that occurred when switching from oral to inhaled steroids, which, in rare cases, has resulted in death.

No one should stop taking any steroids without consulting a physician first, and if steroids are withdrawn, regular follow-up monitoring is necessary. Patients should discuss with their physician measures for preventing adrenal insufficiency during withdrawal, particularly during stressful times, when the risk increases.

Tumor-Necrosis Factor Modifiers

Tumor-necrosis factor (TNF) modifiers are major breakthroughs in the treatment of RA. The current agents (known generally as biologic response modifiers) include infliximab (Remicade), etanercept (Enbrel), and adalimumab (Humira). They are genetically engineered to interfere with specific components of TNF, a powerful immune factor that is important in the disease process. Although they all block TNF, these drugs have some differences:

- Etanercept (Enbrel) is a protein made from the fusion of two TNF receptors. The end product mimics their effects, which neutralize TNF. A 2002 two-year study suggested it is superior to methotrexate in slowing RA disease progression and has fewer side effects. It has been approved for RA, juvenile RA, and psoriatic arthritis.

- Infliximab (Remicade) and adalimumab (Humira) are both monoclonal antibodies (MAbs), which are specially designed antibodies that target TNF. In one study, infliximab was superior to methotrexate, gold, corticosteroids, and an interleukin-1 receptor antagonist. Humira, the latest TNF modifier is the first fully human anti-TNF MAb, which may reduce some of the problems of infliximab.

Studies have reported that all these agents work rapidly and produce significant and sustained improvements. Combinations with methotrexate increase their effectiveness. The combinations may have fewer side effects than using methotrexate alone at higher doses. As with other agents, they do not cure the disease, although some evidence suggests they may slow or even halt joint erosion. For example, in a 1999 study on children with RA taking etanercept, 30% returned to fully normal activities. At this time, however, these agents are very expensive (over $10,000 a year), and many insurers do not cover them.

Side Effects and Complications of Tumor-Necrosis Factor Modifiers

Because TNF modifiers target precise molecular targets, they have fewer widespread effects on the body than general immunosuppressants. Nevertheless, there are concerns and some evidence that suppressing TNF can create long-term problems, including infections and nerve injury.

The side effects of the three agents are similar, but there are some differences between etanercept and the two monoclonal antibodies:

- The most common adverse effects of all three are minor reactions at the injection site, but there are few other immediate side effects.

- Because these agents affect immune factors, there is some risk for severe infections particularly in susceptible individuals, such as those with uncontrolled diabetes, people taking other immunosuppressants, or anyone with a current active infection. For example, cases of tuberculosis and histoplasmosis (a fungal infection in the lungs) have been reported in patients taking TNF-modifiers. (While millions of healthy people unknowingly carry the TB organism, it rarely becomes active in those with healthy immune systems.) RA patients should be tested for TB before initiating treatment. It is not yet known if adalimumab poses as high a risk as infliximab.

- There have been a few reports of aplastic anemia.

- In rare cases, both etanercept and infliximab have been associated with nerve damage that resembles the disease process in multiple sclerosis. This involves demyelination (the loss of myelin, the insulation coat over nerve fibers) and can result in confusion, numbness, changes in vision, and difficulty walking. According to some experts, patients with multiple sclerosis should avoid these agents until further research is complete. (The effects of adalimumab are not known yet.)

- There have been reports of lupus-like symptoms in a few patients taking etanercept, which resolved when the drug was stopped.

- Many patients develop an immune reaction to infliximab itself, which makes the drug less effective overtime. Nevertheless, in one study, benefits persisted for at least two years after stopping the drug. Although adalimumab is a similar agent, it is a fully human molecule and, therefore, may not provoke the immune response that infliximab does. Long-term studies are needed to confirm this.

- Infliximab has been linked to a few deaths in patients with preexisting congestive heart failure.

- There is some suggestion that anti-TNF drugs increase the risk for lymphomas.

Interleukin-1 Antagonists

Drugs that inhibit the interleukin cytokines are also in development. Anakinra (Kineret) is the first of these. It is an intravenous agent that blocks interleukin-1, an important immune factor. It is showing good results when used in combination with DMARDs, such as methotrexate. A 2002 study suggested that it is similar in effectiveness to Remicade and Enbrel—the tumor-necrosis factor modifiers. The decisions to use it will depend on cost and individual side effects. Primary side effects of Kineret include pain at the injection site and leukopenia—a reduction in white blood cell counts that increases the risk for infections.

Investigative Treatments

Investigative Biologic Response Modifiers

A number of other agents that inhibit part of the immune response are being investigated:

- Other tumor necrosis factor blockers.

- Agents that block specific chemical pathways involved with RA. For example, eculizumab (Alexion) is a monoclonal antibody that blocks an immune factor called human complement component C5, which plays a pro-inflammatory role.

- Vaccines that use anti-inflammatory factors to boost the immune system's response against the aberrant immune factors.

Tetracyclines

Tetracycline antibiotics are of interest because they have anti-inflammatory actions and because some cases of RA may be triggered initially by an infection. Minocycline, one of the tetracyclines being studied, has achieved mixed results. In a favorable 2001 study, 60% of patients taking the agent reported improvement compared with 33% taking the DMARD hydroxychloroquine. An earlier study even suggested that many patients may achieve long-term remission if the medication is administered early in the disease. (Studies on doxycycline, another tetracycline, have reported no benefits.)

Thalidomide

Thalidomide inhibits tumor necrosis factors and other cytokines. It also reduces the formation of new blood vessels that allow the disease to progress. Although it was notorious in the past for causing birth defects, it is now being investigated for many diseases, including rheumatoid arthritis. Severe adverse effects, however, may outweigh any benefits.

Oral Collagen Therapy

Oral type II collagen therapy is based on the theory that by consuming a foreign substance orally, the body will slowly become tolerant to it and will not launch an immune attack against it. Oral collagen (which is consumed in tablet form) appeared to slow the autoimmune process in small 2001 studies on adults and young people with juvenile RA. In one of the studies, 90% of recipients reported improvements in symptoms.

Statins

Interesting research is suggesting that compounds derived from statins, the highly regarded cholesterol-lowering drugs, may suppress inflammation responsible for RA damage.

Hormonal Treatments

Some research is investigating the use of dehydroepiandrosterone (DHEA), a mild male hormone, which has anti-inflammatory effects and which is reduced in RA.

Although estrogen is commonly associated with heightened immune factors, some autoimmune diseases, including RA, improve during pregnancy when levels of estriol, a form of estrogen, are high. (Estriol levels are low at other times.) Investigators are testing estriol on patients with autoimmune diseases. Long-term use may have adverse effects, however, and further research is needed.

NO-NSAIDs

Experimental agents are being developed that combine nitric oxide with NSAIDs (NO-NSAIDs). Combining nitric oxide with NSAIDs may prevent gastrointestinal problems and provide benefits similar to the COX-2 inhibitors.

Licofelone

Licofelone is drug that inhibits both the COX enzyme plus an inflammatory substance called Lipoxygenase 5. Early trials indicate they may be effective and safer than either NSAIDs or COX-2 inhibitors, though further study is needed

Kappa Opioids

Opioids are powerful pain relievers but are not regularly used in RA because of their side effects and risk for dependency. Of some interest, however, are specific agents known as kappa opioids, such as asimadoline, that work in the peripheral nervous system (which affects the limbs in the body not the brain). Some evidence now suggests that they are powerful anti-inflammatory agents and in one study a kappa opioid reduced arthritic pain by 80%. More research is warranted.

Chapter 31

How Occupational and Physical Therapy Can Help Arthritis Patients

How Is Arthritis Treated?

Arthritis means inflammation of the joints and it may cause pain, swelling and limited motion of one or many joints in the body. More than 100 different illnesses can cause arthritis.

Treatment begins after diagnosis by a physician who may prescribe medication to reduce inflammation, pain, swelling, and loss of motion. As part of a comprehensive plan for arthritis treatment, your doctor may also prescribe occupational and physical therapy, which can provide additional help in your recovery.

How Can Occupational Therapists Help?

Occupational therapists can teach you how to reduce strain on your joints during daily activities. They can show you how you can modify your home and workplace environments to reduce motions that may aggravate arthritis. Occupational therapists may also provide splints for your hands or wrists and recommend assistive devices to aid in tasks such as driving, bathing, dressing, housekeeping, and certain work activities.

"How Occupational and Physical Therapy Can Help You" ©2003 The Cleveland Clinic Foundation, 9500 Euclid Avenue, Cleveland, OH 44195, 800-223-2273 ext. 48950, www.clevelandclinic.org. Additional information is available from the Cleveland Clinic Health Information Center, 216-444-3771, or www.clevelandclinic.org/health.

How Can Physical Therapists Help?

Physical therapists provide exercises designed to preserve the strength and use of your joints. They can show you the best way to move from one position to another. They can also teach you how to use walking aids such as crutches, a walker, or a cane when needed.

What Are the Goals of Treatment?

These important members of your health care team will work closely with your doctor to tailor a program to your specific needs, whether your arthritic problems are widespread or confined to one joint or body area.

The goals of treatment are to:

- Prevent loss of use of the joints
- Restore abilities that may have been lost
- Help you adapt to new activity levels
- Maintain your fitness
- Maintain your ability to take part in the activities you choose with minimal help from others

Therapy should be started early in order to: reduce painful symptoms of inflammation, prevent deformity and permanent joint stiffness, and maintain strength in the surrounding muscles. When pain and swelling are better controlled, treatment plans may include exercises to increase range of motion and improve muscle strength and endurance.

What Are Some Benefits of Occupational and Physical Therapy Programs?

- Education about your kind of arthritis, so that you can be a well-informed member of your health care team.
- A dietary plan for overweight people, to reduce the stress of excess weight on supporting joints of the back, legs, and feet. (As yet, no specific diet—other than a diet designed for weight loss—has proven helpful for arthritis.)
- Foot care advice, including choice of well-fitting shoes with shock-absorbing outer soles and sculptured (orthotic) insoles molded exactly to the contour of each foot.

- Therapeutic methods to relieve discomfort and improve performance through various physical techniques and activity modifications.

What Are Some Therapeutic Methods?

Rest

Bed rest helps reduce both joint inflammation and pain and is especially useful when multiple joints are affected and fatigue is a major problem.

Individual joint rest is most helpful when arthritis involves one or only a few joints. Custom splints can be made to rest and support inflamed joints, and a soft collar can support the neck while you are sitting or standing.

Thermal Modalities

Applying ice packs or heating pads, as well as deep heat provided by ultrasound and hot packs, help relieve pain locally. Heat also relaxes muscle spasm around inflamed joints.

Heating joints and muscles with a warm bath or shower before exercising may help you exercise more easily.

Exercise

An important part of arthritis treatment that is most effective when done properly every day. Your doctor and therapist will prescribe a program for you that may vary as your needs change.

- Range-of-motion exercise: Gentle movement of each joint through its normal range of motion will help relieve stiffness, improve and maintain joint movement, and increase flexibility.

- Strengthening exercise: Strengthening exercise helps preserve or increase muscle strength.

- Isometric exercises tighten and strengthen the muscle without moving the joint and are most useful when joints are painful.

- Isotonic exercises strengthen the muscle by using it to move a weight.

- Water exercise: Warm water helps relieve pain and relax muscles. Swimming is not necessary, as water exercises may be done while sitting in a shallow pool or standing in shoulder-high water. Support by the water decreases body weight applied to the joints of the spine, legs, and feet. Water support of the arms and legs also helps you move your joints through range of motion exercises more easily.

- Recreational exercise: Recreational exercise does not replace your therapeutic exercise program, but may enhance it with a variety of enjoyable activities. Some examples are games, sports, exercise classes, running and swimming, all of which can benefit muscle strength and joint range of motion. Running and swimming are excellent aerobic activities and will help improve your endurance and lessen fatigue. Any exercise needs to be tailored to the patient's disease and limitations.

Therapy for Joint Surgery Patients

Preoperative programs of education and exercise, started before surgery in the outpatient therapy department, are continued at home. They may be changed in the hospital after surgery to fit new needs in the rehabilitation period. These exercises may be added to your usual exercise regimen and you may find your ability to exercise has improved after surgery.

Joint Protection Techniques

There are ways to reduce the stress on joints affected by arthritis while participating in daily activities. Some of these are:

- Control your weight to avoid putting extra stress on weight-bearing joints such as back, hips, knees, and feet.

- Be aware of body position, using good posture to protect your back and the joints of your legs and feet. Sit down to do a job when you can instead of standing. Change position often since staying in one position for a long time tends to increase stiffness and pain.

- Conserve energy by allowing for rest periods, both during the day and during an activity.

- Respect pain; it is a body signal that is telling you something is wrong. Don't try an activity that puts strain on joints that are already painful or stiff.

A therapist can show you ways to do everyday tasks without worsening pain or producing joint damage. Some joint protection techniques include:

- Use proper body mechanics to get in and out of a car, chair or tub, as well as for lifting objects.

- Use your strongest joints and muscles to reduce the stress on smaller joints. For example, carry a purse or briefcase with a shoulder strap rather than in your hand.

- Distribute pressure to minimize stress on any one joint. Lift dishes with both palms rather than with your fingers, and carry heavy loads in your arms instead of with your hands.

- If your hands are affected by arthritis, avoid tight gripping, pinching, squeezing, and twisting. Ways to accomplish the same tasks with alternate methods or tools can usually be found.

Assistive Devices

Many assistive devices have been developed to make activities easier and less stressful for the joints and muscles. Your therapist will suggest devices that will be helpful for tasks you may have found difficult at home or work.

A few examples of helpful devices include a bath stool in the shower or tub, grab bars around the toilet or tub, and long-handled shoehorns and sock grippers. Your therapist can show you catalogs that have a wide variety of assistive devices you may order.

Summary

As the central member of your treatment team, you are the person responsible for following through with your therapy program. This includes taking medicines as prescribed, and continuing at home with daily exercises and other suggestions made by your therapist. You should discuss questions and problems as they come up, with your doctor and your therapist, so that the program can be adjusted to best meet your needs.

A positive attitude, patience, and persistence will help you to get the greatest benefit from your occupational and physical therapy activities, which are so important in meeting the challenges of arthritis.

Chapter 32

Surgeries Used to Treat Arthritis

Chapter Contents

Section 32.1

Surgery and Arthritis: What You Need to Know

Excerpted from *Surgery & Arthritis: What You Need to Know.* © 2002. Reprinted with permission of the Arthritis Foundation, 1330 W. Peachtree St., Suite 100, Atlanta, GA 30309. To order a free copy of this brochure or other titles from the Arthritis Foundation, call 800-283-7800 or visit www.arthritis.org.

Surgery Pros and Cons

Arthritis is usually a chronic (lifelong) and progressive condition that can cause pain, disability and deformity. However, there are many ways you and your doctor can lessen these problems. One of these ways may be surgery.

Most people with arthritis will never need to have surgery. Instead, their arthritis is managed by proper medication, exercise, physical and occupational therapy, rest, joint protection and alternative therapies.

Benefits of Surgery

Your doctor may recommend that surgery will help your arthritis. The decision to have surgery should not be made quickly or without good reasons. If you are considering joint surgery, it can offer several benefits:

Improved movement and use of a joint are important benefits of joint surgery. Continuous inflammation and damage to bone and cartilage can lead to loss of use of a joint, such as a hip, knee, hand or ankle, and can seriously hamper your activities. When this happens, surgery to replace or stabilize the joint may be suggested. For example, hip or knee surgery can allow you to stand and walk more easily.

Pain relief is also an important benefit of joint surgery. Many people with arthritis have constant pain. Some of this pain can be relieved by rest, heat and cold treatments, exercise, splints and medication. When these therapies don't lessen the pain, surgery may be considered.

Improved alignment of deformed joints, especially in the hand and knee, can be expected with some types of surgery. However, straightening your joints should not be the main reason for having joint surgery.

Your doctor can tell you what to expect from surgery. In the case of severe joint stiffness and deformity, you can usually expect to have better range of motion and relief of pain. But, remember your joint won't be the same as before it was affected by arthritis.

Before you decide to have surgery, be sure to ask your doctor about the risks and benefits of having surgery versus not having surgery.

Section 32.2

Arthroscopy

What Is Arthroscopy?

Arthroscopy is a surgical procedure orthopaedic surgeons use to visualize, diagnose, and treat problems inside a joint.

The word arthroscopy comes from two Greek words, *arthro* (joint) and *skopein* (to look). The term literally means "to look within the joint." In an arthroscopic examination, an orthopaedic surgeon makes a small incision in the patient's skin and then inserts pencil-sized instruments that contain small lenses and lighting systems to magnify and illuminate the structures inside the joint. Light is transmitted through fiber optics to the end of the arthroscope that is inserted into the joint. By attaching the arthroscope to a miniature television camera, the surgeon is able to see the interior of the joint through this very small incision rather than a large incision needed for surgery.

The television camera attached to the arthroscope displays the image of the joint on a television screen, allowing the surgeon to look, for example, throughout the knee—at cartilage and ligaments and under the kneecap. The surgeon can determine the amount or type of injury, and then repair or correct the problem, if it is necessary.

Why Is Arthroscopy Necessary?

Diagnosing joint injuries and disease begins with a thorough medical history, physical examination, and usually x-rays. Additional tests such as an MRI or CT also scan may be needed. Through the arthroscope, a final diagnosis is made which may be more accurate than through open surgery or from x-ray studies.

Disease and injuries can damage bones, cartilage, ligaments, muscles, and tendons. Some of the most frequent conditions found during arthroscopic examinations of joints are:

- Inflammation: Synovitis is an inflamed lining (synovium) in knee, shoulder, elbow, wrist, or ankle.

- Injury (acute and chronic): Shoulder—rotator cuff tendon tears, impingement syndrome, and recurrent dislocations; knee— meniscal (cartilage) tears, chondromalacia (wearing or injury of cartilage cushion), and anterior cruciate ligament tears with instability; and wrist—carpal tunnel syndrome.

- Loose bodies of bone and/or cartilage: Loose bodies can occur in the knee, shoulder, elbow, ankle, or wrist.

Although the inside of nearly all joints can be viewed with an arthroscope, six joints are most frequently examined with this instrument. These include the knee, shoulder, elbow, ankle, hip, and wrist. As advances are made by engineers in electronic technology and new techniques are developed by orthopaedic surgeons, other joints may be treated more frequently in the future.

How Is Arthroscopy Performed?

Arthroscopic surgery, although much easier in terms of recovery than open surgery, still requires the use of anesthetics and the special equipment in a hospital operating room or outpatient surgical suite. You will be given a general, spinal, or a local anesthetic, depending on the joint or suspected problem.

A small incision (about the size of a buttonhole) will be made to insert the arthroscope. Several other incisions may be made to see other parts of the joint or insert other instruments.

When indicated, corrective surgery is performed with specially designed instruments that are inserted into the joint through accessory incisions. Initially, arthroscopy was simply a diagnostic tool for planning standard open surgery. With development of better instrumentation and surgical techniques, many conditions can be treated arthroscopically.

For instance, most meniscal tears in the knee can be treated successfully with arthroscopic surgery.

Some problems associated with arthritis also can be treated. Several disorders are treated with a combination of arthroscopic and standard surgery.

- Rotator cuff procedure

- Repair or resection of torn cartilage (meniscus) from knee or shoulder

- Reconstruction of anterior cruciate ligament in knee

- Removal of inflamed lining (synovium) in knee, shoulder, elbow, wrist, or ankle

- Release of carpal tunnel

- Repair of torn ligaments

- Removal of loose bone or cartilage in knee, shoulder, elbow, ankle, or wrist

After arthroscopic surgery, the small incisions will be covered with a dressing. You will be moved from the operating room to a recovery room. Many patients need little or no pain medications.

Before being discharged, you will be given instructions about care for your incisions, what activities you should avoid, and which exercises you should do to aid your recovery. During the follow-up visit, the surgeon will inspect your incisions; remove sutures, if present; and discuss your rehabilitation program.

The amount of surgery required and recovery time will depend on the complexity of your problem. Occasionally, during arthroscopy, the surgeon may discover that the injury or disease cannot be treated adequately with arthroscopy alone. The extensive open surgery may be performed while you are still anesthetized or at a later date after you have discussed the findings with your surgeon.

What Are the Possible Complications?

Although uncommon, complications do occur occasionally during or following arthroscopy. Infection, phlebitis (blood clots of a vein), excessive swelling or bleeding, damage to blood vessels or nerves, and instrument breakage are the most common complications, but occur in far less than 1 percent of all arthroscopic procedures.

What Are the Advantages?

Although arthroscopic surgery has received a lot of public attention because it is used to treat well-known athletes, it is an extremely valuable tool for all orthopaedic patients and is generally easier on the patient than open surgery. Most patients have their arthroscopic surgery as outpatients and are home several hours after the surgery.

Recovery after Arthroscopy

The small puncture wounds take several days to heal. The operative dressing can usually be removed the morning after surgery and adhesive strips can be applied to cover the small healing incisions.

Although the puncture wounds are small and pain in the joint that underwent arthroscopy is minimal, it takes several weeks for the joint to maximally recover. A specific activity and rehabilitation program may be suggested to speed your recovery and protect future joint function.

It is not unusual for patients to go back to work or school or resume daily activities within a few days. Athletes and others who are in good physical condition may in some cases return to athletic activities within a few weeks. Remember, though, that people who have arthroscopy can have many different diagnoses and preexisting conditions, so each patient's arthroscopic surgery is unique to that person. Recovery time will reflect that individuality.

Section 32.3

Osteotomy and Unicondylar Bone Replacement

Total joint replacement (arthroplasty) is a common and very successful surgery for people with degenerative arthritis (osteoarthritis) of the knee. Two other surgeries can also restore knee function and significantly diminish osteoarthritis pain in carefully selected patients. If osteoarthritis damage to your knee meets certain qualifications, a doctor may recommend either osteotomy or unicompartmental knee arthroplasty (UKA).

Osteoarthritis Damage to the Knee

A normal knee glides smoothly because articular cartilage covers the ends of the bones that form joints. Osteoarthritis damages the cartilage, progressively wearing it away. The ends of the bones become rough like pieces of sandpaper. Damaged cartilage can cause the joint to stick or lock when you use it. Your knee may get painful, stiff, and lose range of motion. See your doctor to diagnose osteoarthritis.

Provide your complete medical history including detailed descriptions of osteoarthritis symptoms and when they began. Have you tried nonsurgical treatments such as rest, weight loss, and nonsteroidal anti-inflammatory medication for pain? Does it hurt too much to get dressed, bathe, or walk upstairs? The doctor will check your knee's range of motion, ligament stability and angular deformity. He or she will observe your knees while you stand and walk, and examine your hips, feet, and ankles. Both knees will probably be x-rayed.

Your doctor's recommendation of a surgical procedure for osteoarthritis knee repair depends in part upon how it is damaged. The knee has three joints (compartments), any or all of which can be impacted by osteoarthritis:

- The inside (medial) compartment (medial tibial plateau and medial femoral condyle) is most commonly involved, producing a bowleg (genu varum) deformity.

- The outside (lateral) compartment (lateral tibial plateau and lateral femoral condyle) is sometimes involved in women or obese people, producing a knock-knee (genu valgum) deformity.

- The kneecap (patellofemoral) compartment (patella and femoral trochlear notch) may also develop osteoarthritis.

If you have early stage arthritis confined to one part of the knee, your doctor may recommend osteotomy or UKA.

Osteotomy

Osteotomy may be appropriate if you are younger than age 60, active, or overweight. There must also be uneven damage to the joint, correctable deformity, and no inflammation. The surgeon reshapes the shinbone (tibia) or thighbone (femur) to improve your knee's alignment. The healthy bone and cartilage is realigned to compensate for the damaged tissue. Knee osteotomy surgically repositions the joint, realigning the mechanical axis of the limb away from the diseased area. This lets your knee glide freely and carry weight evenly on a more normal compartment.

- Proximal tibial valgus osteotomy treats arthritis of the medial compartment, correcting a knee that angles inward (varus deformity).

- Distal femoral varus osteotomy treats arthritis of the lateral compartment, correcting a knee that angles outward (valgus deformity).

The doctor may use one of several techniques to hold the joint in place (i.e., immobilization with a cast, staples, or internal plate devices).

Osteotomy relieves pain and may delay the progression of osteoarthritis. Cosmetically, the knee may not look symmetrical after osteotomy. There's a chance you will eventually need total knee arthroplasty (TKA), which can be a more technically challenging procedure after you've had an osteotomy. Infections and other complications are possible. Depending upon how quickly you heal, you will need to walk with crutches for 1 to 3 months. After that you begin rehabilitative leg strengthening and walking exercises. You may be able to resume your full activities after 3 to 6 months.

Unicompartmental Knee Arthroplasty

Unicompartmental knee arthroplasty (UKA) may be appropriate if you are age 60 or older, not obese, and relatively sedentary. Among other specific qualifications, your knee must have:

- An intact anterior cruciate ligament (ACL)
- No significant inflammation
- No damage to the other compartments, calcification of cartilage, or dislocation

Your doctor will verify that your knee meets the requirements when he or she begins the surgery. (Note: If your knee does not meet the qualifications, you may need TKA.) The surgeon removes diseased bone and puts an implant (prosthesis) in its place. The two small replacement parts are secured to the rest of your knee. You can get UKA surgery on both knees at the same time if you need it.

UKA alleviates pain and may delay the need for TKA. You get better joint motion and function because the procedure preserves both cruciate ligaments and other healthy parts of the knee. You also keep the bone stock in the kneecap joint and the other compartment, which can be helpful if you ever need conversion to TKA in the future. Complications are rare, but the new joint could develop an infection or slip out of place after surgery. For these reasons, your doctor may want to see you for follow-up visits after surgery. You will have to do range of motion and other physical therapy exercises to rehabilitate your knee. Recovery from UKA is faster than from TKA or osteotomy.

Although UKA was a controversial procedure when it was first introduced about 30 years ago, success rates have improved thanks to precise patient selection, refined surgical techniques, and improved implant design. UKA has a higher initial success rate and fewer complications compared with osteotomy. Other advantages include less blood loss during surgery and cheaper cost.

Section 32.4

Total Joint Replacement

What Is Total Joint Replacement?

An arthritic or damaged joint is removed and replaced with an artificial joint called a prosthesis.

What Is a Joint?

A joint is formed by the ends of two or more bones, which are connected by thick tissues. For example, your knee joint is formed by the lower leg bone, called the tibia or shinbone, and your thighbone, called the femur. Your hip is a ball and socket joint, formed by the upper end of the femur, the ball, and a part of the pelvis called the acetabulum, the socket.

The bone ends of a joint are covered with a smooth layer called cartilage. Normal cartilage allows nearly frictionless and pain-free movement. However, when the cartilage is damaged or diseased by arthritis, joints become stiff and painful. Every joint is enclosed by a fibrous tissue envelope or a capsule with a smooth tissue lining called the synovium. The synovium produces fluid that reduces friction and wear in a joint.

Why Is Total Joint Replacement Necessary?

The goal is to relieve the pain in the joint caused by the damage done to the cartilage. The pain may be so severe, a person will avoid using the joint, weakening the muscles around the joint and making it even more difficult to move the joint. A physical examination, possibly some laboratory tests, and x-rays will show the extent of damage to the joint. Total joint replacement will be considered if other treatment options will not relieve your pain and disability.

How Is a Total Joint Replacement Performed?

You will be given an anesthetic and the surgeon will replace the damaged parts of the joint. For example, in an arthritic knee the damaged ends of the bones and cartilage are replaced with metal and plastic surfaces that are shaped to restore knee movement and function. In an arthritic hip, the damaged ball (the upper end of the femur) is replaced by a metal ball attached to a metal stem fitted into the femur, and a plastic socket is implanted into the pelvis, replacing the damaged socket. Although hip and knee replacements are the most common, joint replacement can be performed on other joints, including the ankle, foot, shoulder, elbow, and fingers.

The materials used in a total joint replacement are designed to enable the joint to move just like your normal joint. The prosthesis is generally composed of two parts: a metal piece that fits closely into a matching sturdy plastic piece. Several metals are used, including stainless steel, alloys of cobalt and chrome and titanium. The plastic material is durable and wear-resistant (polyethylene). A plastic bone cement may be used to anchor the prosthesis into the bone. Joint replacements also can be implanted without cement when the prosthesis and the bone are designed to fit and lock together directly.

What Is the Recovery Process?

In general, your orthopaedist will encourage you to use your new joint shortly after your operation. After total hip or knee replacement, you will often stand and begin walking the day after surgery. Initially, you will walk with a walker, crutches, or a cane.

Most patients have some temporary pain in the replaced joint because the surrounding muscles are weak from inactivity and the tissues are healing, but it will end in a few weeks or months.

Exercise is an important part of the recovery process. Your orthopaedic surgeon or the staff will discuss an exercise program for you after surgery. This varies for different joint replacements and for differing needs of each patient.

After your surgery, you may be permitted to play golf, walk, and dance. However, more strenuous sports, such as tennis or running, may be discouraged.

The motion of your joint will generally improve after surgery. The extent of improvement will depend on how stiff your joint was before the surgery.

What Are the Possible Complications?

Tell your orthopaedic surgeon about any medical conditions that might affect the surgery. Joint replacement surgery is successful in more than 9 out of 10 people. When complications occur, most are successfully treatable. Possible complications include:

- Infection—Infection may occur in the wound or deep around the prosthesis. It may happen while in the hospital or after you go home. It may even occur years later. Minor infections in the wound area are generally treated with antibiotics. Major or deep infections may require more surgery and removal of the prosthesis. Any infection in your body can spread to your joint replacement.

- Blood Clots—Blood clots result from several factors, including your decreased mobility, causing sluggish movement of the blood through your leg veins. Blood clots may be suspected if pain and swelling develop in your calf or thigh. If this occurs, your orthopaedic surgeon may consider tests to evaluate the veins of your leg. Several measures may be used to reduce the possibility of blood clots, including: blood thinning medications (anticoagulants); elastic stockings; exercises to increase blood flow in the leg muscles; and plastic boots that inflate with air to compress the muscles in your legs. Despite the use of these preventive measures, blood clots may still occur. If you develop swelling, redness, or pain in your leg following discharge from the hospital, you should contact your orthopaedic surgeon.

- Loosening—Loosening of the prosthesis within the bone may occur after a total joint replacement. This may cause pain. If the loosening is significant, a revision of the joint replacement may be needed. New methods of fixing the prosthesis to bone should minimize this problem.

- Dislocation—Occasionally, after total hip replacement the ball can be dislodged from the socket. In most cases, the hip can be relocated without surgery. A brace may be worn for a period of time if a dislocation occurs. Most commonly, dislocations are more frequent after complex revision surgery.

- Wear—Some wear can be found in all joint replacements. Excessive wear may contribute to loosening and may require revision surgery.

394

- Prosthetic breakage—Breakage of the metal or plastic joint replacement is rare, but can occur. A revision surgery is necessary if this occurs.

- Nerve injury—Nerves in the vicinity of the total joint replacement may be damaged during the total replacement surgery, although this type of injury is infrequent. This is more likely to occur when the surgery involves correction of major joint deformity or lengthening of a shortened limb due to an arthritic deformity. Over time these nerve injuries often improve and may completely recover.

Preparing for Total Joint Replacement

Before surgery, your orthopaedic surgeon will make some recommendations, such as suggesting that you:

- donate some of your own blood so that, if needed, you may receive it during or after surgery

- stop taking some drugs before surgery

- begin exercises to speed your recovery after surgery

- evaluate your need for discharge planning, home therapy, and rehabilitation after surgery

Is Total Joint Replacement Permanent?

Most older people can expect their total joint replacements to last a decade or more. It will give years of pain-free living that would not have been possible otherwise. Younger joint replacement patients may need a second total joint replacement. Materials and surgical techniques are improving through the efforts of orthopaedists working with engineers and other scientists. The future is bright for those who choose to have a total joint replacement to achieve an improved quality of life through greater independence and healthier pain-free activity.

Chapter 33

Hip Replacement

Chapter Contents

Section 33.1

Questions and Answers about Hip Replacement

National Institute of Arthritis and Musculoskeletal and Skin Diseases (NIAMS), January 2001. Available online at http://www.niams.nih.gov; accessed March 2004.

What Is a Hip Replacement?

Hip replacement, or arthroplasty, is a surgical procedure in which the diseased parts of the hip joint are removed and replaced with new, artificial parts. These artificial parts are called the prosthesis. The goals of hip replacement surgery are to improve mobility by relieving pain and improve function of the hip joint.

Who Should Have Hip Replacement Surgery?

The most common reason that people have hip replacement surgery is the wearing down of the hip joint that results from osteoarthritis. Other conditions, such as rheumatoid arthritis (a chronic inflammatory disease that causes joint pain, stiffness, and swelling), avascular necrosis (loss of bone caused by insufficient blood supply), injury, and bone tumors also may lead to breakdown of the hip joint and the need for hip replacement surgery.

Before suggesting hip replacement surgery, the doctor is likely to try walking aids such as a cane, or non-surgical therapies such as medication and physical therapy. These therapies are not always effective in relieving pain and improving the function of the hip joint. Hip replacement may be an option if persistent pain and disability interfere with daily activities. Before a doctor recommends hip replacement, joint damage should be detectable on x-rays.

In the past, hip replacement surgery was an option primarily for people over 60 years of age. Typically, older people are less active and put less strain on the artificial hip than do younger, more active people. In recent years, however, doctors have found that hip replacement surgery can be very successful in younger people as well. New technology has improved the artificial parts, allowing them to withstand more stress and strain. A more important factor than age in determining the success of hip replacement is the overall health and activity level of the patient.

For some people who would otherwise qualify, hip replacement may be problematic. For example, people with chronic diseases such as those that result in severe muscle weakness or Parkinson's disease are more likely than people without chronic diseases to damage or dislocate an artificial hip. Because people who are at high risk for infections or in poor health are less likely to recover successfully, doctors may not recommend hip replacement surgery for these patients.

What Are Alternatives to Total Hip Replacement?

Before considering a total hip replacement, the doctor may try other methods of treatment, such as an exercise program and medication. An exercise program can strengthen the muscles in the hip joint and sometimes improve positioning of the hip and relieve pain.

The doctor also may treat inflammation in the hip with nonsteroidal anti-inflammatory drugs, or NSAIDs. Some common NSAIDs are aspirin and ibuprofen. NSAIDs also include Celebrex and Vioxx, so-called COX-2 inhibitors that block an enzyme known to cause an inflammatory response. Many of these medications are available without a prescription, although a doctor also can prescribe NSAIDs in stronger doses.

In a small number of cases, the doctor may prescribe corticosteroids, such as prednisone or cortisone, if NSAIDs do not relieve pain. Corticosteroids reduce joint inflammation and are frequently used to treat rheumatic diseases such as rheumatoid arthritis. Corticosteroids are not always a treatment option because they can cause further damage to the bones in the joint. Some people experience side effects from corticosteroids such as increased appetite, weight gain, and lower resistance to infections. A doctor must prescribe and monitor corticosteroid treatment. Because corticosteroids alter the body's natural hormone production, patients should not stop taking them suddenly and should follow the doctor's instructions for discontinuing treatment.

If physical therapy and medication do not relieve pain and improve joint function, the doctor may suggest corrective surgery that is less complex than a hip replacement, such as an osteotomy. Osteotomy is surgical repositioning of the joint. The surgeon cuts away damaged bone and tissue and restores the joint to its proper position. The goal of this surgery is to restore the joint to its correct position, which helps to distribute weight evenly in the joint. For some people, an osteotomy relieves pain. Recovery from an osteotomy takes 6 to 12 months. After an osteotomy, the function of the hip joint may continue to worsen and the patient may need additional treatment. The length of time before another surgery is needed varies greatly and depends on the condition of the joint before the procedure.

What Does Hip Replacement Surgery Involve?

The hip joint is located where the upper end of the femur meets the acetabulum. The femur, or thigh bone, looks like a long stem with a ball on the end. The acetabulum is a socket or cup-like structure in the pelvis, or hip bone. This ball and socket arrangement allows a wide range of motion, including sitting, standing, walking, and other daily activities.

During hip replacement, the surgeon removes the diseased bone tissue and cartilage from the hip joint. The healthy parts of the hip are left intact. Then the surgeon replaces the head of the femur (the ball) and the acetabulum (the socket) with new, artificial parts. The new hip is made of materials that allow a natural, gliding motion of the joint. Hip replacement surgery usually lasts 2 to 3 hours.

Sometimes the surgeon will use a special glue, or cement, to bond the new parts of the hip joint to the existing, healthy bone. This is referred to as a cemented procedure. In an uncemented procedure, the artificial parts are made of porous material that allows the patient's own bone to grow into the pores and hold the new parts in place. Doctors sometimes use a hybrid replacement, which consists of a cemented femur part and an uncemented acetabular part.

Is a Cemented or Uncemented Prosthesis Better?

Cemented prostheses were developed 40 years ago. Uncemented prostheses were developed about 20 years ago to try to avoid the possibility of loosening parts and the breaking off of cement particles, which sometimes happen in the cemented replacement. Because each person's condition is unique, the doctor and patient must weigh the advantages and disadvantages to decide which type of prosthesis is better.

For some people, an uncemented prosthesis may last longer than cemented replacements because there is no cement that can break away. And, if the patient needs an additional hip replacement (which is likely in younger people), also known as a revision, the surgery sometimes is easier if the person has an uncemented prosthesis.

The primary disadvantage of an uncemented prosthesis is the extended recovery period. Because it takes a long time for the natural bone to grow and attach to the prosthesis, people with uncemented replacements must limit activities for up to 3 months to protect the hip joint. The process of natural bone growth also can cause thigh pain for several months after the surgery.

Research has proven the effectiveness of cemented prostheses to reduce pain and increase joint mobility. These results usually are noticeable immediately after surgery. Cemented replacements are more frequently used than cementless ones for older, less active people and people with weak bones, such as those who have osteoporosis.

What Can Be Expected Immediately after Surgery?

Patients are allowed only limited movement immediately after hip replacement surgery. When the patient is in bed, the hip usually is braced with pillows or a special device that holds the hip in the correct position. The patient may receive fluids through an intravenous tube to replace fluids lost during surgery. There also may be a tube located near the incision to drain fluid and a tube (catheter) may be used to drain urine until the patient is able to use the bathroom. The doctor will prescribe medicine for pain or discomfort.

How Long Are Recovery and Rehabilitation?

On the day after surgery or sometimes on the day of surgery, therapists will teach the patient exercises that will improve recovery. A respiratory therapist may ask the patient to breathe deeply, cough, or blow into a simple device that measures lung capacity. These exercises reduce the collection of fluid in the lungs after surgery.

A physical therapist may teach the patient exercises, such as contracting and relaxing certain muscles, that can strengthen the hip. Because the new, artificial hip has a more limited range of movement than an undiseased hip, the physical therapist also will teach the patient proper techniques for simple activities of daily living, such as bending and sitting, to prevent injury to the new hip. As early as 1 to 2 days after surgery, a patient may be able to sit on the edge of the bed, stand, and even walk with assistance.

Usually, people do not spend more than 10 days in the hospital after hip replacement surgery. Full recovery from the surgery takes about 3 to 6 months, depending on the type of surgery, the overall health of the patient, and the success of rehabilitation.

How to Prepare for Surgery and Recovery

People can do many things before and after they have surgery to make everyday tasks easier and help speed their recovery.

Before Surgery

- Learn what to expect before, during, and after surgery. Request information written for patients from the doctor or contact one of the organizations listed near the end of this document.

- Arrange for someone to help you around the house for a week or two after coming home from the hospital.

- Arrange for transportation to and from the hospital.

- Set up a recovery station at home. Place the television remote control, radio, telephone, medicine, tissues, waste basket, and pitcher and glass next to the spot where you will spend the most time while you recover.

- Place items you use every day at arm level to avoid reaching up or bending down.

- Stock up on kitchen staples and prepare food in advance, such as frozen casseroles or soups that can be reheated and served easily.

After Surgery

- Follow the doctor's instructions.

- Work with a physical therapist or other health care professional to rehabilitate your hip.

- Wear an apron for carrying things around the house. This leaves hands and arms free for balance or to use crutches.

- Use a long-handled reacher to turn on lights or grab things that are beyond arm's length. Hospital personnel may provide one of these or suggest where to buy one.

What Are Possible Complications of Hip Replacement Surgery?

According to the American Academy of Orthopaedic Surgeons, approximately 120,000 hip replacement operations are performed each year in the United States and less than 10 percent require further surgery. New technology and advances in surgical techniques have greatly reduced the risks involved with hip replacements.

The most common problem that may happen soon after hip replacement surgery is hip dislocation. Because the artificial ball and socket are smaller than the normal ones, the ball can become dislodged from the socket if the hip is placed in certain positions. The most dangerous position usually is pulling the knees up to the chest.

The most common later complication of hip replacement surgery is an inflammatory reaction to tiny particles that gradually wear off of the artificial joint surfaces and are absorbed by the surrounding tissues. The inflammation may trigger the action of special cells that eat away some of the bone, causing the implant to loosen. To treat this complication, the doctor may use anti-inflammatory medications or recommend revision surgery (replacement of an artificial joint). Medical scientists are experimenting with new materials that last longer and cause less inflammation.

Less common complications of hip replacement surgery include infection, blood clots, and heterotopic bone formation (bone growth beyond the normal edges of bone).

When Is Revision Surgery Necessary?

Hip replacement is one of the most successful orthopaedic surgeries performed—more than 90 percent of people who have hip replacement surgery will never need revision surgery. However, because more younger people are having hip replacements, and wearing away of the joint surface becomes a problem after 15 to 20 years, revision surgery is becoming more common. Revision surgery is more difficult than first-time hip replacement surgery, and the outcome is generally not as good, so it is important to explore all available options before having additional surgery.

Doctors consider revision surgery for two reasons: if medication and lifestyle changes do not relieve pain and disability, or if x-rays of the hip show that damage has occurred to the artificial hip that must be corrected before it is too late for a successful revision. This surgery is usually considered only when bone loss, wearing of the joint surfaces, or joint loosening shows up on an x ray. Other possible reasons for revision surgery include fracture, dislocation of the artificial parts, and infection.

What Types of Exercise Are Most Suitable for Someone with a Total Hip Replacement?

Proper exercise can reduce joint pain and stiffness and increase flexibility and muscle strength. People who have an artificial hip should talk to their doctor or physical therapist about developing an appropriate exercise program. Most exercise programs begin with safe range-of-motion activities and muscle strengthening exercises. The doctor or therapist will decide when the patient can move on to more demanding activities. Many doctors recommend avoiding high-impact activities, such as basketball, jogging, and tennis. These activities can damage the new hip or cause loosening of its parts. Some recommended exercises are cross-country skiing, swimming, walking, and stationary bicycling. These exercises can increase muscle strength and cardiovascular fitness without injuring the new hip.

What Hip Replacement Research Is Being Done?

To help avoid unsuccessful surgery, researchers are studying the types of patients most likely to benefit from a hip replacement. Researchers also are developing new surgical techniques, materials, and designs of prostheses, and studying ways to reduce the inflammatory response of the body to the prosthesis. Other areas of research address recovery and rehabilitation programs, such as home health and out-patient programs.

Where Can People Find More Information about Hip Replacement Surgery?

National Institute of Arthritis and Musculoskeletal and Skin Diseases
1 AMS Circle
Bethesda, MD 20892-3675
Toll-Free: (877) 22-NIAMS (226-4267)
Phone: (301) 495-4484
TTY: (301) 565-2966
Fax: (301) 718-6366

Website: http://www.niams.nih.gov
E-mail: niamsinfo@mail.nih.gov

American Academy of Orthopaedic Surgeons (AAOS)
6300 North River Road
Rosemont, IL 60018-4262
Toll-Free: (800) 824-BONE (2663)
Phone: (847) 823-7186
Fax: (847) 823-8125
Website: http://www.aaos.org
E-mail: custserv@aaos.org

Hip Society
951 Old County Road, #182
Belmont, CA 94002
Phone: (650) 596-6190
Fax: (650) 508-2039
Website: http://www.hipsoc.org

American Physical Therapy Association
1111 North Fairfax Street
Alexandria, VA 22314-1488
Toll-Free: (800) 999-2782, X3395
Phone: (703) 684-2782
Fax: (703) 684-7343
TDD: (703) 683-6748
Website: http://www.apta.org

Arthritis Foundation
1330 West Peachtree Street
Atlanta, GA 30309
Toll-Free: (800) 283-7800
Phone: (404) 872-7100
Website: http://www.arthritis.org

Section 33.2

Scientists Identify Risk Factors for Hip Replacement in Women

"Scientists Identify Two Key Risk Factors for Hip Replacement in Women," National Institute of Arthritis and Musculoskeletal and Skin Diseases (NIAMS), June 2003. Available online at http://www.niams.nih.gov; accessed December 2003.

Researchers funded by the National Institute of Arthritis and Musculoskeletal and Skin Diseases have determined that excess body weight and older age increase a woman's chances of needing a total hip replacement to treat osteoarthritis.

Matthew Liang, M.D., M.P.H., Elizabeth Karlson, M.D., and Lisa Mandl, M.D., M.P.H., and their colleagues at Harvard Medical School studied 568 participants from the ongoing Nurses Health Study who received a hip replacement to treat hip osteoarthritis. The researchers examined risk factors—including body mass index, use of hormones after menopause, age, alcohol consumption, physical inactivity and cigarette smoking—for hip replacement. Of these potential risk factors, only body mass index and age were associated with needing a hip replacement. Body mass index is a standard measure of weight in relation to height and is used to estimate body fat. Participants with a high body mass index showed double the risk of having a hip replacement compared with low body mass index participants. The risk from obesity appeared to be established early in life. Participants who had a high body mass index at age 18 showed five times the risk of receiving a hip replacement to treat hip osteoarthritis later in life. Women age 70 and older were nine times more likely to have a hip replacement compared with those under age 55.

According to the authors, this is one of the first long-term prospective studies to show an association between a modifiable risk factor and osteoarthritis. Results suggest that reducing weight may improve quality of life and decrease health care costs related to osteoarthritis.

The Nurses Health Study, from which data were drawn, is one of the largest studies of risk factors for chronic diseases in women. Over 116,000 women are enrolled.

Osteoarthritis is a degenerative joint disease in which cartilage, the slippery tissue that covers the ends of bones in a joint, wears away. This allows bones under the cartilage to rub together, causing pain, swelling, and loss of motion of the joint. Osteoarthritis is one of the most frequent causes of physical disability among adults. It mostly occurs in older people but can also affect younger men and women.

Support for this study was also provided by the National Cancer Institute and the Arthritis Foundation. NIAMS and the National Cancer Institute are part of the National Institutes of Health (NIH), the Federal Government's primary agency for biomedical and behavioral research. NIH is a component of the U.S. Department of Health and Human Services.

Karlson E, Mandl L, Aweh G, Sangha O, Liang M, Grodstein F. Total hip replacement due to osteoarthritis: The importance of age, obesity, and other modifiable risk factors. *Am J Med* 2003;114:93–98.

Chapter 34

Knee Replacement

This chapter provides information for you and your family regarding total knee replacement surgery. The surgical procedure, preoperative and postoperative care, the risks and benefits of surgery, as well as rehabilitation, are explained.

What Is Total Knee Replacement?

Total knee replacement is a surgical procedure in which injured or damaged parts of the knee joint are replaced with artificial parts. The procedure is performed by separating the muscles and ligaments around the knee to expose the knee capsule (the tough, gristle-like tissue surrounding the knee joint). The capsule is opened, exposing the inside of the joint. The ends of the thighbone (femur) and the shinbone (tibia) are removed and often the underside of the kneecap (patella) is removed. The artificial parts are cemented into place. Your new knee will consist of a metal shell on the end of the femur, a metal and plastic trough on the tibia, and if needed, a plastic button in the kneecap.

"Total Knee Replacement: A Patient Guide," produced by the Orthopedic Nursing Division, Department of Nursing, University of Iowa Hospitals and Clinics, Iowa City, Iowa 52242. Copyright protected material used with permission of the authors and the University of Iowa's Virtual Hospital, www.vh.org. Revised December 1999. Reviewed by David A. Cooke, M.D., on February 29, 2004.

Who Is a Candidate for a Total Replacement?

Total knee replacements are usually performed on people suffering from severe arthritic conditions. Most patients who have artificial knees are over age 55, but the procedure is also occasionally performed in younger people.

The circumstances vary somewhat, but generally you would be considered for a total knee replacement if:

- You have daily pain.

- Your pain is severe enough to restrict not only work and recreation but also the ordinary activities of daily living.

- You have significant stiffness of your knee.

- You have significant instability (constant giving way) of your knee.

- You have significant deformity (lock knees or bowlegs).

- Other treatments, such as physical therapy or medication, do not give adequate relief

What Can I Expect from an Artificial Knee?

An artificial knee is not a normal knee, nor is it as good as a normal knee. The operation will usually provide pain relief for at least ten years.

If replacement provides you with pain relief and if you do not have other health problems, you should be able to carry out many normal activities of daily living. The artificial knee rarely allows you to return to active sports or heavy labor, but this will depend on your physician's instructions. Activities that overload the artificial knee must be avoided. About 90 percent of patients with stiff knees before surgery will have better motion after a total knee replacement.

What Are the Risks of Total Knee Replacement?

Total knee replacement is a major operation. About one patient in four develops one or more complications. The effect of most complications is that you must stay in the hospital longer.

The most common complications are not directly related to the knee and usually do not affect the result of the operations. These complications include urinary tract infection, blood clots in a leg, or blood clots in a lung.

Complications affecting the knee are less common, but in these cases the operation may not be as successful. These complications include:

- some knee pain
- loosening of the prosthesis
- stiffness
- infection in the knee

A few complications such as infection, loosening of prosthesis, and stiffness may require reoperation. Infected artificial knees sometimes have to be removed. This is a very serious complication, and usually results in a stiff leg about one to three inches shorter than normal. However, your leg would usually be reasonably comfortable, and you would be able to walk with the aid of a cane or crutches and a shoe lift. After a course of antibiotics, the surgery can often be repeated.

How Long Do Artificial Knees Last?

About 85 to 90 percent of total knee replacements are successful up to ten years. The major long-term problem is loosening. This occurs because either the cement crumbles (as old mortar in a brick building) or the bone melts away (resorbs) from the cement. By ten years, 25 percent of total knee replacements may look loose on x-ray, and about 10 percent will be painful and require reoperation. By ten years, possibly 20 percent may require reoperation.

Loosening is in part related to your weight and activity. For that reason, total knee replacement usually is not performed on very obese or young patients. A loose, painful artificial knee can usually, but not always, be replaced. The results of a second operation are not as good as the first and the risks of complication are higher.

Preparing for Surgery

Preparing for a total knee replacement begins several weeks ahead of the actual surgery date. Sometimes this can be done at your local community hospital. Maintaining good physical health before your operation is important. Activities that will increase upper body strength will improve your ability to use a walker or crutches after the operation.

A blood transfusion is often necessary after knee surgery. You may wish to donate several pints of blood prior to your surgery. Then if you require a transfusion you will receive your own blood. This is called autologous blood donation. The first donation must be given within 42 days of the surgery and the last no less than seven days before your surgery. The usual amount of donation is two to four units, which requires separate visits to the blood center. The first donation must be given at this hospital, but the blood bank personnel will make arrangements to have the rest drawn at a blood center nearer your home. Blood taken elsewhere is transported here automatically, so you will not need to get involved with this.

When donating blood, you must be healthy and without a cold, flu, or infection because you could get this same illness when your blood is transferred at the time of surgery. Eat a nourishing meal two to four hours prior to donation, and avoid strenuous exercise for twelve hours following the procedure.

The blood donor center will check the blood count before drawing additional units. A prescription for iron will be given. Iron may be constipating for some people, so sometimes a stool softener is prescribed. Stool softeners can also be purchased over the counter.

You may be a candidate for autotransfusion after your surgery. Blood collected from the wound drain is filtered and transfused back to the patient early in the postoperative period. The physician will assist you in deciding whether this procedure will be done.

The physician may order blood tests and urinalysis two weeks before surgery to make sure that a urinary tract infection is not present. Urinary tract infections are common, especially in older women, and often go undetected. Teeth need to be in good condition. An infected tooth or gum may also be a possible source of infection for the new knee. The orthopaedic physician may ask you to see your medical doctor, especially if medical problems have been present in the past.

When making preparations for surgery, you should begin thinking about the recovery period following surgery. A patient with a new total knee replacement will need help at home for the first several weeks. Assistance with activities such as dressing and getting meals may be necessary. Most often, discharge from the hospital is anticipated in about one week. Your energy level will not have returned. If assistance from someone at home is not possible, it may be necessary to think about making arrangements to stay a few weeks in an extended care facility. A social worker is available at the hospital to plan an extended period of recovery if necessary.

Preoperative Visit

Most patients need to make a visit to the hospital a few days before their actual surgery date for a preoperative visit. This visit usually lasts several hours, so plan to spend most of the day. The day begins in the clinic, where an interview by the nursing staff concerning past medical history and current medications will be taken, as well as a chest x-ray. You may be instructed to stop taking your anti-inflammatory medications (such as ibuprofen, Naprosyn, Relafen, Daypro, and aspirin) one week before surgery.

Diet. You should follow your regular diet on the day before your surgery. Do not eat or drink after midnight. The day of surgery you may brush your teeth and rinse your mouth without swallowing any water.

Bathing. A shower, bath, or sponge bath should be taken the evening before and morning of surgery. You may be given antiseptic scrub brushes to use. Using the spongy side, scrub your knee for a period of five minutes. This may require assistance from a family member. The brushes contain a special soap that will reduce the risk of infection. If you are allergic to iodine or soap, please inform a nurse. If possible, you should shampoo your hair. Nail polish and makeup should be removed.

Deep breathing exercises. You may be instructed to use deep breathing exercises to minimize the risk of lung complications after surgery. These exercises are necessary to remove any excess secretions that may settle in your lungs while you are asleep during surgery. These exercises are to be done every one or two hours after surgery. An incentive spirometer may be demonstrated. This bedside device assists you in deep breathing exercises.

Blood clot prevention. You may be fitted with elastic support stockings. You should wear them on both legs to the hospital the morning of your surgery. These stockings aid the circulation of your legs and feet to reduce the risk of blood clots.

Anesthesia. You may be scheduled for an appointment with the anesthesiologist to discuss how you will be put to sleep. The anesthesiologist will advise you about taking routine medications on the day of your surgery.

Pain control. Patient-controlled anesthesia (PCA) is the preferred method of pain control for the first two to three days after your surgery. When the PCA is discontinued, your doctor will prescribe pain medication to be taken by mouth. It is important to continue taking the medication because preventing pain is easier than chasing it. If you continue to experience pain after taking the medication, notify your doctor or nurse so alternate methods of pain control can be started.

The physician will also review your medical history and the medications that you take. He or she will listen to your heart and lungs and do a general physical exam. He or she will check for any type of infection. Any blisters, cuts, or boils should be reported. If infection is found, surgery is generally delayed until the infection is cleared.

During your preoperative visit, blood will be drawn and lab tests done to ensure that you are in good general health. X-rays are taken if necessary. Chest x-rays and an electrocardiogram (EKG) are obtained if you have not had one taken for six months or if otherwise indicated. After all of these tests and exams are completed, an anesthesiologist will talk with you to determine the type of anesthesia that is best suited for you. After you see the anesthesiologist, your preoperative evaluation is usually over.

Before you leave the hospital make sure your questions are answered. If at any time you become ill, such as with a cold or flu, you need to call your physician.

Day of Surgery

You will be admitted to the hospital the day of your surgery. You will be taken to a presurgical care unit where an intravenous (IV) is started for the administration of fluids and medications during and after the surgical procedure. From there you will be transported to the operating room by your anesthesiologist.

The actual surgical procedure may take two to four hours. However, preoperative preparation as well as wake-up time may make your operating room and recovery room stay longer.

After Surgery

After surgery you will be taken to the recovery room for a period of close observation, usually one to three hours. Your blood, pressure, pulse, respiration and temperature will be checked frequently. Close attention will be paid to the circulation and sensation in your legs and feet. It is important to tell your nurse if you experience numbness, tingling, or pain in your legs or feet. When you awaken and your condition is stabilized, you will be transferred to your room.

Although circumstances vary from patient to patient, you will likely have some or all of the following after surgery:

- You will find that a large dressing has been applied to the surgical area to maintain cleanliness and absorb any fluid. This dressing is usually changed 2 to 4 days after surgery by the surgeon.

- A hemovac suction container with tubes leading directly into the surgical area enables the nursing staff to measure and record the amount of drainage being lost from the wound following surgery. The hemovac is usually removed by your doctor two to three days after surgery.

- An intravenous (IV) line, started prior to surgery, will continue until you are taking adequate amounts of fluid by mouth. When you are taking fluids well, the IV may be changed to a Heparin Lock, a small sterile tube that will keep a vein accessible for antibiotics and allow for easier movement. Antibiotics are frequently administered every eight hours, for two to three days, to reduce the risk of infection.

- One side effect of anesthesia is often a difficulty in urinating after surgery. For this reason, a sterile tube called a catheter may be inserted into your bladder to insure a passageway for urine. This may remain in place for one to two days.

- Besides the elastic hose, you will also have on compression stocking sleeves. This is a plastic sleeve that is connected to a machine that circulates air in the plastic and around your legs. This is another method of promoting blood flow and decreasing the chances of blood clots. You will also be given medications and exercise instructions (moving your ankles up and down), which also helps to prevent clots.

- Postoperatively you may have temporary nausea and vomiting due to anesthesia or medications. Anti-nausea medication may be given to minimize the nausea and vomiting.

- You will be allowed to progress your diet as your condition permits; starting with ice chips and clear liquids.

- A knee immobilizer will be worn as directed by your physician.

- To help prevent complications, such as congestion or pneumonia, deep breathing and coughing exercises are important. Inhale

415

deeply through your nose; then slowly exhale through your mouth. Repeat this three times and then cough two times. You will be encouraged to use your incentive spirometer.

- In order to speed your rehabilitation, you may be using a continuous passive motion (CPM) machine. It is a device that is fit to your leg and is placed in bed with you. It slowly and smoothly bends and straightens your knee. You will use the machine periodically during the day, and it will be adjusted to increase the bend in your knee.

- You will be assisted into the chair the first day after surgery provided there are no complications. Physical therapy is started one to two days after surgery. It is very important for you to have pain medication 30 minutes before going to physical therapy to help you fully participate in exercises. Please discuss this with your nurse.

How well you regain strength and motion is, in part, dependent upon how well you follow your physical therapy. This part of your rehabilitation is something that you must do for yourself, and not something someone else does for you. If there are no complications after surgery, most patients stay in the hospital approximately one week.

Exercise Program and Physical Therapy

When muscles are not used, they become weak and do not perform well in supporting and moving the body. Your leg muscles are probably weak because you haven't used them much due to your knee problems. The surgery can correct the knee problem, but the muscles will remain weak and will only be strengthened through regular exercise. You will be assisted and advised how to do this, but the responsibility for exercising is yours.

Your overall progress, amount of pain, and condition of the incision will determine when you will start going to physical therapy. If no problems arise, your doctor will have you start one to two days after surgery. You will work with a physical therapist until you are:

- independent in getting in and out of bed.

- independent in walking with crutches or a walker on a level surface.

- independent in walking up and down three stairs.

- independent in your home exercise program.
- able to bend your knee 90 degrees.
- able to straighten your knee.

Your doctor and therapist may modify these goals somewhat to fit your particular condition.

In your physical therapy sessions you will walk, using crutches or a walker, bearing as much weight as indicated by your doctor or physical therapist. You will also work on an exercise program designed to strengthen your leg and increase the motion of your knee.

The continuous passive motion machine may be ordered. The machine is used to maintain motion. However, this is not a substitute for your exercises. You may wear a knee immobilizer at night for comfort and to help keep your knee straight.

Your exercise program may include the following exercises:

Quadriceps Setting

The quadriceps is a set of four muscles located on the front of the thigh and is important in stabilizing and moving your knee. These muscles must be strong if you are to walk after surgery. A quad set is one of the simplest exercises that will help strengthen them.

Lie on your back with legs straight, together, and flat on the bed, arms by your side. Perform this exercise one leg at a time. Tighten the muscles on the top of one of your thighs. At the same time, push the back of your knee downward into the bed. The result should be straightening of your leg. Hold for 5 seconds, relax 5 seconds; repeat 10 times for each leg.

You may start doing this exercise with both legs the day after surgery before you go to physical therapy. The amount of pain will determine how many you can do, but you should strive to do several every hour. The more you can do, the faster your progress will be. Your nurses can assist you to get started.

Terminal Knee Extension

This exercise helps strengthen the quadriceps muscle. It is done by straightening your knee joint.

Lie on your back with a blanket roll under your involved knee so that the knee bends about 30 to 40 degrees. Tighten your quadriceps and straighten your knee by lifting your heel off the bed. Hold 5 seconds, then slowly your heel to the bed. You may repeat 10 to 20 times.

Knee Flexion

Each day you will bend your knee. The physical therapist will help you find the best method to increase the bending (flexion) of your knee. Every day you should be able to flex it a little further. Your therapist will measure the amount of bending and send a daily report to your doctor.

In addition, your therapist may add other exercises as he or she deems necessary for your rehabilitation.

Straight Leg Raising

This exercise helps strengthen the quadriceps muscle also. Bend the uninvolved leg by raising the knee and keeping the foot flat on the bed. Keeping your involved leg straight, raise the leg about 6 to 10 inches. Hold for 5 seconds. Lower the leg slowly to the bed and repeat 10 to 20 times.

Once you can do 20 repetitions without any problems, you can add resistance (such as sandbags) at the ankle to further strengthen the muscles. The amount of weight is increased in one-pound increments.

Use of Heat and Ice

Ice may be used during your hospital stay and at home to help reduce the pain and swelling in your knee. Pain and swelling will slow your progress with your exercises. A bag of crushed ice may be placed in a towel over your knee for 15 to 20 minutes. Your sensation may be decreased after surgery, so use extra care.

If your knee is not swollen, hot, or painful, you may use heat before exercising to assist with gaining range of motion. A moist heating pad or warm damp towels may be used for 15 to 20 minutes. Your sensation may be decreased after surgery, so use extra care.

Guidelines at Home

What happens after I go home?

Medication

- You will continue to take medications as prescribed by your doctor.

- You will be sent home on prescribed medications to prevent blood clots. Your doctor will determine whether you will take a pill (Coumadin or coated aspirin) or give yourself a shot (Enoxaparin). If an injection is necessary, your doctor will discuss it with you, and the nursing staff will teach you or a family member what is necessary to receive this medication.

- You will be sent home on prescribed medications to control pain. Plan to take your pain medication 30 minutes before exercises. Preventing pain is easier than chasing pain. If pain control continues to be a problem, call your doctor.

Activity

- Continue to walk with crutches/walker.

- Bear weight and walk on the leg as much as is comfortable.

- Walking is one of the better kinds of physical therapy and for muscle strengthening.

- However, walking does not replace the exercise program that you are taught in the hospital. The success of the operation depends to a great extent on how well you do the exercises and whether your weakened muscles become stronger.

- If excess muscle aching occurs, you should cut back on your exercises. Continue to wear your knee immobilizer as instructed. It may be worn at night to keep your knee straight.

Other Considerations

- For the next four to six weeks, avoid sexual intercourse. Sexual activity can usually be resumed after your two-month follow-up appointment.

- You can usually return to work within three to six months or as instructed by your doctor.

- You should not drive a car until after the two-month follow-up appointment.

- Continue to wear elastic stockings until your return appointment.

- No shower or tub bath until after the staples are removed.

- When using heat or ice, remember not to get your incision wet before your staples are removed.

Your Incision

Keep the incision clean and dry. Also, upon returning home, be alert for certain warning signs. If any swelling, increased pain, drainage from the incision site, redness around the incision, or fever is noticed, report this immediately to the doctor. Generally, the staples are removed in three weeks.

Prevention of Infection

If at any time (even years after the surgery) an infection develops such as strep throat or pneumonia, notify your physician. Antibiotics should be administered promptly to prevent the occasional complication of distant infection localizing in the knee area. This also applies if any teeth are pulled or dental work is performed. Inform the general physician or dentist that you have had a joint replacement. You will be given a medical alert card. This should be carried in your billfold or wallet. It will give information on antibiotics that are needed during dental or oral surgery or if a bacterial infection develops.

Should I Have a Total Knee Replacement?

Total knee replacement is an elective operation. The decision to have the operation is not made by the doctor, it is made by you.

The physician may recommend the operation, but your decision must be based upon your weighing the benefits of the operation against the risks.

All your questions should be answered before you decide to have the operation.

Chapter 35

Alternative and Complementary Pain Management Techniques

Chapter Contents

421

Section 35.1

Questions and Answers about Glucosamine and Chondroitin

"Questions & Answers—NIH Glucosamine/Chondroitin Arthritis Intervention Trial (GAIT)," National Institutes of Health National Center for Complementary and Alternative Medicine (NCCAM), May 2002. Available online at http://www.nccam.nih.gov; accessed March 2004.

What Is the National Institutes of Health (NIH) Glucosamine/Chondroitin Arthritis Intervention Trial (GAIT)?

GAIT is the first multicenter clinical trial in the United States to test the effects of the dietary supplements glucosamine and chondroitin for treatment of knee osteoarthritis. The study will test whether glucosamine and chondroitin used separately or in combination are effective in reducing pain and improving functional ability in patients with knee osteoarthritis. GAIT includes an additional study (or substudy) that will assess whether glucosamine and chondroitin can reduce or halt the progression of knee osteoarthritis.

The University of Utah School of Medicine was awarded a contract to coordinate this study, which will be conducted at 13 research centers across the United States. The National Center for Complementary and Alternative Medicine (NCCAM) and the National Institute of Arthritis and Musculoskeletal and Skin Diseases (NIAMS) are two components of the National Institutes of Health (NIH) that are responsible for initiating this study.

What Is the Purpose of the Study?

Results of previous studies in the medical literature have yielded conflicting results on the effectiveness of glucosamine and chondroitin as treatments for osteoarthritis. This study will test the short-term (6 months) effectiveness of glucosamine and chondroitin in reducing pain and improving function in a large number of patients with knee osteoarthritis.

The study will also evaluate the impact of glucosamine and chondroitin on progression of knee osteoarthritis following an additional 18-month treatment regimen.

What Prompted the NIH to Study Glucosamine and Chondroitin for Osteoarthritis?

On January 27, 1998, the NCCAM held a meeting to discuss the need, rationale, and feasibility of conducting a Phase III study (a human study involving over 1,000 patients to test the efficacy, safety, and side effects of a substance(s)) of glucosamine and chondroitin for the treatment of knee osteoarthritis. Meeting participants included experts in osteoarthritis, alternative medicine, biostatistics, and family practice and staff of the NIH and the U.S. Food and Drug Administration. The group determined that there is a real and urgent public health need to test these agents in a rigorous way, and that current scientific data support short-term testing of glucosamine and chondroitin for pain control and functional improvement of osteoarthritis.

What Is the Basic Design of the Study?

In this study, patients will be randomly assigned to receive either (1) glucosamine alone, (2) chondroitin alone, (3) glucosamine and chondroitin in combination, (4) celecoxib (brand name Celebrex®), or (5) a placebo (an inactive substance that looks like the study substance). Glucosamine and chondroitin and their combination will be compared to a placebo to verify that these substances significantly improve joint pain and flexibility. Celecoxib, which is an established effective conventional treatment for osteoarthritis, will also be compared to placebo to validate the study design. To reduce the chance of biased results, double-blind research procedures will be used to ensure that neither the researchers nor the patients will know to which of the five treatment groups the patients belong.

In the main or primary study, each patient will be treated for 24 weeks. During this time, patients will be evaluated at 4-, 8-, 16-, and 24-week intervals and closely monitored for improvement of their symptoms as well as for any possible adverse reactions to the agents. Medical evaluations and x-rays will be used to document each patient's diagnosis. The primary outcome will be measured as improvement in pain. Improvement in function will be included as a secondary outcome. All patients will have the option to use acetaminophen (e.g.,

Tylenol®) as required to control severe pain from osteoarthritis throughout the clinical trial.

In the substudy, which will evaluate the progression of knee osteoarthritis, about one-half of the patients enrolled in GAIT will receive blinded treatment for an additional 18 months. As in the primary study, patients will not know to which treatment group they are assigned. Researchers will compare x-rays taken at the beginning of the study and after 1 and 2 years of treatment. Then they will compare and evaluate x-rays from all substudy participants to identify changes in the knee joints as a result of treatment.

How Many Patients Are Needed and When Will the Study Begin?

A total of 1,588 people will be recruited for the study. Recruitment is currently open.

Who Will Be Eligible to Participate in the Study?

Patients with knee pain and x-ray evidence of osteoarthritis are encouraged to consider participation in the study. People who are interested in the study must not have used glucosamine for 3 months and chondroitin for 6 months prior to entering the study.

What Is Osteoarthritis?

An estimated 21 million adults in the United States live with osteoarthritis—one of the most common types of arthritis.

Osteoarthritis, also called degenerative joint disease, is caused by the breakdown of cartilage, which is the connective tissue that cushions the ends of bones within the joint. It is characterized by pain, joint damage, and limited motion. The disease generally occurs late in life, and most commonly affects the hands and large weight-bearing joints. Although the disease can impact several joints, the knees are often affected. Age, female gender, and obesity are risk factors for this condition.

What Are Glucosamine and Chondroitin?

Glucosamine and chondroitin are natural substances found in and around the cells of cartilage. Researchers believe these substances may help in the repair and maintenance of cartilage. In addition, researchers believe that glucosamine inhibits inflammation and stimulates cartilage cell growth, while chondroitin provides cartilage with strength and resilience. Currently, glucosamine and chondroitin are classified as dietary supplements.

What Is a Dietary Supplement?

A dietary supplement is a product (other than tobacco) intended to supplement the diet, which bears or contains one or more of the following dietary ingredients: a vitamin, mineral, amino acid, herb, or other botanical; is intended for ingestion in the form of a capsule, powder, softgel, or gelcap; and is not represented as a conventional food or as a sole item of a meal or the diet (as defined by the U.S. Dietary Supplement Health and Education Act, Oct. 25, 1994).

What Is Celecoxib?

Celecoxib (brand name Celebrex®) is a new type of nonsteroidal anti-inflammatory drug (NSAID), called a COX-2 inhibitor. Like traditional NSAIDs, celecoxib blocks the COX-2 enzyme in the body that stimulates inflammation. Unlike traditional NSAIDs, however, celecoxib does not block the action of COX-1 enzyme, which is known to protect the stomach lining. As a result, celecoxib reduces joint pain and inflammation with reduced risk of gastrointestinal ulceration and bleeding.

Section 35.2

Complementary and Alternative Therapies for Arthritis

This information was written by Michael Loes, MD, and is reprinted with permission from The National Pain Foundation, www.painconnection.org.

Used alone or in combination with other forms of treatment, complementary approaches to arthritis pain relief include:

- Acupuncture—Originating in China, this age-old practice involves inserting long, extremely slender needles into specific points along the body to relieve pain and discomfort.

- Biofeedback—This involves a learning process whereby certain visual or auditory (sound-based) feedback allows you to train yourself to initiate responses that help control or normalize your psychological response to pain.

- Chiropractic—According to the International Chiropractic Association, the primary focus of chiropractic is the detection, reduction, and correction of spinal misalignments and nervous system dysfunction. Doctors of chiropractic attempt to get to the root cause of a health problem, rather than just treat the symptoms. Chiropractic seeks to maximize the natural strengths of the body and its capacity to heal itself without the use of drugs or surgery.

- Hypnosis—This involves entering an altered state of consciousness whereby suggestions inserted while in that state can lead to changes in behavior or, in the case of pain, altered physical sensations. Self-hypnosis involves inducing an altered state of consciousness—and thus controlling pain sensation—by yourself.

- Visual Imagery—The practice of using one's imagination to create mental pictures can help relieve pain—why it works isn't understood. Typically, this involves closing your eyes and imaging something like a healing energy washing over your body or the "wires" to the pain being severed.

Complementary therapies can be used to supplement medications or can be used alone or in combination with other forms of therapy. Complementary techniques to manage pain include diet, exercise, biofeedback, massage, chiropractic care, acupuncture, and self-regulation techniques such as self-hypnosis, relaxation training, yoga, Reiki (a natural healing process using the hands to tap a universal life energy), and Jin Shin Jyutsu (a process to balance the body's energies to bring optimal health and well-being).

The quality of research supporting these approaches varies from therapy to therapy. In some cases, the research is of better quality than that supporting the use of some medications and many surgical procedures. In other cases, the research is not as strong. As with any treatment approach, use of complementary therapies should be discussed with your doctor.

Homeopathic Medicine

Homeopathy is an alternative, non-toxic approach used to treat illness and relieve discomfort in a wide range of health conditions. Founded in Germany in the late 1860s, the practice of homeopathy is based on using the law of similars to stimulate a healing response—a principle that goes back to the days of Hippocrates. The law of similars states that a substance that will cause disease symptoms in a normal person can, when given in homeopathic dilutions to an ill individual, prompt the same set of symptoms to initiate a healing response. Homeopathic preparations, called remedies, must be prepared in a certain way, and the dilution used will depend on the symptoms being treated. Make sure you consult with your physician before taking traditional and homeopathic remedies at the same time. Mixing medications can result in harmful medical interactions.

Complementary Therapies for Arthritis

Following are complementary pain management approaches for the most common types of arthritis.

Osteoarthritis

Diet

Following are some dietary changes people with osteoarthritis have found helpful. However, be patient! Changing your diet may not provide immediate relief.

Fish Oils. These have long been part of arthritis treatment. More than 100 years ago, British doctors gave their patients cod liver oil to alleviate rheumatism. Today, researchers have validated that fish oils are important for relieving arthritis pain. Seafood rich in omega-3 fatty acids, the type of oil shown to be beneficial, include salmon, tuna, sardine, herring, anchovies, and mackerel. Omega-3-enriched eggs, pasta, and other products also are coming on the market.

Vegetarian Diets. In addition to helping to reduce the risk of heart disease and other maladies, vegetarian diets also appear to play a positive role in arthritis, according to several studies. One study found that 90 percent of the patients studied found their grip strength improved, and they had less pain and swelling, morning stiffness, and tenderness after one month on vegetarian diets.

Exercise

Until recently, arthritis sufferers were advised to rest their painful, inflamed joints. But gradually, doctors have learned that exercise can be beneficial. Exercise strengthens muscles, ligaments, and tendons, which compensates for weakened joints; flushes fluids cartilage, drawing nutrients in and toxins out; stimulates healthy cell regeneration; and limbers and tones the entire body. Many forms of exercise are beneficial, including stretching, bicycling, low-impact aerobics, dancing, golf, walking, water calisthenics, yoga, tai chi, and even climbing stairs.

Go slowly but consistently. Three to four times a week, for a total of three to four hours, is the ultimate goal. Start easy. Build up gradually. Listen to your body and don't force it to do something that is painful, such as sitting cross-legged for yoga. If you are suffering from severe arthritis, heart disease, or other health problems, work with your health care professional to develop a safe exercise program. Most experts agree that if exercise causes pain that lasts more than one hour, you have exercised too much.

Topical Analgesics

Salves, creams, and ointments can provide relief for muscle aches or mild pain in a few joints, according to the Arthritis Foundation. They also can be an adjunct to oral arthritis medications. The active ingredients in such preparations include: counterirritants, such as menthol, eucalyptus oil, or wintergreen oil, which essentially distract the brain from feeling arthritis pain; salicylates, which like salicylates (aspirin) found in oral painkillers, inhibit prostaglandins, the substances that contribute to inflammation and pain; and capsaicin, extracted from cayenne peppers, which acts on the substance that sends pain messages to the brain.

Rheumatoid Arthritis

Diet

Avoiding certain foods—such as dairy products, wheat, corn, and tomatoes and their relatives—may help prevent rheumatoid arthritis attacks. As a result, many doctors suggest that their arthritis patients eliminate milk, cheese, and other dairy products from their diets. Tofu cheeses and soy milk can be substituted. Wheat and corn, used as main ingredients, additives, and fillers in food and over-the-counter and medical drugs, can be hard to avoid, but eliminating them from the diet also helps some rheumatoid arthritis sufferers. It's important to check all food labels and medical packages for wheat and corn ingredients. Some rheumatoid arthritis patients also feel better and have fewer flare-ups when they eliminate from their diets members of the nightshade family, which includes tomatoes, eggplants, and bell peppers.

Foods also may help arthritis sufferers. Fish oils have long been part of arthritis treatment. More than 100 years ago, British doctors gave their patients cod liver oil to alleviate rheumatism. Today, researchers have validated that certain fish oils help relieve rheumatoid arthritis pain. Seafoods rich in omega-3 fatty acids, the type of oil shown to be beneficial, include salmon, tuna, sardine, herring, anchovies, and mackerel. Omega-3-enriched eggs, pasta, and other products also are coming on the market.

Vegetarian diets, in addition to reducing the risk of heart disease and other maladies, also appear to play a positive role in relieving arthritis pain, according to several studies. One report found that 90 percent of the patients studied had better grip strength and less pain and swelling, morning stiffness, and tenderness after one month on vegetarian diets.

Exercise

Gentle exercise can help rheumatoid arthritis patients stay healthy and flexible. The Arthritis Foundation recommends putting joints through their full range of motion once a day, with periods of rest during acute systemic or local joint arthritis flare-ups. Consult your doctor about what type and how much exercise is best for your particular condition.

Ankylosing Spondylitis

Early diagnosis and treatment of this condition is critical to controlling pain and stiffness and perhaps plays a part in preventing the bones in the neck and back from fusing. In women, ankylosing spondylitis (AS), or spinal arthritis, often is mild and difficult to diagnose. Treatment is tailored to the individual.

Diet

AS patients may be helped by eating less starchy foods (bread, pasta, and potatoes) and more protein.

Exercise

Deep breathing exercises and aerobic conditioning help keep the rib cage and chest flexible. Swimming is often recommended for AS patients, as is sleeping on a firm mattress.

Gout

To help prevent recurrences, gout patients should drink plenty of fluids, avoid alcohol, and eat less protein and purines (found in yeast extracts, fish roe and herrings).

Some overweight individuals find that if they lose weight, their uric acid levels decrease.

Systemic Lupus Erythematosus (SLE)

SLE patients may benefit from fish oil and from diets that are low calories and low fat. Avoiding animal proteins can help protect the kidneys. Researchers also are investigating compounds called indoles, also known as mustard oil, which are found in broccoli, cabbage, Brussels sprouts, cauliflower, kale, kohlrabi, collard and mustard greens, rutabaga, turnips and bok choy. Indoles stimulate enzymes that convert estrogen—which has been linked to SLE flare-ups—to a more benign type.

Chapter 36

Integrative Medicine Treatments and Lifestyle Changes to Help Arthritis

Exercise

It is important to maintain a balance between rest (which will reduce inflammation) and exercise (which will relieve stiffness and weakness). Studies have suggested that even as little as three hours of physical therapy over six weeks will help people with rheumatoid arthritis (RA), and that these benefits are sustained.

The goal of exercise is the following:

- To maintain a wide range of motion.
- To increase strength, endurance, and mobility.
- To improve general health.
- To promote well-being.

In general, some patients recommend the following approaches:

- Start with the easiest exercises, stretching and tensing of the joints without movement.
- Next attempt mild strength training. (One study found that people with RA who exercised with machines that use compressed air for gentle resistance experienced less pain and increased muscle tone.)

Excerpted from "Rheumatoid Arthritis" © 2003 A.D.A.M., Inc. Reprinted with permission.

- Aerobic exercises may then be tried, for example, walking, dancing, or swimming, particularly in heated pools.

- Avoid heavy impact exercises such as running, downhill skiing, and jumping.

- Tai chi, which uses graceful slow sweeping movements, is an excellent method for combining stretching and range-of-motion exercises with relaxation techniques. It is of particularly value for elderly RA patients who report significantly less pain after practicing this technique.

While traditional guidelines have restricted RA patients to only gentle exercise, recent research suggests that more intense exercise may not only be safe, but may actually produce greater muscle strength and overall functioning. Common sense is the best guide:

- If exercise is causing sharp pain, stop immediately.

- If lesser aches and pains continue for more than two hours afterwards, then a lighter exercise program should be tried for a while.

- Using large joints instead of small ones for ordinary tasks can help relieve pressure, for instance, closing a door with the hip or pushing buttons with the palm of the hand.

Diet

Fad diets for RA are common. Some claims include the following:

- Some people claim that foods from the nightshade family (tomatoes, potatoes, green peppers, and eggplant) can exacerbate arthritis.

- The Dong Diet eliminates all additives, preservatives, fruits, red meat, herbs, alcohol, and dairy.

- A few studies have reported that vegetarian diets may be helpful for some patients. In one study, 40% of patients who were on a vegetarian diet and avoided foods containing gluten (found in wheat, barley, and rye) reported improved scores.

- In another study high total caloric intake correlated with worse symptoms.

Little scientific evidence of benefits for RA exists for any of these diets, and some may result in deficiencies of important nutrients. On the other hand, one interesting study in England found that 10 out of 17 people benefited from any diet recommended by their doctor.

Mediterranean Diet

Perhaps the best recommendation is for the Mediterranean Diet. A 2003 study reported that RA patients who followed it experienced reduced inflammatory activity, improved physical function and improved vitality compared to those on a standard Western diet. The Mediterranean diet is also rich in heart-healthy fiber and nutrients, omega-3 fatty acids, and antioxidants. The diet recommends the following:

- A relatively high fat intake (about 35% to 45% of daily calories), but mostly from monounsaturated and polyunsaturated oils. The Mediterranean diet is known specifically for its use of olive oil. One 1999 study found some evidence that high intake of olive oil and cooked vegetables reduced the risk of RA.

- Daily glass or two of wine.

- Protein source with this diet is primarily fish, which might be specifically helpful for RA patients. Fish (particularly—but not only—oily fish) have anti-inflammatory effects. It should be noted that protein is lost during the inflammatory process, and one study indicated that high amounts of protein might be protective. Either fish or soy should, in any case, be the primary sources of protein. (Although not included in the Mediterranean diet, soy may have specific benefits for RA.) Some evidence also suggests that fish oil supplements might be helpful.

- Carbohydrate choices emphasize fresh fruits, vegetables, nuts, legumes, beans, and whole grains.

- Foods seasoned with garlic, onions, and herbs.

Coffee and Tea

A 2002 study reported an association between RA and decaffeinated coffee but not regular coffee. Furthermore, drinking tea was associated with a lower risk.

Vitamins

Certain vitamin supplements may be beneficial. For example, certain drugs used for RA deplete folic acid, a critical vitamin B. Some patients take antioxidant supplements, such as vitamins C and E and selenium, although there is no strong evidence supporting their benefits. (Some studies have reported some possible benefits with vitamin E or other antioxidant combinations when used with standard medications.) Patients should check with their physicians about the need for supplements.

Miscellaneous Supportive Treatments

Various ointments, including Ben Gay and capsaicin (a cream that use the active ingredient in chilies) may help soothe painful joints.

Orthotic devices are specialized braces and splints that support and help align joints. Many such devices made from a variety of light materials are available and can be very beneficial when worn properly.

A number of specially designed appliances and devices are available to ease daily activities.

Managing Psychological and Emotional Conditions

Although the influence of stress or emotions on the progression of RA is not fully known, having a history of major depression that persists or reoccurs seems to increase the pain, disability, and fatigue. Stress management alone cannot reduce pain, but it may be very helpful in helping people deal with their condition. One interesting 1999 study found that people with RA reported significant clinical improvement after writing about their pain, stress, or other traumatic experiences. Writing for 20 minutes, just a few days a week, resulted in improvement that lasted for months. A 2001 study found that spirituality (defined as "a belief in a power outside oneself and one's own existence," as opposed to the practice of any specific religion) is associated with better health, happiness and well-being among RA patients. (Spiritual healing does not appear to offer any advantages.)

Alternative and Integrative Medicine

People often turn to alternative therapies or nontraditional remedies to relieve the pain of rheumatoid arthritis. Some alternative procedures, such as acupuncture, therapeutic touch, massage, relaxation techniques, biofeedback, and hypnosis, are nearly always harmless as long as they are not used as substitutes for proven treatments. Some examples are the following:

- In one small 2001 British study, acupuncture reduced pain by a third in 73% of patients, and more than half reported at least a

50% improvement in pain. Patients reduced their use of pain medications from 17 to six tablets per week on average.

- Balneotherapy, also known as hydrotherapy or spa therapy, is an ancient form of therapy that involves mineral baths to soothe pain, and some patients have reported relief using such baths.

A number of herbal remedies have been used traditionally in treating RA, including boswellia, equisetum arvense (horsetail), devil's claw, and many others. Herbal or other remedies can be of some concern, however, as the ingredients in over-the-counter herbal or natural remedies are not regulated or controlled.

Part Five

Coping with Arthritis

Chapter 37

Caring for Yourself When You Have Arthritis

Chapter Contents

Section 37.1

Health-Related Quality of Life among People with Arthritis

Arthritis is the leading cause of disability in the U.S. In 2003, arthritis and other rheumatic conditions affected 70 million people—a number that is expected to climb as the baby boom generation ages. That's almost 33 percent of the population.

Arthritis conditions don't usually cause death, but they do worsen health-related quality of life. Arthritis is the leading cause of disability in the United States, limiting the everyday activities of more than 7 million Americans. Arthritis results in 39 million physician visits and almost 2.5 million hospitalizations each year.

Findings on the impact of arthritis by the Centers for Disease Control and Prevention (CDC) show people with arthritis have worse health-related quality of life than people without it, regardless of sex, age or education level. From 1996 to 1998, the CDC interviewed more than 32,000 people in 11 states about:

- their general self-rated health.
- the frequency of days in which their physical health was not good.
- the frequency of days in which their mental health was not good.
- the frequency of days in which their usual activities were limited.

Overall, the CDC found about 29 percent of people with arthritis. Doctors had diagnosed most of these people (75 percent). Others had symptoms of pain, aching, stiffness, or swelling in or around a joint on most days for at least a month.

The prevalence of arthritis among the respondents having either chronic joint symptoms or doctor-diagnosed arthritis was:

- Sex: women—33%; men—25%

- Age group: 18- to 44-year-olds—16%; 45- to 64-year-olds—39%; 65 years and older—53%

- Education level: Less than high school—41%; High school graduate or some college—30%; College graduate—21%

People with arthritis reported having fair or poor health about three times more often than did people without arthritis. The CDC says "unhealthy days" are days in which physical and/or mental health was not good. Among arthritis sufferers, the most unhealthy days were experienced by:

- women

- younger people

- people with less than a college education

Depression is common in people with all types of arthritis, especially rheumatoid arthritis. For people with less education, unhealthy days may reflect less access to health care or more physical labor, the CDC says.

Prevailing myths have portrayed arthritis as an inevitable part of aging that can only be endured. But the CDC says there are effective interventions that are available to prevent or reduce arthritis-related pain and disability. These include early diagnosis and appropriate management, including weight control, physical activity, physical and occupational therapy, and joint replacement, when necessary.

Section 37.2

Protecting Your Joints

Joint protection involves using them wisely to preserve them and help reduce the risk of damage—or further damage if you already have damage due to arthritis or injuries. This may require finding new ways to do things and using helpful equipment—or asking other people for help.

Respect Pain

- Perform activities only up to the point of slight fatigue or discomfort. Then take a break—at least until pain disappears before starting again.

- Recognize that pain lasting more than two hours after an activity is a warning sign. Don't push yourself that far again.

- Use a warm heating pad for morning pain and stiffness, or use ice packs on warm and swollen joints.

- Ask your physician about alternate activities if your exercise regimen is causing you significant pain. For example, if playing tennis exacerbates your pain, try swimming instead.

- Discuss any persistent pain with your physician.

Plan Ahead—Balance Your Activities

- Prioritize your daily activities, making sure to include rest and relaxation, as well as work and exercise.

- Spread out light and heavy tasks throughout the day.

- Be realistic about what you can do. Delegate tasks that will put you at risk for injury, or just ask for help.

- Do the exercises your physician recommends for your specific condition. Get involved in additional exercise—as long as it's appropriate for you—since building muscle around the joints protects them.

- Conserve your energy. Make sure the supplies you use most are the easiest to reach, which may require the installation of lower shelves. Sit often. Eliminate unnecessary tasks. Use electric appliances rather than your own muscle power whenever possible.

- Enhance flexibility and mobility by changing your position frequently. Stretch every 15 minutes when writing or using a computer. Avoid long periods of standing, sitting, and lying down.

Distribute Work over Your Body, Using Your Largest, Strongest Joints

- Avoid placing excessive weight or strain on any single joint. Spread the weight of an object or task over several joints to limit the stress on a single joint. Get the shoulder, elbow, and wrist involved in lifting—not just the fingers. For example, lift, carry, and hold items with both hands or arms. Use both hands or the side of your body to open heavy doors. Hold small items in the palm of your hand, not your fingers.

- Keep items close to your body. "Hugging" packages is safer than carrying them on one side or in one hand.

- Use a bag with shoulder straps rather than holding it in your hand, if it is heavy.

- When using stairs, lead with your strong leg as you go up the stairs and with your weaker leg as you go down. This will limit the stress on the weaker joints. Use a hand rail.

Use Joints in Their Most Stable Position

- For example, if you have wrist problems, don't stir by rotating your wrist. Instead, grip the spoon in your fist, with the spoon end exiting on the pinky side of your hand, and stir (thumb up) using your whole arm and keeping the wrist stable.

- Avoid twisting motions. This is especially important for people who have back or hip pain—and for those with hand problems. Wringing motions stress fingers and encourage deformities.

443

Don't wring out washcloths; just drape them over the faucet to dry. This also may require a little home redecorating to replace your doorknobs with lever door opening devices.

Maintain Correct Posture

- Keep your back straight, especially important when lifting large objects.

- Bend at the knees and hips, not at the waist.

- Separate feet to widen your base of support.

- Keep the item you are lifting close to your body.

- Stand on a low, stable footstool when reaching for high objects.

- Use a firm chair with good arms and back support. Use a tall chair to make sitting down and standing easier.

- Seek exercises that strengthen your posture.

- Get familiar with ergonometrics, especially if your work requires constant sitting or repetitive motion. Your company's human resources department may be able to help.

Control Your Weight

- Losing extra pounds can make a difference in your prognosis. For example, your knees sustain an impact three to five times your body weight when you descend stairs. If you weigh 200 pounds, that means up to 1,000 pounds banging on your knees. If you are very overweight, any loss of weight will be beneficial.

- Get advice from your physician about a healthy diet for you. Remember that excess weight contributes to additional, more threatening diseases, which could, in turn, further limit your mobility—diabetes, heart disease, stroke.

Use Adaptive Devices and Techniques

- Use built-up handles made of foam or plastic for holding toothbrushes, pencils, and pens.

- Alternate hands when opening and closing jars or use a special device designed for people with limited strength or motion in their hands.

- Use reachers or other devices to pick up items from the floor or to retrieve them from a high shelf.

- Wear proper safety equipment, e.g., knee or wrist pads.

- Use a spiked cutting board for preparing vegetables to keep them stable and you safe.

- Check out Web sites, catalogs and stores that sell products specifically designed for people with arthritis or other conditions that limit movement.

Chapter 38

Questions and Answers about Arthritis and Exercise

This chapter answers general questions about arthritis and exercise. The amount and form of exercise recommended for each individual will vary depending on which joints are involved, the amount of inflammation, how stable the joints are, and whether a joint replacement procedure has been done. A skilled physician who is knowledgeable about the medical and rehabilitation needs of people with arthritis, working with a physical therapist also familiar with the needs of people with arthritis, can design an exercise plan for each patient.

What is arthritis?

There are over 100 forms of arthritis and other rheumatic diseases. These diseases may cause pain, stiffness, and swelling in joints and other supporting structures of the body such as muscles, tendons, ligaments, and bones. Some forms can also affect other parts of the body, including various internal organs.

Many people use the word arthritis to refer to all rheumatic diseases. However, the word literally means joint inflammation; that is, swelling, redness, heat, and pain caused by tissue injury or disease in the joint.

National Institute of Arthritis and Musculoskeletal and Skin Diseases (NIAMS), May 2001. Available online at http://www.niams.nih.gov; accessed March 2004.

The many different kinds of arthritis comprise just a portion of the rheumatic diseases. Some rheumatic diseases are described as connective tissue diseases because they affect the body's connective tissue—the supporting framework of the body and its internal organs. Others are known as autoimmune diseases because they are caused by a problem in which the immune system harms the body's own healthy tissues. Examples of some rheumatic diseases are:

- osteoarthritis
- rheumatoid arthritis
- fibromyalgia
- systemic lupus erythematosus
- scleroderma
- juvenile rheumatoid arthritis
- ankylosing spondylitis
- gout

In this chapter, the term arthritis will be used as a general term to refer to arthritis and other rheumatic diseases.

Should people with arthritis exercise?

Yes. Studies have shown that exercise helps people with arthritis in many ways. Exercise reduces joint pain and stiffness and increases flexibility, muscle strength, cardiac fitness, and endurance. It also helps with weight reduction and contributes to an improved sense of well-being.

How does exercise fit into a treatment plan for people with arthritis?

Exercise is one part of a comprehensive arthritis treatment plan. Treatment plans also may include rest and relaxation, proper diet, medication, and instruction about proper use of joints and ways to conserve energy (that is, not waste motion) as well as the use of pain relief methods.

What types of exercise are most suitable for someone with arthritis?

Three types of exercise are best for people with arthritis:

- Range-of-motion exercises (e.g., dance) help maintain normal joint movement and relieve stiffness. This type of exercise helps maintain or increase flexibility.

- Strengthening exercises (e.g., weight training) help keep or increase muscle strength. Strong muscles help support and protect joints affected by arthritis.

- Aerobic or endurance exercises (e.g., bicycle riding) improve cardiovascular fitness, help control weight, and improve overall function. Weight control can be important to people who have arthritis because extra weight puts extra pressure on many joints. Some studies show that aerobic exercise can reduce inflammation in some joints.

Most health clubs and community centers offer exercise programs for people with physical limitations.

How does a person with arthritis start an exercise program?

People with arthritis should discuss exercise options with their doctors and other health care providers. Most doctors recommend exercise for their patients. Many people with arthritis begin with easy, range-of-motion exercises and low-impact aerobics. People with arthritis can participate in a variety of, but not all, sports and exercise programs. The doctor will know which, if any, sports are off-limits.

The doctor may have suggestions about how to get started or may refer the patient to a physical therapist. It is best to find a physical therapist who has experience working with people who have arthritis. The therapist will design an appropriate home exercise program and teach clients about pain-relief methods, proper body mechanics (placement of the body for a given task, such as lifting a heavy box), joint protection, and conserving energy.

Try these tips to get started:

- Discuss exercise plans with your doctor.

- Start with supervision from a physical therapist or qualified athletic trainer.

- Apply heat to sore joints (optional; many people with arthritis start their exercise program this way).

- Stretch and warm up with range-of-motion exercises.

- Start strengthening exercises slowly with small weights (a 1- or 2-pound weight can make a big difference).

- Progress slowly.

- Use cold packs after exercising (optional; many people with arthritis complete their exercise routine this way).

- Add aerobic exercise.

- Consider appropriate recreational exercise (after doing range-of-motion, strengthening, and aerobic exercise). Fewer injuries to joints affected by arthritis occur during recreational exercise if it is preceded by range-of-motion, strengthening, and aerobic exercise that gets your body in the best condition possible.

- Ease off if joints become painful, inflamed, or red, and work with your doctor to find the cause and eliminate it.

- Choose the exercise program you enjoy most and make it a habit.

What are some pain relief methods for people with arthritis?

There are known methods to help stop pain for short periods of time. This temporary relief can make it easier for people who have arthritis to exercise. The doctor or physical therapist can suggest a method that is best for each patient. The following methods have worked for many people:

- **Moist heat** supplied by warm towels, hot packs, a bath, or a shower can be used at home for 15 to 20 minutes three times a day to relieve symptoms. A health professional can use short waves, microwaves, and ultrasound to deliver deep heat to noninflamed joint areas. Deep heat is not recommended for patients with acutely inflamed joints. Deep heat is often used around the shoulder to relax tight tendons prior to stretching exercises.

- **Cold** supplied by a bag of ice or frozen vegetables wrapped in a towel helps to stop pain and reduce swelling when used for 10 to 15 minutes at a time. It is often used for acutely inflamed joints. People who have Raynaud phenomenon should not use this method.

- **Hydrotherapy** (water therapy) can decrease pain and stiffness. Exercising in a large pool may be easier because water takes some weight off painful joints. Community centers, YMCAs, and YWCAs have water exercise classes developed for people with arthritis. Some patients also find relief from the heat and movement provided by a whirlpool.

- **Mobilization therapies** include traction (gentle, steady pulling), massage, and manipulation (using the hands to restore normal movement to stiff joints). When done by a trained professional, these methods can help control pain and increase joint motion and muscle and tendon flexibility.

- **TENS** (transcutaneous electrical nerve stimulation) and biofeedback are two additional methods that may provide some pain relief, but many patients find that they cost too much money and take too much time. In TENS, an electrical shock is transmitted through electrodes placed on the skin's surface. TENS machines cost between $80 and $800. The inexpensive units are fine. Patients can wear them during the day and turn them off and on as needed for pain control.

- **Relaxation therapy** also helps reduce pain. Patients can learn to release the tension in their muscles to relieve pain. Physical therapists may be able to teach relaxation techniques. The Arthritis Foundation has a self-help course that includes relaxation therapy. Health spas and vacation resorts sometimes have special relaxation courses.

- **Acupuncture** is a traditional Chinese method of pain relief. A medically qualified acupuncturist places needles in certain sites. Researchers believe that the needles stimulate deep sensory nerves that tell the brain to release natural painkillers (endorphins).

- **Acupressure** is similar to acupuncture, but pressure is applied to the acupuncture sites instead of using needles.

How often should people with arthritis exercise?

- Range-of-motion exercises can be done daily and should be done at least every other day.

- Strengthening exercises should be done every other day unless you have severe pain or swelling in your joints.

- Endurance exercises should be done for 20 to 30 minutes three times a week unless you have severe pain or swelling in your joints. According to the American College of Rheumatology, 20- to 30-minute exercise routines can be performed in increments of 10 minutes over the course of a day.

What type of strengthening program is best?

This varies depending on personal preference, the type of arthritis involved, and how active the inflammation is. Strengthening one's muscles can help take the burden off painful joints. Strength training can be done with small free weights, exercise machines, isometrics, elastic bands, and resistive water exercises. Correct positioning is critical, because if done incorrectly, strengthening exercises can cause muscle tears, more pain, and more joint swelling.

Are there different exercises for people with different types of arthritis?

There are many types of arthritis. Experienced doctors, physical therapists, and occupational therapists can recommend exercises that are particularly helpful for a specific type of arthritis. Doctors and therapists also know specific exercises for particularly painful joints.

There may be exercises that are off-limits for people with a particular type of arthritis or when joints are swollen and inflamed. People with arthritis should discuss their exercise plans with a doctor. Doctors who treat people with arthritis include rheumatologists, orthopaedic surgeons, general practitioners, family doctors, internists, and rehabilitation specialists (physiatrists).

How much exercise is too much?

Most experts agree that if exercise causes pain that lasts for more than 1 hour, it is too strenuous. People with arthritis should work with their physical therapist or doctor to adjust their exercise program when they notice any of the following signs of strenuous exercise:

- unusual or persistent fatigue
- increased weakness
- decreased range of motion
- increased joint swelling
- continuing pain (pain that lasts more than 1 hour after exercising)

Should someone with rheumatoid arthritis continue to exercise during a general flare? How about during a local joint flare?

It is appropriate to put joints gently through their full range of motion once a day, with periods of rest, during acute systemic flares or local joint flares. Patients can talk to their doctor about how much rest is best during general or joint flares.

Are researchers studying arthritis and exercise?

Researchers are looking at the effects of exercise and sports on the development of musculoskeletal disabilities, including arthritis. They have found that people who do moderate, regular running have low, if any, risk of developing osteoarthritis. However, studies show that people who participate in sports with high-intensity, direct joint impact are at risk for the disease. Examples are football and soccer.

Sports involving repeated joint impact and twisting (such as baseball and soccer) also increase osteoarthritis risk. Early diagnosis and effective treatment of sports injuries and complete rehabilitation should decrease the risk of osteoarthritis from these injuries.

Researchers also are looking at the effects of muscle strength on the development of osteoarthritis. Studies show, for example, that strengthening the quadriceps muscles can reduce knee pain and disability associated with osteoarthritis. One study shows that a relatively small increase in strength (20 to 25 percent) can lead to a 20 to 30 percent decrease in the chance of developing knee osteoarthritis. Other researchers continue to look for and find benefits from exercise to patients with rheumatoid arthritis, spondyloarthropathies, systemic lupus erythematosus, and fibromyalgia. They are also studying the benefits of short- and long-term exercise in older populations.

Where can people find more information on arthritis and exercise?

National Institute of Arthritis and Musculoskeletal and Skin Diseases
1 AMS Circle
Bethesda, MD 20892-3675
Toll-Free: (877) 22-NIAMS (226-4267); Phone: (301) 495-4484
TTY: (301) 565-2966; Fax: (301) 718-6366
Website: http://www.niams.nih.gov
E-mail: niamsinfo@mail.nih.gov

American Academy of Orthopaedic Surgeons (AAOS)
6300 North River Road
Rosemont, IL 60018-4262
Toll-Free: (800) 824-BONE (2663)
Phone: (847) 823-7186
Fax: (847) 823-8125
Website: http://www.aaos.org
E-mail: custserv@aaos.org

American College of Rheumatology
1800 Century Place, Suite 250
Atlanta, GA 30345-4300
Phone: (404) 633-3777
Fax: (404) 633-1870
Website: http://www.rheumatology.org

American Physical Therapy Association
1111 North Fairfax Street
Alexandria, VA 22314-1488
Toll-Free: (800) 999-2782, X3395
Phone: (703) 684-2782
Fax: (703) 684-7343
TDD: (703) 683-6748
Website: http://www.apta.org

Arthritis Foundation
1330 West Peachtree Street
Atlanta, GA 30309
Toll-Free: (800) 283-7800
Phone: (404) 872-7100
Website: http://www.arthritis.org

Lupus Foundation of America (LFA), Inc.
2000 L Street, N.W.
Suite 710
Washington, DC 20036
Toll-Free: (800) 558-0121
Phone: (202) 349-1155
Website: http://www.lupus.org

SLE Foundation, Inc.
149 Madison Avenue
Suite 205
New York, NY 10016
Phone: (212) 685-4118
Website: http://www.lupusny.org

National Fibromyalgia Partnership, Inc.
P.O. Box 160
Linden, VA 22642-0160
Toll-Free: (866) 725-4404
Fax: (866)666-2727
Website: http://www.fmpartnership.org
E-mail: mail@fmpartnership.org

Spondylitis Association of America
P.O. Box 5872
Sherman Oaks, CA 91413
Toll-Free: (800) 777-8189
Website: http://www.spondylitis.org
E-mail: info@spondylitis.org

Chapter 39

Water Exercise and Arthritis

Regular exercise is an important part of improving and maintaining your health. However, for people who have arthritis, regular exercise may not only be painfully difficult, but nearly impossible.

Arthritis is a general term used to describe inflammation of the joints. This disease causes the joints to ache, stiffen, weaken, and swell. Everyday activities, such as using your hands, walking, going up and down stairs, and standing up from a seated position may be difficult. Your doctor may prescribe a treatment plan comprising medication, rest, proper diet, stress relief, and exercise. Proper exercise keeps joints mobile, keeps muscles strong, helps you regain lost motion and strength, makes daily activities easier, and improves general physical and mental fitness. However, if activities such as walking in the park or participating in aerobics classes are too painful, you may be able to exercise in a warm water pool.

Exercising in warm water has many benefits. The warm temperature of many therapeutic pools (95 degrees Fahrenheit to 98 degrees Fahrenheit) increases blood flow to muscles, which helps the muscles relax. As your muscles relax, you will be able to exercise more comfortably. The buoyancy (what causes you to float) helps support the arms as you slowly move them through the water in an almost effortless fashion. Buoyancy also greatly decreases the amount of body

"Aquatic Exercise for People with Arthritis," by Dana Bridges, P.T., A.T.C., Hughston Health Alert, Winter 1997. © Hughston Sports Medicine Foundation. For additional information, visit http://www.hughston.com/hha/hha.htm. Reviewed by David A. Cooke, M.D., on February 29, 2004.

weight placed on the back, hips, knees and feet. When you stand in waist-deep water, only 50% of your body weight is put on the lower part of your body; in neck-deep water, only 10%. Therefore, walking and leg exercises may be done with little or no weight on the painful joints of your lower body.

Water is 600 to 700 times more resistive than air. The even distribution of water's resistance affords a safe means to exercise to gain strength without soreness or risk of serious injury to arthritic joints. Strengthening and range of motion exercises performed in a warm pool are less painful and safer than other forms of exercise.

Many rehabilitation and community facilities offer organized aquatic arthritis programs. These exercise programs offer a support-group atmosphere that fosters increased self-esteem, socialization, and emotional well-being. People who exercise regularly look and feel better. Many times, the group activity will encourage you to continue exercise on a regular basis.

If you are involved in a supervised exercise program, you don't have to know how to swim. Swimming is not the only form of exercise you can do in the water. An aquatic arthritis exercise program can include exercises, such as gentle range of motion; gentle strengthening; and cardiovascular activities, such as walking laps.

Before you begin any exercise program, talk with your doctor. This consultation is especially important if you have severe cardiovascular disease, a history of seizures, uncontrolled high or low blood pressure, severe respiratory problems, or allergies to chlorine or bromine. Together, you and your doctor can create the best program for you.

Don't forget that rest and proper hydration are important parts of an aquatic exercise program. A general guideline to follow is to drink a glass of water before and after exercising in a warm pool. Including regular aquatic exercise can be a very important part of the treatment of all types of arthritis.

Exercise will help you maintain or improve your quality of life and sense of well-being. The warmth and comfort of the water will keep you coming back for more.

Chapter 40

Yoga and Arthritis

Penny Rickhoff lives with pain that never ends. It began in 1985 when she ruptured a disk in her lower back, and it worsened several years later when a file cabinet fell on her. "Basically, on a scale of one to 10, my pain averages about a five, which is moderate," says Rickhoff, a substitute teacher in her early 50s who lives in Scottsdale, Arizona. "In the evening, it goes to a six. And periodically, I have flare-ups that send it up to an eight or nine."

The intense flare-ups in her lower back, which occur a few times a year when she lifts something heavy or suddenly moves the wrong way, are excruciating. "My muscles contract, and they become hard and immobile. Sometimes I can hardly even turn in bed. It's like a constant, heated, deep pain—and if I move, it becomes a stabbing pain," she says. "Then I feel faint, and if I try to get up and move too much, my blood pressure goes up and sometimes I feel nauseous." Even after the flare-up subsides, she still hurts nonstop. "It's a constant aching feeling that is always there and never goes away."

Rickhoff's suffering has made a huge impact on her life. After the file-cabinet injury, she was forced to give up her job as a corporate pilot. Her condition contributed to marital problems. (She and her husband eventually got divorced.) Even going out with friends has become difficult, because her back often hurts more late in the day.

"Team Up to Fight Pain" by Alice Lesch Kelly, *Yoga Journal,* September/October 2003. Reprinted by permission. © 2003 *Yoga Journal.* LLC. All rights reserved.

Rickhoff is one of 50 million Americans who suffer from chronic pain, including pain from lower back problems, arthritis, cancer, repetitive stress injuries, headaches, fibromyalgia, and other ailments, as well as from botched surgeries and industrial accidents. "The individual with chronic pain is not comfortable while awake, and usually doesn't sleep well at night," says Steven D. Feinberg, M.D., clinical adjunct professor of anesthesiology at the Stanford University School of Medicine and director of the Bay Area Pain Program in Los Gatos, California. "Weight gain and sexual difficulties occur," he continues. "Anger, depression, despair, and irritability are common. Chronic pain is often accompanied by loss of hope and self-esteem. It saps the individual's energy and the ability to think straight."

Chronic pain, defined as continuous pain for more than six months, can trigger a cycle of disability. Those who suffer from it often retreat into themselves, becoming inactive and minimizing contact with other people; lack of social interaction contributes to feelings of depression and isolation. They may rely on medications to get through the day, and then to sleep, and those medications may cause side effects—dizziness, nausea, and drowsiness—that immobilize them further. Inactivity causes their muscles to weaken; deconditioned muscles make them feel even more infirm. Over time, despair may set in, and the pain may seem even worse; studies show that depressed people feel pain more acutely than nondepressed people. Feeling worse, they may ask their doctor for more medication, and when they take it, they may feel even groggier, debilitated, and depressed. And the cycle progresses downward.

Because chronic pain is such a complicated problem, managing it requires a multidimensional approach. Although chronic pain is the most common reason people seek medical attention in the United States, physicians admit they often feel powerless when it comes to easing it. The typical Western approach—bed rest and trial-and-error treatments—is far too narrow to help many people.

Some patients look for alternative solutions, such as traditional Chinese medicine or acupuncture. These treatments sometimes help lessen pain, but they offer little in the way of easing psychological, social, or occupational burdens; they're only part of the solution. That's why physicians and complementary-care providers alike are heralding a new option: the pain-team approach.

Developing a Game Plan

A pain team works like this: Instead of an individual practitioner using a single Eastern remedy or Western therapy, a multidisciplinary squad of physicians, physical therapists, psychologists, occupational therapists, family therapists, and other conventional-care providers joins forces with acupuncturists, yoga and qi gong instructors, massage therapists, biofeedback practitioners, nutritionists, relaxation therapists, or other complementary-care givers. All of them work together to create a whole-body, East-meets-West approach.

"Treatment of pain by one therapy or a single approach is just not appropriate," says James N. Dillard, M.D., assistant clinical professor of rehabilitation medicine at the Columbia University College of Physicians and Surgeons and author of *The Chronic Pain Solution: Your Personal Path to Pain Relief* (Bantam, 2002). "We get better results in people from combining the best of conventional medicine with the best of complementary and alternative therapies."

Enthusiasm for the pain-team approach is growing among both complementary-care providers and conventional physicians. "There is increasing interest in this approach because people are not doing well just taking tons of medications," says Dillard, who directs a course on integrative pain medicine at Columbia each year that is attended by hundreds of physicians and complementary-care providers.

The multidisciplinary pain-team philosophy is the guiding force at the Bay Area Pain Program, where chronic-pain sufferers take part in an eight-week program led by a pain team. Participants, many of whom have industrial injuries and have undergone repeated surgeries, get various treatments. Along with being immersed in physical therapy; wellness, yoga, tai chi, and qi gong classes; psychological and job counseling; art therapy; and peer support, they also learn anger management, assertiveness training, coping strategies, and relaxation techniques.

Yoga is a crucial part of the program, says coordinator Bridget Flynn. "A lot of these people have been completely sedentary for years," she explains. "They're petrified to move. They're afraid to even bend over." Stiff muscles and impaired range of motion amplify their pain; yoga helps them relax and begin to embrace the notion of moving again after so much physical stagnancy. As they become more active physically, they begin to break the cycle of pain, muscle weakness, and isolation. Many find that when they begin to move again, they require less medication and are able to do other activities, such as biking and swimming. Their pain may not completely disappear, but they feel more optimistic and proactive, and they find ways to manage their pain and improve their quality of life.

Flynn describes a patient with a degenerative disk disease that left her so bent that her ear touched her shoulder: "For her, the big thing was to stand straight. She would become nauseous trying to hold her head up." With the support of her yoga teacher and her fellow classmates, the woman challenged herself week after week. "She got to the point where she stood in Mountain Pose, and the whole group was cheering," Flynn recalls. "It was such a huge deal for her just to stand straight—it was a perfect Mountain Pose. What a great metaphor for her life. If she can conquer that mountain, she can do other things too."

Working with the Pain

Similar successes are found at the UCLA Pediatric Pain Program. It combines acupuncture, biofeedback, massage, yoga, psychology, and other therapies with cutting-edge Western medical treatments to help children and teens with arthritis, headaches, irritable bowel syndrome, and other chronic-pain conditions.

Iyengar Yoga is an essential part of the UCLA program, according to director Lonnie Zeltzer, M.D., who is also a professor of pediatrics, anesthesiology, psychiatry, and biobehavioral sciences at the UCLA School of Medicine. "For people with chronic pain, Iyengar is particularly good," Zeltzer says, "because B.K.S. Iyengar has researched and understood the therapeutic benefits of the poses." Iyengar Yoga's use of bolsters, blocks, straps, blankets, and other supportive props also lets them modify the postures for optimal effectiveness.

"Using props allows students to work with their pain instead of avoiding it," Zeltzer says. Props also allow people to do poses that would otherwise aggravate rather than help their condition.

"For kids with headaches, just sitting cross-legged and resting their foreheads on a bolster is so calming," says Beth Sternlieb, a certified Iyengar teacher and the staff yoga instructor for the UCLA program. "And for those who are depressed—a common side effect of chronic pain—we do a lot of backbends and chest openers. These poses make them feel alive and confident and optimistic."

Other postures give them a sense of satisfaction: With props, for example, children with arthritis in their hands and shoulders can learn to do Handstand, which many of their friends can't do.

Sternlieb's duties extend beyond the yoga studio. Each week, she meets with all the other care providers of the UCLA pain team to share information about each patient's progress, sleep patterns, medication changes, eating habits, and pain levels. Sternlieb says this information-sharing process is crucial in treating each patient as a whole, individual person, and it is one of the most important components of the pain-team approach. "People are complex, especially the kinds of kids who come to the pain clinic," she says. "They come to us after long periods of searching. Because of that complexity, it takes a variety of approaches to help them. As a team, we gather a lot more information than we would individually. Each practice opens up a different window of observation."

Eddie Cohn, a 29-year-old songwriter and recruiter for a market research firm in Santa Monica, California, is one of Sternlieb's students outside the program. At the age of 12, he was diagnosed with rheumatoid arthritis, a persistent and painful inflammation of the joints. It went into remission when he was 18 but then returned five years later. He relied mainly on medications during his first bout with the disease, but the second time around, he was determined to expand his treatment options. "I wanted to be more proactive as to what I could do rather than just going to a doctor and getting medication," Cohn says.

He faced considerable challenges. In addition to joint pain and swelling, he suffered from pericarditis, a painful inflammation around the heart. With Sternlieb as his teacher, he practiced mainly restorative poses and inversions for about a year. "It gave me a lot of strength, both physically and mentally," he says.

He gradually worked up to four or five Iyengar classes a week, and over time, he reduced and then eliminated his many medications. He then added active poses—standing poses and backbends—to his practice. Now he is in remission again, and he credits his good health to continued yoga practice and an overall commitment to maintaining balance in his life. "I am careful—no alcohol, no smoking; I eat fish three times a week and lots of fruits and vegetables," Cohn says. "I believe you need to nurture your immune system as if it's a precious thing. For me, it's all about not being overextended."

Why Yoga Helps

Experts believe there are many reasons yoga helps people with chronic pain. First and foremost are the physical ones: Yoga loosens muscles that have been tightened by inactivity, stress, and tension. It helps release muscle spasms, corrects postural problems, increases range of motion, and enhances flexibility.

Yoga also delivers psychological benefits. Many people in continual pain shut themselves down emotionally as a way of coping. They take sleeping pills, always keep the television on, or do other things that help block out their own consciousness. Many feel angry and bitter.

"Patients come in with so much psychological baggage," Flynn says. "Reflection is hard, because they are so uncomfortable with their own thoughts. Yoga gives them a safe, positive way to become more conscious. It's a personal, private journey, and they can take it as slowly as they want."

Engaging in physical activity can also empower a person who has felt mistreated by the health care system. "It makes the person feel less like a victim, because they're taking control," Dillard says. "It gives the person something to do besides pop pills and go to the doctor."

And there's more. Zeltzer believes—and she is busy working on research to support her case—that yoga can bring about physiological changes in the central nervous system that relieve pain. Here's her theory: Intense pain causes pain-processing pathways in the brain to function abnormally, allowing pain to persist even after the disease or injury heals. How does this happen? Zeltzer believes that severe pain throws the nervous system off-kilter, and as a result, the body's pain-control system "gets out of whack" and doesn't turn itself off.

"Yoga helps get the central nervous system back in service," she says. "And I think there are changes in the body's inflammatory process with yoga. It's more than just increasing flexibility and strength."

Perhaps the most important advice for those with chronic pain is not to give up. It may take time to find caregivers who can truly help, but those who continuously search, learn, and take a proactive approach will find them. "It's really important that people know there is help for their chronic-pain problems," says Sternlieb, "that their suffering can be transformed into insight and a sense of mastery."

Alice Lesch Kelly is a regular contributor to *YJ*.

Chapter 41

Nutritional Concerns of People with Arthritis

Can the foods you eat affect your arthritis? Given the varied nature of the symptoms of arthritis, it's natural to think that the food you ate yesterday caused or reduced the pain you feel today. While this may or may not be the case, one thing is for sure—eating a nutritious, well-balanced diet is a good idea for everyone and can be especially important for those with arthritis. In fact, there is good evidence that excessive weight and the type of diet you follow may influence symptoms of certain types of arthritis and related conditions.

On the other hand, one needs to be wary of special diets and nutritional supplements that claim to cure arthritis. Unfortunately, most of the claims for these cure-all diets or nutritional supplements have not been scientifically tested to determine if they work and are safe.

Arthritis is a complicated autoimmune disease without simple answers. Because there are more than 100 types of arthritis and related diseases, there isn't one single diet plan that will help everyone. What medical and nutrition experts do generally recommend, however, is that people with arthritis follow a diet based on variety, balance, and moderation.

Consuming a variety of different kinds of fruits, vegetables, and whole grains is important in addition to moderating the amount of foods high in sugar, salt, and saturated fat. Eating a well-balanced

"Nutrition Advice for People with Arthritis" by Pat Kendall, Ph.D., R.D., August 2003, is reprinted with permission from the author and Colorado State University Cooperative Extension, http://www.ext.colostate.edu. © 2003 Colorado State University Cooperative Extension.

diet may help you feel better overall, aid in weight control, and help prevent other chronic diseases such as heart disease and cancer.

Recent research also suggests that consuming omega-3 fatty acids found in cold-water fish and other seafood may reduce joint inflammation in people with rheumatoid arthritis. In addition, an adequate intake of both vitamin D and calcium is necessary to prevent osteoporosis. Arthritis patients tend to develop osteoporosis as a result of a lack of exercise and, in the case of rheumatoid arthritis, from the inflammation. Further, eating foods rich in zinc and selenium (lean ground beef, chicken, whole-wheat bread, eggs, almonds, milk, and tofu) may be beneficial because both of these minerals have anti-inflammatory properties.

Certain medications also may affect your body's nutrient needs. For example, antacids, taken sometimes to reduce stomach irritation, can contain high levels of calcium, sodium, and magnesium. Glucocorticoids prescribed to treat rheumatoid arthritis can cause your body to lose potassium and retain sodium. Penicillamine, also used for rheumatoid arthritis, may lower blood levels of copper. Methotrexate used for rheumatoid arthritis, myositis, and psoriatic arthritis may lower levels of folic acid. Colchicine, used for gout, may affect how well vitamin B12 is absorbed. In many cases, eating a variety of foods will provide sufficient levels of these minerals without added supplementation. However, it is a good idea to ask your doctor how the medication prescribed for you may affect your nutrient needs and whether a vitamin and mineral supplement may be appropriate for you.

For arthritis patients, good nutrition can sometimes be challenging. Joint pain, inflammation, and fatigue can make food preparation difficult. Certain arthritis medications can lower your appetite or cause stomach upset. Likewise, the depression that sometimes affects people with chronic illnesses may alter eating habits and appetite. The key is to educate yourself, make gradual changes, and seek the guidance of your doctor or a registered dietitian.

Chapter 42

Arthritis on the Job

Arthritis is the number one cause of disability in the United States, making up nearly 20 percent of all disabilities among people aged 15 and over. An estimated 43 million Americans are affected by the disease. Many face work-related physical limitations. The total cost of arthritis, including medical care and lost productivity, is nearly $65 billion per year.

A Brief Overview of Arthritis

It is important to note that there are more than 100 different types of arthritis, each producing different symptoms and levels of impairment. Some of the most common forms of arthritis include osteoarthritis, rheumatoid arthritis, fibromyalgia, and lupus.

Osteoarthritis, often called degenerative arthritis, involves the breakdown of bones and cartilage, causing pain and stiffness. Osteoarthritis commonly affects the movement and function of fingers, knees, feet, hips, and back.

Rheumatoid arthritis is an abnormality in the immune system causing inflammation of the lining in the joints and/or internal organs.

"Workplace Accommodations for Individuals with Arthritis" is part of a brochure series on reasonable accommodation in the implementation of the Americans with Disabilities Act. © 2001 Program on Employment and Disability, Cornell University. Reprinted with permission. For additional information, contact the Program on Employment and Disability at 607-255-2906 (Voice), 607-255-2891 (TDD), or visit their website at http://www.ilr.cornell.edu/ped.

Rheumatoid arthritis often affects the same joints on both sides of the body and can affect the hands, wrists, feet, knees, ankles, shoulders, neck, jaw, and elbows. The disease may also cause inflammation of internal organs, leading to significant organ damage. Individuals with rheumatoid arthritis are likely to experience times when they have few symptoms and other times when they have very severe symptoms causing significant limitations.

Fibromyalgia has become a more common diagnosis during the past several years. It is a condition that affects muscles and their attachments to bone and is characterized by widespread pain, fatigue, stiffness, sleep disturbance, and psychological distress.

Lupus is a rheumatic disease affecting skin and body tissue. Additionally, some people experience involvement of organs such as kidneys, lungs, or heart. Lupus is generally diagnosed between age 18 and 45. Symptoms include skin rashes, abnormal sun sensitivity, and joint pain, inflammation, and stiffness. Lupus is treatable, but can be a very serious impairment. Individuals with lupus will experience flares and remissions. A flare is a period of worsening symptoms. A remission is a period with few or no symptoms of the disease.

Regardless of the specific diagnosis, individuals with arthritis need appropriate rest and exercise. It is important that they learn to pace their activities and maintain appropriate self-care skills to minimize pain and functional loss. With reasonable accommodations from employers, many people with arthritis continue to be productive employees.

Who Is Considered an Individual with a Disability?

Many people with arthritis would meet the definition of an "individual with a disability" under the Americans with Disabilities Act (ADA). Under the ADA, an individual with a disability is a person who: has a physical or mental impairment that substantially limits one or more major life activities, has a record of such an impairment, or is regarded as having such an impairment.

An impairment is substantially limiting if it prevents or significantly restricts the performance of a major life activity. The nature, severity, duration, and long-term impact of the condition are all factors that go into determining whether an impairment rises to the level of an ADA disability. Mitigating measures, such as medication, must also be considered. Thus, if an individual's arthritis is completely or substantially controlled with medication all the time, s/he would not be considered to have an ADA disability because the condition does not substantially limit a major life activity.

The ADA does not cover impairments that are relatively minimal in nature and severity or that are considered short-term (e.g., mild arthritis in a finger causing only occasional discomfort). Many forms of arthritis (e.g., rheumatoid, lupus) can be controlled with proper treatment. However, even when properly treated, an individual with arthritis may have periods of severe pain and functional limitation. In this situation, the ADA would apply even when the arthritis is in remission. Chronic conditions that are substantially limiting when active or have a high likelihood of recurrence in substantially limiting forms are covered under the ADA.

What Are Reasonable Accommodations?

The ADA requires employers to provide reasonable accommodations to qualified disabled individuals in three areas of employment: 1) the job application process, 2) job functions, and 3) benefits and privileges of employment. A reasonable accommodation is any modification to a job, employment practice or process, or a work environment that makes it possible for an individual with a disability to successfully fulfill the duties of a job. Employers are not required to provide items primarily for personal use, such as purchasing a wheelchair.

Reasonable accommodations are not nearly as costly as many employers fear. A study conducted by the Job Accommodation Network (JAN) in 1990 showed that one third of all accommodations were accomplished with no cost to the employer and more than half cost $1,000.00 or less; eighty percent of the accommodations that JAN suggests cost less than $500.00. Additionally, most employers surveyed indicated that their company had benefited overall financially as a result of making job accommodations.

How Do I Know the Requested Accommodation Is Necessary and Is the Most Appropriate Accommodation?

The individual with a disability will likely have a great deal of experience modifying tasks. It is logical to use his/her expertise. It is also important to consider the individual's preferences as well as the employer's needs.

Working together to outline various options for accommodating the individual will likely be the most beneficial approach. Occupational therapists can also help by completing evaluations of the workstation and the employee's functioning. The therapist can offer suggestions for modifying the workstation or the process the employee uses to complete a task. S/he will work with the employer and employee to find accommodations that are both effective and reasonable. Assistance is also available through organizations such as the regional ADA Disability and Business Technical Assistance Center, the Job Accommodation Network, and the local Vocational Rehabilitation office.

What Types of Accommodations Should Be Considered?

Accommodations for employees with arthritis may be administrative or mechanical in nature. Administrative accommodations may include reassigning or reallocating marginal duties, being flexible about how or when tasks are performed, and allowing a flexible work schedule or telecommuting. Reassignment to a different, available job is also an option if no other accommodation is effective.

Mechanical accommodations include modifying the employee's workstation, modifying or providing special tools or equipment, and ensuring that the building, the work area, and other non-work areas used by employees, such as restrooms and break rooms, are accessible.

For example, an employee with osteoarthritis of the hips or knees may have difficulty standing all day. Providing a stool of the appropriate height would allow the individual to alternate between sitting and standing at a workstation without interrupting production. Another person may have difficulty sitting for long periods. If s/he works at a desk, a podium could be used to raise the work surface allowing the employee to change positions as needed.

More significant accommodations for an individual with arthritis in the lower extremities could include moving a workstation to a ground floor to alleviate the need to climb stairs, or providing another employee to assist with lifting or other physically demanding non-essential tasks.

Arthritis in the hands and arms can be particularly problematic for an individual whose job requires repetitive hand function such as factory assembly or typing. There are a number of adaptive tools available to assist individuals with grasping and manipulating objects. These tools may be especially effective if the individual has arthritis in only one hand. Moving the individual from a job requiring finger manipulations to one requiring gross handling may be an alternative for some individuals. Computer technology provides a number of alternatives for individuals with arthritis in the upper extremities. Adaptive keyboards that reduce stress on the arms are available through most computer dealers. Additionally, a number of voice-activated computer software packages are available to reduce the amount of actual typing the individual must perform. These programs are fairly inexpensive and user-friendly.

Some individuals with arthritis have more difficulty in the morning. Providing a flexible work schedule allowing the employee to start work later in the morning may significantly improve the individual's ability to perform work functions. Many employers allow employees to work from home. This allows employees to set a schedule that best fits their needs and provides the opportunity to change positions and take breaks when needed.

These are only a few examples of appropriate accommodations for employees with arthritis. Many accommodations can be achieved with little cost to the employer and minimal disruption of the work site. Generally, the cost of the accommodation is far less than the cost of disability payments.

Who Can I Contact for More Information?

For answers to specific questions regarding the ADA or arthritis, please contact the sources listed below.

Disability & Business Technical Assistance Centers
Toll-Free: (800) 949-4232
Website: http://www.adata.org

Americans with Disabilities Act
Toll-Free: (800) 514-0301
TTY: (800) 514-0383
Website: http://www.usdoj.gov/crt/ada/adahom1.htm

Access Board
Toll-Free: 800-872-2253
TTY: (800) 993-2822
Website: http://www.access-board.gov

Access Board offers technical assistance on ADA accessibility guidelines.

Internal Revenue Service
Toll-Free: (800) 829-1040
TTY: (800) 829-4059
Website: http://www.irs.gov

The IRS provides information on tax credits and deductions that can assist businesses in complying with ADA.

Disability Rights Education and Defense Fund Hotline
Toll-Free: (800) 466-4232
Website: http://www.dredf.org

This organization provides technical assistance, education, advocacy, and legal assistance relative to the ADA and individuals with disabilities.

U.S. Equal Employment Opportunity Commission
Toll-Free: (800) 669-4000
TTY: (800) 669-6820
Website: http://www.eeoc.gov

This agency offers technical assistance on the ADA provisions governing employment.

Chapter 43

Stress and Arthritis

Understanding Arthritis

The word arthritis literally means joint inflammation (*arth* = joint; *itis* = inflammation). It refers to more than 100 forms of arthritis and related conditions. Arthritis affects the joints and tissues around the joints, such as muscles and tendons. Some forms of arthritis also can affect other parts of the body, including the skin and internal organs.

Arthritis usually causes stiffness, pain and fatigue. The severity varies from person to person, and even from day to day. In some types of arthritis, only a few joints are affected and the impact may be small. In others, systems in the entire body may be affected. Arthritis may be chronic, which means it could last for many months or years, or even a lifetime.

Nearly 43 million Americans have arthritis. While arthritis brings many challenges, there are ways you can meet them and continue to lead a fulfilling life.

This chapter is for people who have stress due to arthritis and related diseases. It provides basic information about stress as well as tips on how you can effectively manage it.

Excerpted from *Managing Your Stress*. © 2002. Reprinted with permission of the Arthritis Foundation, 1330 W. Peachtree St., Suite 100, Atlanta, GA 30309. To order a free copy of this brochure or other titles from the Arthritis Foundation, call 800-283-7800 or visit www.arthritis.org.

471

How Does the Body React to Stress?

When you feel stressed, your body's muscles become tense. This muscle tension can increase your pain and fatigue and may limit your abilities, which can make you feel helpless. This can cause you to become depressed. A cycle of stress, pain, fatigue, limited/lost abilities and depression may develop. If you understand your reaction and learn how to manage stress, you can help break that cycle.

How to Manage Your Stress

The key to managing stress is to make it work for you instead of against you. A complete program for managing your stress has six parts:

1. Learn your body's signals of stress.
2. Learn to identify what causes your stress.
3. Learn changes you can make to help reduce stress.
4. Learn how to manage what you can't change.
5. Learn how to reduce the effects of stress on your body.
6. Maintain a lifestyle that can build your resistance to stress.

Reduce the Effects of Stress on Your Body

Learning how to relax is one of the most important ways to cope with stress in a healthy way. Relaxation is more than just sitting back and being quiet. It is an active process using methods to calm your body and mind. Learning how to relax takes practice. As you learn new ways to relax, keep these principles in mind:

- Stress is caused by many things, which means there are many ways to manage stress. The better you understand what causes your stress, the more successfully you can manage it.
- Not all relaxation techniques work for everyone. Try out different methods until you find one or two you like best. You may learn that some techniques work well for specific situations.
- Remember that learning these new skills will take time. Practice new techniques for at least two weeks before you decide if they work well for you.

If you need help learning how to relax, see a mental-health professional or contact your local Arthritis Foundation chapter.

Chapter 44

Arthritis and Sleep

When Pain and Sleep Problems Arise

When you can't sleep and your head aches or your back hurts, you are also likely to lose a lot of sleep. In fact, 20% of American adults (42 million people) report that pain or physical discomfort disrupts their sleep a few nights a week or more. That was the finding of a 2000 National Sleep Foundation (NSF) Sleep in America poll. Yet many people don't recognize how large the problem is. Nor do they consider the possible consequences, which may include difficulty maintaining alertness, lack of energy, impaired mood, and trouble handling stress. Lack of sleep, so often due to pain or discomfort, can also put you at risk for injury, poor health, and accidents.

How Pain Affects Sleep

Pain is a leading cause of insomnia. When pain makes it hard to sleep, falling asleep is often the greatest problem. However, 65 percent of those with pain and sleep problems in a 1996 NSF Gallup survey indicated that they were awakened during the night by pain.

And 62 percent woke up too early because of pain. Difficulty falling asleep, staying asleep, and waking earlier than desired are all symptoms of insomnia. In addition, many people who experience pain wake up feeling unrefreshed. Insomnia may be a short-term problem experienced for only a night or two now and then, or it may be chronic, lasting for a month or more.

Headache, Arthritis, and Other Medical Conditions

Headache is the second most common pain. Of those who experience the onset of headaches during sleep, 55% report having sleep disorders. In particular, there is a sleep connection with tension or migraine headaches (throbbing pain with blood vessels tightening and opening.) For example, migraine headaches can occur following sleep deprivation or too much sleep. Headaches have also been associated with such sleep disorders as sleep apnea, (frequent pauses in breathing accompanied by loud snoring during sleep), especially upon awakening and sleep movement disorders. In some cases (e.g. snoring and sleep apnea), treatment of the sleep disorder reduced the headaches. Another type of headache that is even worse, cluster headaches, strike one after another in cycles. Blood vessel activity appears to play a role, too. Cluster headaches may be related to sleep and sleep disorders as well.

Of people with rheumatic or arthritic disorders, as many as 75% often suffer from sleep problems. For example, people with osteoarthritis, especially of the hips and knees, tend to sleep lighter or have restless sleep. People with rheumatoid arthritis often have disturbed sleep with morning stiffness along with a decrease in energy, weakness, and function. Sleep arousals are often associated with flares, or an increase in inflammation and tenderness. Individuals with fibromyalgia, a condition of aches and pains throughout the body and many tender points, usually suffer from light and unrefreshing sleep, daytime fatigue, and difficulty with thinking and mood. Frequently, such people share many similar features with people that have chronic fatigue syndrome. They may suffer from chronic headaches, irritable bowel syndrome, and sometimes jaw pain or temporomandibular disorder.

Often they have an arousal disturbance in their brain wave pattern during sleep, which may occur alone or accompany restless legs (an unpleasant, tingling feeling in the legs) and sometimes sleep apnea (pauses in breathing during sleep accompanied by snoring). Because the poor quality of sleep contributes to the persistent muscle pain, tenderness, and low energy of rheumatic illnesses, people with osteoarthritis, rheumatoid arthritis, and fibromyalgia should be evaluated for primary sleep disorders.

In general, there is a high prevalence of sleep problems in various medical conditions with pain often altering the sleep process, and at the same time, the sleep problem interacts with the disease process. For example, patients with heart disease tend to have less deep sleep, more fragmented, and less efficient sleep. This poor sleep can affect their well-being. Gastrointestinal problems, such as heartburn, ulcers, and irritable bowel syndrome with their associated discomfort, often lead to difficulty obtaining a good night's sleep. In a recent Gallup poll, 75% of respondents reported that nighttime heartburn made it difficult to fall asleep and wakes them during the night. All of these problems may be associated with psychological distress, which also contributes to poor, inadequate sleep.

Managing Pain and Sleep Problems

Pain is often considered one of the most poorly treated health problems in America. Sleep problems and disorders are often not recognized or treated properly either. However, medication that appropriately addresses both the pain and sleep problem, exercise, and psychological approaches may help. The psychological methods include:

- learning to relax one's muscles and free your mind of stress (relaxation training)

- learning to control specific body functions involved in headaches or other sources of pain, such as temperature or muscle tension (biofeedback)

- therapies that focus on changing your way of thinking about the pain experienced (cognitive therapy) or changing the behavior or attitudes related to the pain (behavioral therapy)

These approaches take time and practice with a specialist, may add considerably to healthcare costs, and may not be covered by individual health insurance plans. However, these methods have no known side effects, drug interactions, or concerns about long-term use. In fact, there may be more long-term benefits.

What You Can Do to Get Good Sleep

Practicing healthy sleep habits can help improve the quantity and quality of your sleep.

Steps to better sleep:

- Establish a relaxing bedtime routine such as listening to soft music or taking a warm bath. Avoid alerting activities before bedtime.

- Avoid heavy meals or feeling hungry before bed. A light, healthy snack is best.

- Create a conducive environment that is cool, quiet, and dark.

- Go to sleep at the same time every night and awaken at the same time each morning.

- Avoid caffeinated drinks (coffees, teas, cola drinks, etc.) and foods (chocolate) in the afternoon and in the evening.

- Avoid the regular use of alcoholic drinks to help you sleep.

- Avoid or give up smoking. Nicotine, like caffeine, makes you more alert, but can lead to fragmented sleep.

- Exercise regularly, but not within three hours of bedtime. A gentle, preferably supervised, aerobic fitness program (e.g. walking, aquatic aerobics, stationary bicycle riding) carried out on a regular basis is very helpful for improving the quality of sleep and controlling aching muscles.

- Use the bed only for sleep and sex.

- Get out of bed if you can't fall asleep within 15 minutes.

- Avoid regular naps. If you need to take a nap, do so by mid-afternoon and for 15 to 30 minutes only.

When these approaches don't help, or when the sleep and pain problems don't go away, it may be time to try medications.

Chapter 45

Arthritis and Pregnancy

Chapter Contents

Section 45.1

Preparing to Become a Parent When You Have Arthritis

Overcoming the Difficulties

Whether or not to have a baby is a major decision for any woman. The decision is made even more complicated if the woman has arthritis and must deal daily with physical pain and limitation. Some important questions to be considered include: Am I ready to have a baby?, Will my arthritis go away?, Will my child inherit arthritis?, Will arthritis affect my pregnancy?, Will pregnancy affect my arthritis?, How can I plan ahead and make it easier?

Am I Ready?

Since arthritis affects physical ability, strength, and endurance, it is imperative to honestly judge whether you would be able to care for a baby. A newborn is wholly dependent on its mother and it is valid to question your capabilities. The Self-Test for Strength and Endurance can help assess your potential limitations:

- Can you lift a 10 lb. bag of potatoes from the height of your bed?

- Can you hold a 10 lb. bag of potatoes in one arm while sitting for at least 10 minutes?

- Can you go up and down stairs easily while carrying a 10 lb. bag?

- Can you walk around the house carrying the 10 lb. bag for up to 10 minutes?

- Do you get increased pain in the hips, knees, or feet when carrying the 10 lb. bag?

- Can you screw on and off the top of a baby bottle?

- Can you get through an average day without taking a nap?

- Can you bend your neck, chin to chest, to see the baby if you were holding it close?

Will My Arthritis Go Away?

In some cases, the symptoms of rheumatoid arthritis are relieved during pregnancy. This can occur at any time during the pregnancy. In most women, the improvement occurs by the end of the fourth month. Although joint swelling may decrease, joint pain and stiffness can still persist due to existing joint damage. Unfortunately, the improved symptoms do not continue after the pregnancy is over. A flare in the disease can occur approximately two to eight weeks after the baby is born.

During pregnancy lupus may stay the same, improve, or get worse. Ideally, to minimize the chances of a flare, the lupus should be in remission for six months prior to becoming pregnant. The remission should be reflected in both how you feel as well as normal blood test results.

Research on scleroderma and other types of arthritis is not as definitive. Some studies indicate that scleroderma flares, and other studies report that it improves with pregnancy.

Having an abortion does not prevent a flare. Any type of delivery, spontaneous abortion, therapeutic abortion, or stillbirth can result in a flare.

Will My Child Inherit Arthritis?

The cause of most forms of arthritis is not known. Scientists have found certain genetic markers that may be indicative of whether people are at higher risk for developing particular types of arthritis. The relationship between these markers and the actual development of arthritis is indistinct. Having these markers does not guarantee passing on the disease to your child. There is no definite way to know if your child will develop arthritis.

Heredity is not regarded as the single factor in developing arthritis. Environment is viewed as a contributor as well. Currently, there are some who believe that a person may be born with a susceptibility to the disease, but that it still requires something to trigger the disease.

Will Arthritis Affect My Pregnancy?

In most women the actual course of pregnancy is not affected by arthritis. However, individuals with rheumatoid arthritis have a statistically greater chance of premature births and neonatal complications. There is a greater chance of miscarriage and a small possibility of congenital abnormalities.

The forms of arthritis that affect internal organs may cause problems during pregnancy. Pregnancy can be life-threatening for women who have lupus, scleroderma, or other rheumatic diseases, especially if the disease has caused kidney problems or high blood pressure.

If the rib joints are affected by arthritis, the pregnancy may be uncomfortable possibly because it is more difficult to breathe abdominally. If the hips have been affected by arthritis it may complicate normal delivery and a cesarean section may be needed. If lungs are affected, more shortness of breath may be experienced.

Will Pregnancy Affect My Arthritis?

The joints and muscles may be affected by the physical changes that occur during pregnancy. Problems with weight-bearing joints (hips, knees, ankles, and feet) may become worse due to increased weight. Muscle spasms in the back may occur because as the uterus grows, the spine curves slightly to support it. This can also sometimes cause pain, numbness, and tingling in the legs.

If there is any problem with pericarditis, inflammation of the sac around the heart, or with myocarditis, inflammation of the heart muscle, pregnancy would further complicate the problem. Blood flow through the body is increased during pregnancy so it is important that the heart is functioning normally.

Arthritis Medications and Pregnancy

Ideally it would be best to be off all medications during pregnancy. This is not always possible however. Some medications are considered more safe than others if medication must be continued. Aspirin has been used by many women during pregnancy without any damage to the fetus. Gold and prednisone also have been used during pregnancy, but should be avoided if possible. Immunosuppressive drugs should not even be considered during pregnancy.

Whether or not to continue or stop medications is a decision to be made with the advice of a physician. Some medications can be stopped abruptly but a flare may result from their discontinued use.

Planning Ahead

All points of concern should be brought into open discussion between the pregnant woman and her partner, doctor, obstetrician, and rheumatologist. In most cases, pregnancy should not be a problem at all especially if the disease is mild.

- Know what arthritis medication is safe for you to continue taking.
- Exercise to keep muscles strong and joints flexible.
- Eat a balanced diet and maintain good nutrition.
- Learn ways to protect joints from stress and strain.
- Adopt stress management techniques.

Section 45.2

Sharp Drop in Stress Hormones May Set Stage for Arthritis after Pregnancy

"Sharp Drop In Stress Hormones May Set Stage For Arthritis, Multiple Sclerosis After Pregnancy," National Institute of Arthritis and Musculoskeletal Diseases (NIAMS), October 30, 2001. Available online at http://www.niams.nih.gov; accessed November 2003.

A sharp drop in stress hormones after giving birth to a child may predispose some women to develop certain conditions in which the immune system attacks the body's own tissues, according to researchers at the National Institutes of Health.

The study was conducted by researchers at the National Institute of Child Health and Human Development (NICHD) and the National Institute of Arthritis and Musculoskeletal and Skin Diseases. The study appeared in the October issue of *The Journal of Clinical Endocrinology and Metabolism.*

"This finding has important implications for understanding why immune disorders may subside during pregnancy, but flare up again

481

after birth," Duane Alexander, M.D., director of the NICHD. "Understanding the immune processes involved may provide important new therapies for each of these conditions."

Rheumatoid arthritis (RA) is a disorder in which the immune system apparently causes pain, swelling, stiffness, and loss of function in the joints. In multiple sclerosis, the immune system attacks the brain and nervous system.

The immune hormones Interleukin 12 (IL-12) and tumor necrosis factor alpha TNF alpha hormones are involved in triggering the body's immune cells to ward off disease causing invaders, explained the study's senior investigator, George P. Chrousos, M.D., chief of NICHD's Pediatric and Reproductive Endocrinology Branch. Both hormones also seem to be involved in the swelling and tissue destruction seen in rheumatoid arthritis and multiple sclerosis. Similarly people with these conditions also have higher-than-normal amounts of the two immune hormones.

In pregnant women who have either multiple sclerosis or rheumatoid arthritis, symptoms may ease up or even disappear during the third trimester of pregnancy, Dr. Chrousos said. After the women give birth, however, their symptoms often return. Similarly, pregnant women who do not have either disorder may develop one of them within a year of giving birth.

The researchers recruited 18 women with normal, healthy pregnancies for their study. Next, the researchers charted the women's levels of IL-12 and TNF alpha in the third trimester of pregnancy as well as within the weeks following the birth of their child. The investigators found that, during the third trimester of pregnancy, the women's levels of IL-12 were about three times lower than it was after they had given birth. Similarly, the women's TNF alpha levels were 40 percent lower during the third trimester than it was after birth.

The researchers also found, however, that the women's levels of the stress hormones cortisol, norepinephrine (formerly adrenalin), and 1,25 hydroxyvitamin D3 were two to three times higher than they were after the women had given birth. All three hormones are produced to help the body respond to a stress. The most well known of these, norepinephrine, is involved in the "fight or flight" response, in which strength and reflexes are enhanced, to escape or deal with a possible threat. Other research has shown that all three of these stress hormones serve to hinder the production of immune system hormones.

The increase in these stress hormones is probably caused by the master stress hormone, corticotropin releasing hormone (CRH). This hormone is produced in the pituitary gland in response to stress, and ultimately signals the production of cortisol, norepinephrine, and 1,25 hydroxyvitamin D3. Similarly, CRH is also produced by the placenta.

"It appears as if suppression of IL-12 and TNF alpha results indirectly from the CRH the placenta produces," Dr. Chrousos said. "After birth, the supply of CRH plummets and the levels of the two immune hormones rise sharply. This appears to result in a 'rebound' effect that could exacerbate disorders like rheumatoid arthritis and multiple sclerosis."

In one earlier study, Dr. Chrousos and his coworkers found that an abrupt drop in CRH after birth resulted in post partum depression in some women. In a more recent study, they showed that production of CRH by the placenta and the uterine lining played a role in preventing the mother's immune system from rejecting the early embryo.

Chapter 46

Sex and Arthritis

How Does Arthritis Affect Sexuality?

Arthritis is a chronic illness that causes joint pain, inflammation or redness of joints, and fever. It can change the way you feel about yourself. It may increase your dependence on others. The fear of hurting or being hurt may also limit the ability of you and your partner to share physical closeness.

How much arthritis affects your sex life depends on:

- how severe the disease is
- how much discomfort you suffer
- how much you can do physically
- how much pain is caused by touch, movement, and weight bearing
- side effects of medication
- effects of surgery or radiation on movement

The fear of hurting or being hurt can indirectly cause sexual problems by:

- decreasing vaginal lubrication and orgasm in women

"Arthritis and Sexuality," is reprinted from Clinical Reference Systems Senior Health Advisor, 2002.1 with permission from McKesson Health Solutions. Copyright 2003 McKesson Health Solutions, LLC.

- causing the man to lose his erection

Aware of the possibility of causing pain, partners make avoiding pain the top priority. Thus, with the first wince, moan, or word, desire shifts to compassion and the sexual encounter ends.

What Can Be Done about It?

To control the pain of arthritis, the condition must be diagnosed and treated. The solutions for each couple will depend upon how much they value physical intimacy in their relationship. A person of any age may have little interest in sex. It may be the result of years of frustration or become a problem only after a crisis appears. Couples who had sexual problems or little interest in sex before the onset of arthritis often use the disease as an excuse to avoid sex.

While arthritis may cause one couple to avoid sex, it may increase the need for closeness and touch in another. Those who have always needed to share emotionally and physically will find ways to meet those needs.

Your doctor or therapist can help you by:

- talking to you about your needs as a couple

- making suggestions to help you cope with the disability

- helping you understand the physical and emotional changes caused by aging, and any side effects of medications or surgery

To overcome the frustration of both partners during sexual activity you may:

- Use a simple signal, such as a touch or a cough, before the pain is too severe.

- Use a lubricant such as Astroglide, K-Y, or Lubrin during foreplay.

- Take the emphasis off having intercourse and focus on touch, sharing, and closeness by using: sex play; mutual pleasuring to orgasm; or masturbation with fantasy to orgasm.

- Find positions that are comfortable.

- Use pillows to support and protect joints.

- Look at the diagrams of sexual positions in publications from the Arthritis Foundation.

- Avoid weight-bearing positions for the partner with arthritis:
  - If the man is on top and the woman has arthritis, he should support his own weight with his hands and knees.
  - If the man has arthritis, the woman should sit astride him or lie beside him supported by pillows.

The partner with arthritis should:

- Avoid sex after a heavy meal.
- Attempt intercourse only when well rested.
- Take a hot shower or bath before sex.
- Use medicines such as acetaminophen, aspirin, ibuprofen, or COX-2 inhibitors to reduce pain. Ask your doctor which medicine would work best for you.

Chapter 47

Mobility and Arthritis

Chapter Contents

Section 47.1

Adapting Your Car to Your Arthritis

Do you find yourself avoiding your car because of your arthritis? Is it hard to manage the hand controls, painful to get in and out, or uncomfortable to sit? These and other problems can be vastly improved by making simple changes to your current car—or looking for specific features in a new one.

Remember that comfort isn't the only issue. When a particular movement in the car is awkward or painful, or the stress of coping with arthritis and driving results in exhaustion—often a big problem with fibromyalgia, lupus, and rheumatoid arthritis—your reactions can be delayed. And that can lead to accidents.

Car Comfort Tune-Up

Here's how to make handling your car more comfortable, less tiring, and safer.

- For a surer grip and to give hand joints more cushioning, pad the steering wheel with a shearling cover.

- To make keys easier to hold and turn, buy some slip-on plastic key covers that enlarge the end you grip and make it less slippery.

- If you have neck, back, or hip problems, install a panoramic rear-view mirror to minimize twisting.

- In car seats that have a tilt adjuster, be sure it's set so that your knees are slightly higher than your buttocks; if they're lower, it can stress your back.

- For aid getting in and out, get a rotating portable pad that's kind of a lazy Susan device for your car.

Shopping for a New Car

Newer cars often have seats that can be adjusted in any direction and many have adjustable back supports. Here are some other helpful features to put on your sopping checklist:

- Seats that are flat enough to make sliding in and out easy because deep bucket seats can be troublesome;

- Controls that are all within comfortable reach and aren't manipulated by tiny knobs or stiff levers;

- A central armrest to take weight off your shoulder—and extra padding to add height may also help;

- A telescoping wheel to make getting in and out less cumbersome;

- A four-door model because doors on two-door cars are often heavier and harder on hands, arms, and shoulders;

- Power everything—steering, brakes, windows, side mirrors, door-locking systems, and seat-adjusting controls;

- A trunk with a low lip so you don't have to heave things in and out.

But don't stop with what's available on the showroom floor. You may be able to have modifications made to a new car at the factory or, if you've recently bought a car, be reimbursed by the manufacturer for subsequent installations of helpful equipment. Options range from easier-to-reach seatbelts to a fold-up or slide-out entry step. Check manufacturer's Web sites to find out about the various modifications available.

Section 47.2

Traveling with Arthritis

"How to Travel with Your Arthritis," by Carol Page, PT, CHT, is reprinted with permission from the Rheumatology Division of the Hospital for Special Surgery, New York, NY. ©2003 Hospital for Special Surgery. All rights reserved. For additional information, visit http://www.rheumatology .hss.edu.

Do you worry about arthritis spoiling your vacation or business trip? What to take with you, what you do en route, and how you settle in to your vacation digs can have a big impact on whether you have joint trouble on a trip. Try these travel-smart tips.

- Pack your medications first—in labeled containers that go in your carry-on luggage. And take an extra copy of your prescriptions with you in case your medications get lost. Nothing can spoil your trip worse than not having your medications at hand.

- Get a suitcase with wheels or use a wheeled luggage cart. Try to get a model that you can push rather than pull. Pushing (preferably with two hands) places the load squarely in front of you. This helps to conserve energy and avoid the joint-twisting strain of pulling with one hand. Models that are designed for pulling can usually be pushed if the handle locks in an upright position.

- Don't over-pack nor over-lift. Even though your suitcase is on wheels, there are all too many occasions when you will have to lift it—onto the x-ray platform, into the overhead bin, etc. When those occasions arise, don't be shy about asking someone else to do the lifting—preferably someone else in a uniform whose job it is to help but if someone like that is not available, just someone who looks strong. People are more willing to help than you might think.

- Don't sit for hours at a time in a plane, bus, or car. Standing and walking for even two minutes every hour can make a huge difference in how you feel when you arrive. On planes and buses,

492

try to get an aisle seat, which makes it easier to regularly stretch your arms and legs as well as stand up and walk around. If you're driving, allow time for hourly five-minute stops.

- Sit way back, making sure your rear end touches the seat back. Slouching leads to back pain, whether or not you have arthritis. If you're short and stuck in a deep seat, stick something behind you for comfortable back support—a pillow, folded airplane blanket, or your own coat or sweater.

- Try a bath at the end of the day. When hours of sightseeing or shopping have left you tired and achy, a deep, soothing soak can relax and revive you. If you have osteoarthritis, ease into a moderately hot bath. But for inflammatory types such as rheumatoid arthritis or lupus, you may want a cool bath or simply want to put cool compresses on hot, complaining joints. You can buy cold packs that will chill in the hotel mini bar.

- Pack a plug-in night-light. In unfamiliar surroundings, it can help prevent stumbles or falls. If you forget to bring one along, just leave the bathroom light on when you go to bed.

- Pack a small emergency kit in your carry-on bag. Your own levels of concern and where you're going will determine what you pack. But at the least it should include: bottled water to take your medicine; one meal's worth of calories, such as from a health-food bar; a flashlight; in winter, a Kevlar blanket, available online or at hardware stores.

Chapter 48

Housekeeping and Arthritis

Chapter Contents

Section 48.1

Making Chores Easier When You Have Arthritis

Performing daily activities and chores is painful and tiring for many arthritis sufferers. The good news is there are many ways to help you to continue to perform your daily activities and chores without as much pain and tiredness.

Proper body mechanics are important to reducing pain. Begin by using good posture to protect the neck, back, hips, and knees. If standing for long periods is painful, lean against a wall or put one foot up on a stool. When lifting something that is low or on the ground, bend your knees and lift by straightening your legs. Do not use your back to lift. Use a device to reach with instead of bending to get something from the floor or cupboards. These devices can be bought from a medical supply store. If you have to bend, keep your back straight. Sit properly with your back straight to do work such as sorting, folding, and ironing clothing.

Organize your work and storage areas so that all equipment and tools can be kept within easy reach and at a comfortable level. Use a lazy Susan or plastic bins to keep things close by. Use lightweight tools with built-up or extended handles for gardening and other yard work.

Wear good walking shoes that fit and provide good support. Elastic shoelaces or Velcro closures make putting on shoes easier.

Self-help devices make tasks easier and more efficient. But always try to use your own body's range of motion and strength first. Self-help devices can provide leverage to give more force. Use a pizza cutter instead of a knife to cut. If your range of motion is limited, long-handled shoehorns and bath brushes can extend your reach.

When working in the kitchen and baking, place the mixing bowl in the sink while stirring. A damp cloth underneath will help keep it from slipping. Hold mixing spoons like a dagger to take stress off your hands. Use lightweight baking dishes, plates, pots, and pans, and serve from them. Use a wheeled cart to move heavy items from place to place. It also helps to sit on a high stool while cooking or washing dishes.

See a healthcare provider to learn how to use your body with minimal joint stress to have less pain, easier movement, and even more energy.

Section 48.2

Caring for Your Home and Yourself When You Have Arthritis

Excerpted with permission from *Your Home and Arthritis,* a booklet from the Arthritis Research Campaign, United Kingdom. © 2003 Arthritis Research Campaign. All rights reserved. To view the complete text of this booklet, or to find other information, visit the Arthritis Research Campaign website at http://www.arc.org.uk.

This information is for people who have any kind of arthritis or rheumatic disease and who wish to find out what equipment and adaptations might help overcome problems with everyday activities at home. These problems may include:

- getting up from a chair or out of the bath
- getting dressed, shaving, or putting on makeup
- doing jobs in the kitchen, workshop, or garage
- shopping and housework.

How Can I Adapt My Home?

Few people have a perfect home, but minor changes can make life easier and safer for you. For example:

To avoid trips and falls:

- Remove loose mats.
- Have well-lit stairs, hall, and landing.
- Have enough space to get between your furniture.

497

- Fix a second banister on the stairs and a grab rail by the door-step.

To avoid bending down:

- Attach a basket to the inside of your letter box.
- Raise electrical sockets higher up the wall.

To make switches, dials, and plugs easier to grip:

- Light switches are easier to use if they are the large rocker-type, pull-cord, or touch-operated type.
- Central heating rarely needs to be adjusted and is less effort than an open fire.
- Electric or gas fires are easier to turn on if the control knob is located at the top.
- If you have difficulty turning dials or knobs, a contour grip will help.
- Handiplugs and stick-on plug grips can make plugs easier to take out of sockets.

To make using the TV and phone easier:

Remote controls have made operating the TV, video, and music system easier. There are many styles of phones; choose one which suits your needs. For example:

- Some phones have a hands-free option, which enables you to use the phone without having to keep the receiver pressed to your ear.
- A cordless phone is easy to grip and handy to keep by you. It will save you getting up when you are relaxing and will allow you to call help in an emergency—for example, should you have difficulty getting out of the bath.
- A phone-alarm system has an alarm button which can be kept in a pocket, hung around the neck, or pinned to clothing. When the button is pressed it activates the phone to call for help. Many agencies operate a phone-alarm system for which you pay a small rental fee.
- Mobile phones give you peace of mind when you are out and about.

What Can I Do If I Have Difficulty Reaching Things?

Arthritis causes restricted movement in joints—such as shoulders, back, and hips—which can make reaching for things difficult. Long-handled gadgets to assist with washing and dressing are discussed later in this chapter. Try reorganizing storage in drawers and cupboards to make it easier to reach the things you need most often. A reaching stick enables you to pick things up from the floor without reaching down.

What about Getting out of a Chair?

If you have stiff and painful joints, particularly in your back, hips or knees, you may find it difficult to get up from a low armchair. It can help in the short term to raise the height of your seat using an extra cushion. An armchair raiser unit is a series of four interlinked blocks which fit under the chair legs to raise the height of the chair—or you may prefer to sit on your dining chair or plastic garden chair.

When you buy an easy chair consider the following:

- Is it high enough? Can you get up from it easily?
- When seated, are your feet flat on the floor?
- Does it have comfortable arm and back rests to fully support you?

You may wish to consider an electrically operated riser-recliner chair, which will eliminate all effort on your part. It also allows you to relax fully while seated.

What about Reading and Writing?

Gripping things tightly for a long time, such as a book or pen, can make hands and wrists painful. Look for pens which have a chunky or sticky grip which is easy to hold. Rest your book or newspaper in your lap or on the table to avoid straining your fingers. Many people with arthritis find that resting their book on a beanbag or bookrest is helpful.

What about Using My Computer?

Sitting for a long time and adopting a bad posture will make aches and pains worse. The following tips may help:

- Take frequent breaks and change your position often.

499

- Sit squarely facing the computer, with your back and arms supported.

- Find a table and chair which enable you to sit comfortably.

- Wear wrist splints for support, or try resting your wrists on a sponge bar in front of the keyboard.

- Be aware that using bifocal glasses at the computer can force you to tilt your head back and cause neck strain.

- Voice-activated software can be easier to use than a mouse and keyboard if you have pain in your hands.

What Can I Do to Make Life Easier in the Kitchen?

Many of us dream of our ideal kitchen! If you have decided to have your kitchen redesigned, or to adapt another part of your home, or if you are moving to a completely new place, seek advice from your occupational therapist. You will receive professional advice and be able to see, and try out, some helpful equipment.

Most people, however, will adapt and improve their present kitchen.

Choosing Kitchen Equipment

When buying a cooker, microwave, washing machine, dishwasher, fridge-freezer, coffee machine or kettle, shop around to make sure the equipment you are buying is easy to use and maintain.

Ask yourself the following questions when choosing kitchen equipment.

- Are the control knobs easy to reach, grip and turn, push, or pull?

- Is it the right height for you to work at or reach into?

- Can you open the doors or remove the lid?

- Will you be able to clean and maintain it easily?

Consider the ways some equipment can save you considerable time and effort.

- Microwave cooker: Cooking with a microwave is often quicker and the dishes used are lighter than traditional saucepans. Some combine an oven and grill. If situated on a work surface they can often be easier to reach into than a conventional cooker oven. A microwave can be used for more complex cooking as well as defrosting and reheating food.

- Dishwasher: Dishwashers are available in different sizes to suit your household. When buying new kitchenware, check it is dishwasher-proof and cut down even further on your washing-up.

- Fridge-freezer: You can choose between different sizes and whether to have the fridge or the freezer compartment at the top. The freezer compartment usually has pull-out drawers which, if not overfilled, are easier to use than a chest-type freezer.

- Electric jug kettle: This is generally easier to grip and pour from than the traditional kettle. Designs vary, and some pour more easily than others. The cordless design is easier to use. However, if you wish to use a kettle tipper you will need a corded kettle. A useful tip is to bring water to the kettle in a light-weight plastic jug to avoid having to unplug or move the kettle.

Work Surfaces and Cupboards

Find the work surface in your kitchen at which you are most comfortable and avoid standing for long periods. You may find it helpful to sit at the kitchen table or perch on a high stool.

If your work surfaces are on the same level and with no gaps in between, you will be able to slide pans and groceries along them to avoid lifting.

People with arthritis often find it difficult to reach into very low or high cupboards, particularly if they are cluttered or stacked several layers deep. You may find the following helpful:

- Rearrange how you store things and remove items no longer in use.

- Store frequently used items within easy reach on the work surface or at the front of cupboards at a convenient height.

- Move wall-mounted cupboards to a lower position.

- Fit large handles or sliding doors.

- Have shelves which slide or rotate out when you open the door.

- Have drawers mounted on rollers which run more easily.

Preparing Food

Cutting, cleaning, peeling, grating or mixing food can be hard if you find it difficult to grip things. Other common problems are opening tins, jars, and bottles, lifting saucepans, and carrying food from the kitchen to the room where you eat.

Ready-made meals, stored in the freezer, can be reheated in the microwave. Supermarkets sell ready prepared food such as chopped vegetables, grated cheese, and roasted potatoes. Even if you prefer to prepare and cook your own meal, having a few prepared ingredients and ready-made meals in the freezer means you can avoid struggling on days when your arthritis is particularly troublesome.

Cooking and Serving

Using a microwave is often the quickest and easiest way to cook food. However, if you are using a conventional cooker the following will help you to reduce the strain on painful hands and wrists:

- a lightweight, two-handled saucepan
- a vegetable steamer (lighter than a saucepan, as less water is required)
- a slotted spoon to remove boiled vegetables from the saucepan
- a wire chip basket, placed in the saucepan (this lifts out when vegetables are cooked, leaving the water behind)
- a colander, placed in the sink to drain the vegetables (the saucepan is placed on the draining board and tilted to allow the contents to fall into the colander)
- a flat-bottomed ladle to remove soups and stews from the saucepan.

A serving trolley can be useful for moving food from the cooker to the table, and can double as a walking aid.

At the Kitchen Sink

Lever taps are the easiest to use; you can buy these, or fit tap turners onto existing taps.

To avoid stooping while washing up, raise your washing-up bowl by putting it on blocks or another upturned bowl in the sink (if the tap height allows). Wringing out dishcloths can be painful for hands. Experiment using different types of sponges, which you can squeeze out with the heel of your hand.

Eating and Drinking

You may find padding the handles of cutlery helpful if your fingers do not bend easily. There is also a wide range of specialist cutlery

502

available. Use lightweight crockery and cups with large handles which can be gripped with several fingers. Insulated or pedestal mugs can be held with both hands because you can support them underneath without burning yourself.

Can I Make Jobs Easier in the Workshop and Garage?

To organize storage in your workshop, potting shed, or garage, use the same ideas as suggested for the kitchen. Countertops should be at a comfortable height and you should sit or perch to work. Pad the handles of tools to make them easier to grip, and buy lightweight, power-assisted tools such as drills or screwdrivers.

What Can I Do to Make Housework Easier?

Plan to do small amounts of housework often rather than doing it all in one go. Pace yourself, taking regular breaks, to avoid making joints painful. You may find your energy lasts longer if you organize tasks to cut down on too many trips upstairs. Wearing wrist splints while polishing and sweeping can ease. Using a long-handled dust-pan and brush will mean less bending down.

Making Beds

The main problem when making a bed is shifting the weight of the mattress. This can make tucking in bedclothes painful and difficult. You may find it helpful to have a lightweight mattress with fitted sheets and duvet. These need little alteration between linen changes once they are in place.

Washing, Drying, and Ironing Clothes

When buying clothes, look for fabrics which are lightweight and don't need ironing. You may find it easier to do half-loads when washing. A reaching gadget may help to get the clothes out of the machine, and raising a clothes basket on a block or box will make it easier to pick up. Tumble-drying clothes avoids the need to hang them out and cuts down on ironing. For the ironing you do need to do, it will help to sit down to iron.

How Can I Wash Myself More Easily?

Just as in the kitchen, you will find lever taps easier to use on the handbasin and bath. Liquid soap in a push-button dispenser can also

503

be useful. Some other helpful things to assist you to grip and reach include a:

- long-handled sponge
- long-handled hairbrush
- long flannel strap with hand rings
- long-handled toe-wipe
- long-handled makeup sponge.

Drying yourself can be difficult if your shoulders and elbows are stiff and painful. A thick toweling dressing gown put on straight from the shower or bath is much easier than struggling to dry yourself with a bath towel.

Reaching up to shave or put on makeup often makes arms and shoulders ache. Resting your elbow on a table or shelf at the appropriate height will rest your arm and reduce aching. You may also find some of the following helpful:

- lightweight electric razor
- electric toothbrush
- choosing eyeliner pencils and mascara with chunky grips—or try fattening the grip by wrapping an elastic band around it
- using a small make-up sponge to apply face cream if you find it difficult to do with your fingertips. This can be mounted on a long handle to improve reach.

Is There Anything to Help Me Get out of the Bath?

Getting in and out of a bath can be extremely difficult, particularly if you have a painful back, hips, or knees. It is not advisable for someone to lift you in and out, as it could easily injure his or her back.

You may find a non-slip mat in the bath useful to give you more grip. The following aids may also help you:

- grab rail
- bath board and seat
- powered bath seat lift.

Another possible option is a special walk-in bath, but installing one of these will be expensive.

Taking a Shower

Many people find it easier to take a shower. A grab rail and seat will help you to shower comfortably and safely. If your shower is over the bath you may find it safer to sit on a bath board (a slatted board placed across the top of the bath). There are large-size, level-access showers for people whose mobility is more severely restricted and these are often cheaper to install than a walk-in bath.

Using the Toilet

If your shoulders, hips, and knees are stiff or painful, getting up from the toilet and reaching to clean yourself can be difficult. The following equipment can help:

- grab rail beside the toilet
- raised toilet seat
- frame surrounding the toilet to push up from
- bottom-wiping gadget
- portable bidet which fits onto a standard toilet pan
- automatic-flushing toilet which incorporates a bidet which washes and dries you.

Are There Gadgets to Help Me Dress?

With rheumatoid arthritis, joints are often stiff and aching first thing in the morning. This can make dressing time-consuming and tiring.

It is usually easiest to sit down to dress. Choose loose-fitting clothes with simple fastenings, clip-on ties, and front-fastening bras. These can all help, especially on days when the pain is worse. An alternative to tights are full- or half-length stay-up stockings with elastic tops to hold them up.

Clothing can be adapted by replacing some fastenings with Velcro. Try placing a keyring or tag on a zip to hook your finger through. There are a wide variety of gadgets designed to help:

- dressing stick
- buttonhook for fastening buttons
- long-handled shoehorn
- sock aid

Slip-on shoes are the easiest to put on; however, lace-ups allow you to loosen them when feet swell. Some people find Velcro fastenings or elastic laces helpful.

What Can I Do to Make Shopping Easier?

People with arthritis often find shopping is difficult and tiring. Many have found ways round this problem, for example:

- Friends or neighbors may be able to shop for you.
- Social Services may arrange for someone to help.
- You can shop by phone or Internet with home delivery, or by using mail-order catalogs.

What If I Want to Do the Shopping?

Try some of the following suggestions:

- Plan to shop on a day when you don't have other things to do so you don't become too tired.
- Don't attempt to carry too much in one trip.
- Plastic bags with firm handle-grip inserts are easier to carry (you can buy these at some supermarkets).
- Take someone with you to help.
- Ask for help at the supermarket.
- For short trips on foot, consider using a shopping basket on wheels.
- Many large stores provide wheelchairs and scooters for customers' use.

Part Six

Additional
Help and Information

Chapter 49

Glossary of Arthritis-Related Terms

Analgesic: A compound capable of producing analgesia, i.e., one that relieves pain by altering perception of nociceptive stimuli without producing anesthesia or loss of consciousness.[1]

Ankylosing spondylitis: Arthritis of the spine, resembling rheumatoid arthritis, that may progress to bony ankylosis with lipping of vertebral margins; the disease is more common in the male.[1]

Antinuclear antibody test (ANA): This test checks blood levels of antibodies that are often present in people who have connective tissue diseases or other autoimmune disorders, such as lupus. Since the antibodies react with material in the cell's nucleus (control center), they are referred to as antinuclear antibodies. There are also tests for individual types of ANAs that may be more specific to people with certain autoimmune disorders. ANAs are also sometimes found in people who do not have an autoimmune disorder. Therefore, having ANAs in the blood does not necessarily mean that a person has a disease.[2]

Arthritis: Inflammation of a joint or a state characterized by inflammation of joints.[1]

Definitions in this chapter were compiled from several sources. Terms marked 1 are from *Stedman's Medical Dictionary, 27th Edition.* © 2000, Lippincott Williams & Wilkins. All rights reserved. Terms marked 2 are from various publications produced by the National Institute of Arthritis and Musculoskeletal and Skin Diseases.

Arthropathy: Any disease affecting a joint.[1]

Arthroplasty: Creation of an artificial joint to correct advanced degenerative arthritis or an operation to restore as far as possible the integrity and functional power of a joint.[1]

Behçet disease: A syndrome characterized by simultaneously or successively occurring recurrent attacks of genital and oral ulcerations (aphthae) and uveitis or iridocyclitis with hypopyon, often with arthritis.[1]

Biologic response modifier: Agent that modifies host responses to neoplasms by enhancing immune systems or reconstituting impaired immune mechanisms.[1]

Bursitis: Inflammation of a bursa.[1]

Complement: This test measures the level of complement, a group of proteins in the blood. Complement helps destroy foreign substances, such as germs, that enter the body. A low blood level of complement is common in people who have active lupus.[2]

Complete blood count (CBC): This test determines the number of white blood cells, red blood cells, and platelets present in a sample of blood. Some rheumatic conditions or drugs used to treat arthritis are associated with a low white blood count (leukopenia), low red blood count (anemia), or low platelet count (thrombocytopenia). When doctors prescribe medications that affect the CBC, they periodically test the patient's blood.[2]

Corticosteroids: A steroid produced by the adrenal cortex (i.e., adrenal corticoid); a corticoid containing a steroid.[1]

C-reactive protein test: This is a nonspecific test used to detect generalized inflammation. Levels of the protein are often increased in patients with active disease such as rheumatoid arthritis, and may decline when corticosteroids or nonsteroidal anti-inflammatory drugs (NSAIDs) are used to reduce inflammation.[2]

Creatinine: This blood test is commonly ordered in patients who have a rheumatic disease, such as lupus, to monitor for underlying kidney disease. Creatinine is a breakdown product of creatine, which is an important component of muscle. It is excreted from the body entirely by the kidneys, and the level remains constant and normal when kidney function is normal.[2]

Erythrocyte sedimentation rate (sed rate): This blood test is used to detect inflammation in the body. Higher sed rates indicate the presence of inflammation and are typical of many forms of arthritis, such as rheumatoid arthritis and ankylosing spondylitis, and many of the connective tissue diseases.[2]

Fibromyalgia: A syndrome of chronic pain of musculoskeletal origin but uncertain cause. The American College of Rheumatology has established diagnostic criteria that include pain on both sides of the body, both above and below the waist, as well as in an axial distribution (cervical, thoracic, or lumbar spine or anterior chest); additionally there must be point tenderness in at least 11 of 18 specified sites.[1]

Giant cell arteritis: A subacute, granulomatous arteritis involving the external carotid arteries, especially the temporal artery; occurs in elderly persons and may be manifested by constitutional symptoms, particularly severe headache, and sometimes sudden unilateral blindness. Shares many of the symptoms of polymyalgia rheumatica.[1]

Glucosamine and chondroitin: Glucosamine and chondroitin are natural substances found in and around the cells of cartilage. Researchers believe these substances may help in the repair and maintenance of cartilage. In addition, researchers believe that glucosamine inhibits inflammation and stimulates cartilage cell growth, while chondroitin provides cartilage with strength and resilience. Currently, glucosamine and chondroitin are classified as dietary supplements.[2]

Gout: A disorder of purine metabolism, occurring especially in men, characterized by a raised but variable blood uric acid level and severe recurrent acute arthritis of sudden onset resulting from deposition of crystals of sodium urate in connective tissues and articular cartilage.[1]

Hematocrit (PCV, packed cell volume): This test and the test for hemoglobin (a substance in the red blood cells that carries oxygen throughout the body) measure the number of red blood cells present in a sample of blood. A decrease in the number of red blood cells (anemia) is common in people who have inflammatory arthritis or another rheumatic disease.[2]

Hydrotherapy: Therapeutic use of water by external application, either for its pressure effect or as a means of applying physical energy to the tissues.[1]

Juvenile rheumatoid arthritis: Chronic arthritis beginning in childhood, most cases of which are pauciarticular, i.e., affecting few joints. Several patterns of illness have been identified: in one subset, primarily affecting girls, iritis is common and antinuclear antibody is usually present; another subset, primarily affecting boys, frequently includes spinal arthritis resembling ankylosing spondylitis; some cases are true rheumatoid arthritis beginning in childhood and characterized by the presence of rheumatoid factor and destructive deforming joint changes, often undergoing remission at puberty.[1]

Lyme disease: A subacute inflammatory disorder caused by infection with *Borrelia burgdorferi,* a nonpyogenic spirochete transmitted by *Ixodes scapularis,* the deer tick, in the eastern U.S. and *I. pacificus,* the western black-legged tick, in the western U.S.; the characteristic skin lesion, erythema chronicum migrans, is usually preceded or accompanied by fever, malaise, fatigue, headache, and stiff neck; neurologic, cardiac, or articular manifestations may occur weeks to months later. Residual articular or neurologic symptoms, which may persist for months or years after the initial infection, probably represent an immune response to the organism.[1]

Myositis: Inflammation of a muscle.[1]

Non-steroidal anti-inflammatory drugs: A large number of drugs exerting anti-inflammatory (and also usually analgesic and antipyretic) actions; examples include aspirin, acetaminophen, diclofenac, indomethacin, ketorolac, ibuprofen, and naproxen. A contrast is made with steroidal compounds (such as hydrocortisone or prednisone) exerting anti-inflammatory activity.[1]

Osteoarthritis: Arthritis characterized by erosion of articular cartilage, either primary or secondary to trauma or other conditions, which becomes soft, frayed, and thinned with eburnation of subchondral bone and outgrowths of marginal osteophytes; pain and loss of function result; mainly affects weight-bearing joints, is more common in older persons.[1]

Osteoporosis: Reduction in the quantity of bone or atrophy of skeletal tissue; an age-related disorder characterized by decreased bone mass and increased susceptibility to fractures.[1]

Paget disease: A generalized skeletal disease, frequently familial, of older persons in which bone resorption and formation are both increased, leading to thickening and softening of bones (e.g., the skull), and bending of weight-bearing bones.[1]

Pauciarticular: A joint condition in which only a few (greater than 1, less than 5) joints are involved.[1]

Polyarticular: Relating to or involving many joints.[1]

Polymyalgia rheumatica: A syndrome within the group of collagen diseases different from spondylarthritis or from humeral scapular periarthritis by the presence of an elevated sedimentation rate; much commoner in women than in men.[1]

Polymyositis: Inflammation of a number of voluntary muscles simultaneously.[1]

Pseudogout: Acute episodic synovitis caused by deposits of calcium pyrophosphate crystals rather than urate crystals as in true gout.[1]

Psoriasis: A common multifactorial inherited condition characterized by the eruption of circumscribed, discrete and confluent, reddish, silvery-scaled maculopapules; the lesions occur predominantly on the elbows, knees, scalp, and trunk.[1]

Reiter syndrome: The association of urethritis, iridocyclitis, mucocutaneous lesions, and arthritis, sometimes with diarrhea; one or more of these conditions may recur at intervals of months or years, but the arthritis may be persistent.[1]

Rheumatoid arthritis: A generalized disease, occurring more often in women, which primarily affects connective tissue; arthritis is the dominant clinical manifestation, involving many joints, especially those of the hands and feet, accompanied by thickening of articular soft tissue, with extension of synovial tissue over articular cartilages, which become eroded; the course is variable but often is chronic and progressive, leading to deformities and disability.[1]

Rheumatoid factor: This test detects the presence of rheumatoid factor, an antibody found in the blood of most (but not all) people who have rheumatoid arthritis. Rheumatoid factor may be found in many diseases besides rheumatoid arthritis, and sometimes in people without health problems.[2]

Rheumatologist: A specialist in rheumatology.[1]

Rheumatology: The medical specialty concerned with the study, diagnosis, and treatment of rheumatic conditions.[1]

Scleroderma: Thickening and induration of the skin caused by new collagen formation, with atrophy of pilosebaceous follicles.[1]

Septic (infectious) arthritis: Acute inflammation of synovial membranes, with purulent effusion into a joint, due to bacterial infection; the usual route of infection is hemic to the synovial tissue, causing destruction of the articular cartilage, and may become chronic, with sinus formation, osteomyelitis, deformity, and disability.[1]

Still disease: A form of juvenile chronic arthritis (formerly called juvenile rheumatoid arthritis) characterized by high fever and signs of systemic illness that can exist for weeks or months before the onset of arthritis.[1]

Synovial fluid examination: Synovial fluid may be examined for white blood cells (found in patients with rheumatoid arthritis and infections), bacteria or viruses (found in patients with infectious arthritis), or crystals in the joint (found in patients with gout or other types of crystal-induced arthritis). To obtain a specimen, the doctor injects a local anesthetic, then inserts a needle into the joint to withdraw the synovial fluid into a syringe. The procedure is called arthrocentesis or joint aspiration.[2]

Synovium: The connective tissue membrane that lines the cavity of a synovial joint and produces the synovial fluid; it lines all internal surfaces of the cavity except for the articular cartilage of the bones.[1]

Systemic lupus erythematosus: An inflammatory connective tissue disease with variable features, frequently including fever, weakness and fatigability, joint pains or arthritis resembling rheumatoid arthritis, diffuse erythematous skin lesions on the face, neck, or upper extremities, lymphadenopathy, pleurisy or pericarditis, glomerular lesions, anemia, hyperglobulinemia, and a positive LE cell test.[1]

Tendinitis: Inflammation of a tendon.[1]

Total joint arthroplasty: Arthroplasty in which both joint surfaces are replaced with artificial materials, usually composed of metal and high-density plastic; currently being performed for hip, knee, shoulder, and elbow.[1]

Transcutaneous electrical nerve stimulation (TENS): TENS has been found effective in modifying pain perception. TENS blocks pain messages to the brain with a small device that directs mild electric pulses to nerve endings that lie beneath the painful area of the skin.[2]

Urinalysis: In this test, a urine sample is studied for protein, red blood cells, white blood cells, and bacteria. These abnormalities may indicate kidney disease, which may be seen in several rheumatic diseases, including lupus. Some medications used to treat arthritis can also cause abnormal findings on urinalysis.[2]

White blood cell count (WBC): This test determines the number of white blood cells present in a sample of blood. The number may increase as a result of infection or decrease in response to certain medications or in certain diseases, such as lupus. Low numbers of white blood cells increase a person's risk of infections.[2]

Chapter 50

Directory of Arthritis Organizations and Resources

Government Agencies and Organizations

Agency for Healthcare Research and Quality
540 Gaither Road
Rockville, MD 20850
Phone: (301) 427-1364
Website: http://www.ahrq.gov
E-mail: info@ahrq.gov

Centers for Disease Control and Prevention
1600 Clifton Road
Atlanta, GA 30333
Toll-Free: (800) 311-3435
Phone: (404) 639-3311
Website: http://www.cdc.gov
E-mail: ccdinfo@cdc.gov

National Center for Alternative and Complementary Medicine
P.O. Box 7923
Gaithersburg, MD 20898
Toll-Free: (888) 644-6226
Phone: (301) 519-3153
TTY: (866) 464-3615
Fax: (866) 464-3616
Website: http://nccam.nih.gov
E-mail: info@nccam.nih.gov

Resources in this chapter were compiled from several sources deemed reliable; all contact information was verified and updated in March 2004.

National Heart, Lung, and Blood Institute
Building 31, Room 5A52
31 Center Drive, MSC 2486
Bethesda, MD 20892-2480
Phone: (301) 592-8573
Fax: (301) 592-8563
TTY: (240) 629-3255
Website: http://www.nhlbi.nih.gov
E-mail: nhlbiinfo@nhlbi.nih.gov

National Institute of Allergy and Infectious Disease
6610 Rockledge Drive, MSC 6612
Bethesda, MD 20892-6612
Phone: (301) 402-1663
Fax: (301) 402-0120
Website: http://www.niaid.nih.gov

National Institute of Arthritis and Musculoskeletal and Skin Diseases
1 AMS Circle
Bethesda, MD 20892-3675
Toll-Free: (877) 22-NIAMS (226-4267)
Phone: (301) 495-4484
TTY: (301) 565-2966
Fax: (301) 718-6366
Website: http://www.niams.nih.gov
E-mail: niamsinfo@mail.nih.gov

National Institute on Aging
Building 31, Room 5C27
31 Center Drive, MSC 2292
Bethesda, MD 20892
Phone: (301) 496-1752
Website: http://www.nia.nih.gov
E-mail: webmaster@nia.nih.gov

Osteoporosis and Related Bone Diseases–National Resource Center
2 AMS Circle
Bethesda, MD 20892-3676
Toll-Free: (800) 624-BONE
Phone: (202) 223-0344
TTY: (202) 466-4315
Fax: (202) 293-2356
Website: http://www.osteo.org
E-mail: OsteoInfo@osteo.org

U.S. Food and Drug Administration
5600 Fishers Lane
Rockville, MD 20857-0001
Toll-Free: (888) 463-6332
Website: http://www.fda.gov

Private and Nonprofit Organizations

AllAboutArthritis.com/ DePuy Orthopaedics
700 Orthopaedic Drive
P.O. Box 988
Warsaw, IN 46581
Phone: (574) 372-7333
Website: http://www.allaboutarthritis.com
E-mail: allaboutarthritis@dpyus.jnj.com

American Academy of Physical Medicine and Rehabilitation
One IBM Plaza, Suite 2500
Chicago, IL 60611-3604
Phone: (312) 464-9700
Fax: (312) 464-0227
Website: http://www.aapmr.org
E-mail: info@aapmr.org

American Academy of Orthopaedic Surgeons (AAOS)
6300 North River Road
Rosemont, IL 60018-4262
Toll-Free: (800) 824-BONE (2663)
Phone: (847) 823-7186
Fax: (847) 823-8125
Website: http://www.aaos.org
E-mail: custserv@aaos.org

American Academy of Pain Management
13947 Mono Way #A
Sonora, CA 95370
Phone: (209) 533-9744
Fax: (209) 533-9750
Website: http://www.aapainmanage.org
E-mail: aapm@aapainmanage.org

American Behçet's Disease Association
P.O. Box 19952
Amarillo, TX 78114
Toll-Free: (800) 723-4238
Website: http://www.behcets.com

American Chronic Pain Association
P.O. Box 850
Rocklin, CA 95677
Toll-Free: (800) 533-3231
Phone: (916) 632-0922
Fax: (916) 632-3208
Website: http://www.theacpa.org
E-mail: ACPA@pacbell.net

American College of Foot and Ankle Surgeons
515 Busse Highway
Park Ridge, Illinois 60068
Toll-Free: (800) 421-2237
Phone: (847) 292-2237
Website: http://www.acfas.org
E-mail: info@acfas.org

American College of Rheumatology
1800 Century Place
Suite 250
Atlanta, GA 30345-4300
Phone: (404) 633-3777
Fax: (404) 633-1870
Website: http://www.rheumatology.org

American Juvenile Arthritis Organization
1330 West Peachtree Street
Atlanta, GA 30309
Toll-Free: (800) 283-7800
Phone: (404) 872-7100
Website: http://www.arthritis.org
E-mail: arthritis@finelinesolutions.com

American Medical Association/Medem
649 Mission Street, 2nd Floor
San Francisco, CA 94105
Toll-Free: (877) 926-3336
Phone: (415) 644-3800
Fax: (415) 644-3950
Website: http://www.medem.com
E-mail: info@medem.com

American Occupational Therapy Association
4720 Montgomery Lane
P.O. Box 31220
Bethesda, MD 20824-1220
Phone: (301) 652-2682
TTY: (800) 377-8555
Fax: (301) 652-7711
Website: http://www.aota.org

American Orthopaedic Foot and Ankle Society
2517 Eastlake Avenue East, Suite 200
Seattle, WA 98102
Toll-Free: (800) 235-4855
Phone: (206) 223-1120
Website: http://www.footcaremd.com
E-mail: footcaremd@ideabank.com

American Pain Foundation
201 N. Charles Street
Suite 710
Baltimore, MD 21201-4111
Toll-Free: (888) 615-PAIN (7246)
Website: http://www.painfoundation.org
E-mail: info@painfoundation.org

American Pain Society
4700 West Lake Avenue
Glenview, IL 60025-1485
Phone: (847) 375-4715
Fax (Toll-Free): (877) 734-8758
http://www.ampainsoc.org
E-mail: info@ampainsoc.org

American Physical Therapy Association
1111 North Fairfax Street
Alexandria, VA 22314-1488
Toll-Free: (800) 999-2782, X3395
Phone: (703) 684-2782
Fax: (703) 684-7343
TDD: (703) 683-6748
Website: http://www.apta.org

American Podiatric Medical Association
9312 Old Georgetown Road
Bethesda, MD 20814
Toll-Free: (800) ASK-APMA
Phone: (301) 571-9200
Fax: (301) 530-2752
Website: http://www.apma.org
E-mail: askapma@apma.org

Arthritis Foundation
1330 West Peachtree Street
Atlanta, GA 30309
Toll-Free: (800) 283-7800
Phone: (404) 872-7100
Website: http://www.arthritis.org
E-mail: arthritis@finelinesolutions.com

Arthritis National Research Foundation
200 Oceangate, Suite 830
Long Beach, CA 90802
Toll-Free: (800) 588-CURE (2873)
Fax: (562) 983-1410
Website: http://www.curearthritis.org
E-mail: anrf@ix.netcom.com

Arthritis Research Campaign

Copeman House, St. Mary's
Court, St. Mary's Gate
Chesterfield, Derbyshire S41 7TD
UNITED KINGDOM
Toll-Free: 011-44-0870-850-5000
Phone: 011-44-0-1246-558033
Fax: 011-44-0-1246 558007
Website: http://www.arc.org.uk
E-mail: Info@arc.org.uk

Arthritis Society

393 University Avenue
Suite 1700
Toronto, Ontario M5G 1E6
CANADA
Toll-Free: (800) 321-1433
Phone: (416) 979-7228
Fax: (416) 979-8366
Website: http://www.arthritis.ca
E-mail: info@arthritis.ca

Arthritis Source

University of Washington
Department of Orthopaedics
and Sports Medicine
1959 N.E. Pacific Street
P.O. Box 356500
Seattle, WA 98195-6500
Phone: (206) 543-3690
Fax: (206) 685-3139
Website: http://www.orthop
.washington.edu/arthritis
E-mail: sportsmd@u.washington
.edu

American Society for Surgery of the Hand

6300 North River Road
Suite 600
Rosemont, IL 60018
Phone: (847) 384-8300
Fax: (847) 384-1435
Website: http://www.
hand-surg.org
E-mail: info@assh.org

Cleveland Clinic

9500 Euclid Avenue
Cleveland, OH 44195
Toll-Free: (800) 223-2273, ext.
48950
Phone: (216) 444-2200
TTY: (216) 444-0261
Website: http://
www.clevelandclinic.org

Fibromyalgia Network

P.O. Box 31750
Tucson, AZ 85751-1750
Toll-Free: (800) 853-2929
Website: http://
www.fmnetnews.com

Hip Society

951 Old County Road, #182
Belmont, CA 94002
Phone: (650) 596-6190
Fax: (650) 508-2039
Website: http://www.hipsoc.org

521

Hospital for Special Surgery—Rheumatology Division
535 East 70th Street
New York, NY 10021
Toll-Free: (866) 749-7047
Phone: (212) 606-1753
Website: http://www.rheumatology.hss.edu

International Still's Disease Foundation
1123 S. Kimbrel Avenue
Panama City, FL 32404
Fax: (850) 871-6656
Website: http://www.stillsdisease.org
E-mail: webmaster@stillsdisease.org

Johns Hopkins Arthritis Center
Johns Hopkins University Division of Rheumatology
5501 Hopkins Bayview Circle
Baltimore, MD 21224
Phone: (410) 550-2400
Fax: (410) 550-5601
Website: http://www.hopkins-arthritis.org

Kids on the Block, Inc.
9385-C Gerwig Lane
Columbia, MD 21046
Toll-Free: (800) 368-KIDS (5437)
Phone: (410) 290-9095
Fax: (410) 290-9358
Website: http://www.kotb.com
E-mail: kotb@kotb.com

Myositis Association
1233 20th St. NW
Suite 402
Washington, DC 20036
Phone: (202) 887-0088
Fax: (202) 466-8940
Website: http://www.myositis.org
E-mail: tma@myositis.org

National Ankylosing Spondylitis Society
P.O. Box 179
Mayfield, East Sussex TN20 6ZL
UNITED KINGDOM
Phone: 011-44-01435 873527
Fax: 011-44-01435 873027
Website: http://www.nass.co.uk
E-mail: nass@nass.co.uk

National Chronic Pain Outreach Association, Inc.
7979 Old Georgetown Road,
Suite 100
Bethesda, MD 20814-2429
Phone: (301) 652-4948
Fax: (301) 907-0745
Website: http://neurosurgery.mgh.harvard.edu/ncpainoa.htm

National Fibromyalgia Association
2200 Glassell Street
Suite A
Orange, CA 92865
Phone: (714) 921-0150
Fax: (714) 921-6920
Website: http://fmaware.org
E-mail: NFA@fmaware.org

National Osteoporosis Foundation
1232 22nd Street NW
Washington, DC 20037-1292
Toll-Free: (877) 868-4520
Phone: (202) 223-2226
Fax: (770) 442-9742
Website: http://www.nof.org
E-mail: customerservice@nof.org

National Pain Foundation
3511 S. Clarkson Street
Englewood, CO 80113
Website: http://
www.painconnection.org
E-mail:
aardrup@painconnection.org

National Psoriasis Foundation
6600 SW 92nd Avenue
Suite 300
Portland, OR 97223-7195
Toll-Free: (800) 723-9166
Phone: (503) 244-7404
Fax: (503) 245-0626
Website: http://
www.psoriasis.org
E-mail: getinfo@psoriasis.org

National Scoliosis Foundation
5 Cabot Place
Stoughton, MA 02072
Toll-Free: (800) 673-6922
Fax: (781) 341-8333
Website: http://www.scoliosis.org
E-mail: NSF@scoliosis.org

National Sleep Foundation
1522 K Street, NW
Suite 500
Washington, DC 20005
Phone: (202) 347-3471
Fax: (202) 347-3472
Website: http://
www.sleepfoundation.org
E-mail: nsf@sleepfoundation.org

Scleroderma Foundation
12 Kent Way
Suite 101
Byfield, MA 01922
Toll-Free: 800-722-HOPE (4673)
Phone: (978) 463-5843
Fax: (978) 463-5809
Website: http://
www.scleroderma.org
E-mail: sfinfo@scleroderma.org

Scleroderma Research Foundation
2320 Bath Street
Suite 315
Santa Barbara, CA 93105
Toll-Free: (800) 441-CURE
Phone: (805) 563-9133
Website: http://www.srfcure.org

Scoliosis Association, Inc.
P.O. Box 811705
Boca Raton, FL 33481-1705
Toll-Free: (800) 800-0669
Phone: (561) 991-4435
Fax: (561) 994-2455
Website: http://www.scoliosis-assoc.org

Scoliosis Research Society
611 East Wells Street
Milwaukee, WI 53202-3892
Phone: (414) 289-9107
Fax: (414) 276-3349
Website: http://www.srs.org

Sjögren's Syndrome Foundation
8120 Woodmont Avenue
Suite 530
Bethesda, MD 20814
Toll-Free: (800) 475-6473
Fax: (301) 718-0322
Website: http://sjogrens.com

Spondylitis Association of America
P.O. Box 5872
Sherman Oaks, CA 91413
Toll-Free: (800) 777-8189
Website: http://www.spondylitis.org
E-mail: info@spondylitis.org

Surviving Scleroderma
Website: http://sclerodermasupport.com
E-mail: webmaster@sclerodermasupport.org

Chapter 51

Organizations That Provide Information and Assistance for People Disabled by Arthritis or Taking Arthritis Medications

Agencies and Organizations That Provide Information and Assistance for People Disabled by Arthritis

Americans with Disabilities Act Home Page
U.S. Department of Justice
950 Pennsylvania Avenue, NW
Civil Rights Division
Disability Rights Section–NYAV
Washington, DC 20530
Toll-Free: (800) 514-0301
Fax: (202) 307-1198
TTY: (800) 514-0383
Website: http://www.ada.gov

Center for Assistive Technology & Environmental Access
490 Tenth Street NW
Atlanta, GA 30332-0156
Toll-Free: (800) 726-9119
Phone: (404) 894-1414
Fax: (404) 894-9320
Website: http://www.assistivetech.net
E-mail: info@assistivetech.net

Job Accommodation Network
P.O. Box 6080
Morgantown, WV 26506-6080
Toll-Free V/TTY: (800) 526-7234
Phone V/TTY: (304) 293-7186
Fax: (304) 293-5407
Website: http://www.jan.wvu.edu
E-mail: jan@jan.wvu.edu

Resources in this chapter were compiled from several sources deemed reliable; all contact information was verified and updated in March 2004.

Medicare Rights Center
1460 Broadway
17th Floor
New York, NY 10036
Phone: (212) 869-3850
Fax: (212) 869-3532
Website: http://
www.medicarerights.org/
index.html
E-mail: info@medicarerights.org

**National Center on
Physical Activity and
Disability**
1640 W. Roosevelt Road
Chicago, IL 60608-6904
Toll-Free V/TTY: (800) 900-8086
Fax: (312) 355-4058
Website: http://www.ncpad.org

**National Organization of
Social Security Claimants'
Representatives**
6 Prospect Street
Midland Park, NJ 07432-1691
Toll-Free: (800) 431-2804
Website: http://www.nosscr.org
E-mail: webmaster@nosscr.org

**National Organization on
Disability**
910 Sixteenth Street, NW
Suite 600
Washington, DC 20006
Phone: (202) 293-5960
TTY: (202) 293-5968
Fax: (202) 293-7999
Website: http://www.nod.org
E-mail: ability@nod.org

**Office of Disability
Employment Policy**
Website: http://disabilityinfo.gov

**Rehabilitation Services
Administration**
400 Maryland Avenue, SW
Washington, DC 20202-2551
Phone: (202) 205-5482
Website: http://www.ed.gov/
about/offices/list/osers/rsa

Patient Assistance Programs for People Taking Arthritis Medications

Acetaminophen (Tylenol®)
Ortho-McNeil Patient
Assistance Program
P.O. Box 938
Somerville, NJ 08876
Toll-Free: (800) 577-3788
http://www.ortho-mcneil.com/
about/patientprogram.html

Adalimumab (Humira®)
Abbott Immunology
Toll-Free: (866) 4-HUMIRA
http://www.abbottimmunology
.com/ab.asp

Alendronate (Fosamax®)
Merck Patient Assistance
Program
Toll-Free: (800) 727-5400
Toll-Free: (800) 994-2111 (health
care professionals only)
http://www.merck.com/pap/pap/
consumer/index.jsp

Celecoxib (Celebrex®)
Pfizer for Living Share Card
Program
Toll-Free: (800) 459-4156
Website: http://
www.pfizersharecard.com

Connection to Care
Toll-Free: (800) 707-8990
Website: http://www.pfizer.com/
subsites/philanthropy/access/
connection.care.index.html

Sharing the Care
Toll-Free: (800) 984-1500
Website: http://www.pfizer.com/
subsites/philanthropy/access/
sharing.care.index.html

Cyclosporine (Neoral®)
Novartis Pharmaceuticals
Patient Assistance Program
P.O. Box 8609
Somerville, NJ 08876
Toll-Free: (800) 277-2254
Website: http://
www.pharma.us.novartis.com/
novartis/pap/pap.jsp?checked=y

Dicyclomine (Bentyl®)
Aventis Pharmaceuticals
Patient Assistance Program
P.O. Box 759
Somerville, NJ 08876
Toll-Free: (800) 221-4025
Website: http://
www.aventispharma-us.com/
contactus/PatientAssistance.jsp

Etanercept (Enbrel®)
Encourage Foundation™
Toll-Free: (888) 4-ENBREL
Website: http://www.enbrel.com

Etidronate (Didronel®)
Procter & Gamble
Pharmaceuticals
c/o Express Scripts
P.O. Box 6553
St. Louis, MO 63166-6553
Toll-Free: (800) 830-9049
Website: http://
www.pgpharma.com

Gamimunc®
Bayer Indigent Program
P.O. Box 29209
Phoenix, AZ 85038-9209
Toll-Free: (800) 998-9180
Toll-Free: (800) 468-0894 X 2765
Website: http://www.bayer.com

Infliximab (Remicade®)
Remicade® Patient Assistance
Program
P.O. Box 221709
Charlotte, NC 28222-1709
Phone: (866) 489-5957
Fax: (866) 489-5958
Website: http://www.remicade
.com/pdf/IN03292.pdf

Lansoprazole (Prevacid®)
TAP Pharmaceuticals, Inc.
Toll-Free: (800) 621-1020
Website: http://www.tap.com

Leflunomide (Arava®)
Aventis Pharmaceuticals
Patient Assistance Program
P.O. Box 759
Somerville, NJ 08876
Toll-Free: (800) 221-4025
Website: http://
www.aventispharma-us.com/
contactus/PatientAssistance.jsp

527

Meloxicam (Mobic®)
Boehringer Ingelheim Cares
Foundation, Inc.
c/o ESI/SDS
P.O. Box 66555
St. Louis, MO 63166-6773
Toll-Free: (800) 556-8317
Website: http://us.boehringer-
ingelheim.com/about/
philanthropy/Patient_Assistance
_Program.html

**Mycophenolate Mofetil
(CellCept®)**
Roche Medical Needs Program
Roche Laboratories, Inc.
340 Kingsland Street
Nutley, NJ 07110
Toll-Free: (800) 285-4484
Website: http://www.roche.com

Nabumetone (Relafen®)
SmithKline Beecham
Foundation Access to Care
c/o Express Scripts/SDS
P.O. Box 2564
Maryland Heights, MO 63043-
8564
Toll-Free: (800) 546-0420
Fax: (800) 729-4544
Website: http://www.gsk.com

Naproxen (Naprosyn®)
Roche Medical Needs Program
Roche Laboratories, Inc.
340 Kingsland Street
Nutley, NJ 07110
Toll-Free: (800) 285-4484
Website: http://www.roche.com

**Nitrofurantoin
(Macrodantin®, Macrobid®)**
Procter & Gamble
Pharmaceuticals
c/o Express Scripts
P.O. Box 6553
St. Louis, MO 63166-6553
Toll-Free: (800) 830-9049
Website: http://
www.pgpharma.com

Omeprazole (Prilosec®)
Patient Assistance Program
Astrazeneca Foundation
P.O. Box 15197
Wilmington, DE 19850-5197
Toll-Free: (800) 959-5432
Website: http://
www.astrazeneca-us.com/con-
tent/drugAssistance/
patientAssistanceProgram/
default.asp

Paroxetine (Paxil®)
SmithKline Beecham Founda-
tion Access to Care
c/o Express Scripts/SDS
P.O. Box 2564
Maryland Heights, MO 63043-
8564
Toll-Free: (800) 546-0420
Fax: (800) 729-4544
Website: http://www.gsk.com

Raloxifene (Evista®)
Eli Lilly and Company
Toll-Free: (877) 795-4559
Website: http://
www.lillyanswers.com

Risedronate (Actonel®)
Procter & Gamble
Pharmaceuticals
c/o Express Scripts
P.O. Box 6553
St. Louis, MO 63166-6553
Toll-Free: (800) 830-9049
Website: http://
www.pgpharma.com

Rituximab (Rituxan®)
Genentech Access to Care
Foundation
1 DNA Way
South San Francisco, CA 94080-4990
Toll-Free: (800) 530-3083
Fax: (650) 225-1366
Website: http://www.gene.com/
gene/about/community/
uninsured-prog.jsp

Rofecoxib (Vioxx®)
Merck Patient Assistance
Program
Toll-Free: (800) 727-5400
Toll-Free: (800) 994-2111 (health
care professionals only)
Website: http://www.merck.com/
pap/pap/consumer/index.jsp

Teriparatide (Forteo®)
Eli Lilly and Company
Toll-Free: (877) 795-4559
Website: http://
www.lillyanswers.com

Tramadol (Ultram®, Ultracet®)
Ortho-McNeil Patient
Assistance Program
P.O. Box 938
Somerville, NJ 08876
Toll-Free: (800) 577-3788
Website: http://www.ortho-mcneil.com/about/
patientprogram.html

Valdecoxib (Bextra®)
Pfizer for Living Share Card
Program
Toll-Free: (800) 459-4156
Website: http://
www.pfizersharecard.com

Connection to Care
Toll-Free: (800) 707-8990
Website: http://www.pfizer.com/
subsites/philanthropy/access/
connection.care.index.html

Sharing the Care
Toll-Free: (800) 984-1500
Website: http://www.pfizer.com/
subsites/philanthropy/access/
sharing.care.index.html

Chapter 52

Additional Reading about Arthritis

Books about Arthritis and Rheumatology

Adderly, Brenda D. *The Arthritis Cure Cookbook*. Washington, DC: Lifeline Press, 2000. ISBN 0895262193.

Allen, Ronald J.; Brander, Victoria Anne; Stulberg, S. David. *Arthritis of the Hip & Knee: The Active Person's Guide to Taking Charge*. Atlanta, GA: Peachtree Publishers, 1998. ISBN 1561451495.

Arthritis Foundation. *All You Need to Know about Joint Surgery: Preparing for Surgery, Recovery, and an Active New Lifestyle*. Atlanta, GA: Arthritis Foundation, 2002. ISBN 0912423331.

Arthritis Foundation. *Let's Get Active: Just Six Weeks to Better Flexibility, Strength, and Fitness with Arthritis*. Atlanta, GA: Arthritis Foundation, 2004. ISBN 0912423447.

Arthritis Foundation. *The Arthritis Foundation's Guide to Good Living with Fibromyalgia*. Atlanta, GA: Arthritis Foundation, 2001. ISBN 0912423269.

Arthritis Foundation. *The Arthritis Foundation's Guide to Good Living with Osteoarthritis*. Atlanta, GA: Arthritis Foundation, 2000. ISBN 0912423250.

Resources listed in this chapter were compiled from several sources. Inclusion does not constitute endorsement. This list is not considered complete; it is merely intended to serve as a starting point for readers interested in pursuing additional information. Websites were all verified and accessed in March 2004.

Arthritis Foundation. The *Arthritis Foundation's Guide to Good Living with Rheumatoid Arthritis*. Atlanta, GA: Arthritis Foundation, 2000. ISBN 0912423218.

Bernstein, Susan; Klippel, John H. *The Arthritis Foundation's Guide to Pain Management*. Atlanta, GA: Arthritis Foundation, 2003. ISBN 0912423390.

Brown, Ellen Hodgson. *Healing Joint Pain Naturally: Safe and Effective Ways to Treat Arthritis, Fibromyalgia, and Other Joint Diseases*. New York, NY: Broadway Books, 2001. ISBN 076790561X.

Bruce, Debra Fulghum; McIlwain, Harris H. *Pain-Free Arthritis: A 7-Step Plan for Feeling Better Again*. New York, NY: Henry Holt and Company, LLC, 2003. ISBN 0805073256.

Cram, David L. *Coping with Psoriasis: A Patient's Guide to Treatment*. Omaha, NE: Addicus Books, 2000. ISBN 188603947X.

Dunkin, Mary Anne. *The Arthritis Foundation's Guide to Managing Your Arthritis*. Atlanta, GA: Arthritis Foundation, 2001. ISBN 0912423285.

Horstman, Judith. *The Arthritis Foundation's Guide to Alternative Therapies*. Atlanta, GA: Arthritis Foundation, 1999. ISBN 0912423234.

Kazanowski, Mary K.; Laccetti, Margaret Saul. *Pain*. Thorofare, NJ: Slack, 2002. ISBN 1556425228.

Klein, Arthur C. *Chronic Pain: The Complete Guide to Relief.* New York, NY: Carroll and Graf, 2001. ISBN 0786708344.

Klippel, John H.; Crofford, Leslie; Stone, John H. (Eds.) *The Pocket Primer on the Rheumatic Diseases*. Atlanta, GA: Arthritis Foundation, 2003. ISBN 0912423382.

Klippel, John H.; Dieppe, Paul A. *Rheumatology, 2nd Edition*. St. Louis, MO: Mosby, 2000. ISBN 0723424055.

Lahita, Robert. *Rheumatoid Arthritis: Everything You Need to Know*. New York, NY: Penguin Putnam, 2001. ISBN 1583331018.

Lorig, Kate; Fries, James F.; Gecht, Maureen R. *The Arthritis Helpbook: A Tested Self-Management Program for Coping with Arthritis and Fibromyalgia, 5th Edition*. New York, NY: HarperCollins Publishers, 2000. ISBN 073820224X.

Mayes, Maureen D. *The Scleroderma Book: A Guide for Patients and Families.* New York, NY: Oxford University Press, 1999. ISBN 0195115074.

McIlwain, Harris H; Fulghum, Debra. *The Fibromyalgia Handbook, 3rd Edition: A 7-Step Program to Halt and Even Reverse Fibromyalgia.* New York, NY: Henry Holt and Company, LLC, 2003. ISBN 0805072411.

Nelson, Miriam E., Baker, Kristin R.; Roubenoff, Ronenn; Lindner, Lawrence. *Strong Women and Men Beat Arthritis: The Scientifically Proven Program That Allows People with Arthritis to Take Charge of Their Disease.* New York, NY: Perigee, 2003. ISBN 0399528563.

Paget, Steven A.; Lockshin, Michael D.; Loebl, Suzanne. *The Hospital for Special Surgery Rheumatoid Arthritis Handbook: Everything You Need to Know to Lead a Full Life.* New York, NY: John Wiley & Sons, Inc., 2001. ISBN 0471410454.

Sayce, Valerie; Fraser, Ian. *Exercise Beats Arthritis: An Easy-to-Follow Program of Exercises, 3rd Edition.* Boulder, CO: Bull Publishing Company, 1998. ISBN 0923521453.

Shlotzhauer, Tammi; McGuire, James L. *Living with Rheumatoid Arthritis, 2nd Edition.* Baltimore, MD: Johns Hopkins University Press, 2003. ISBN 0801871468.

Tucker, Lori B.; DeNardo, Bethany A.; Stebulis, Judith A; Schaller, Jane D. *Your Child with Arthritis: A Family Guide for Caregiving.* Baltimore, MD: Johns Hopkins University Press, 2000. ISBN 0801865344.

Wallace, Daniel J. *The Lupus Book: A Guide for Patients and Their Families, Revised and Expanded Edition.* New York, NY: Oxford University Press, 2000. ISBN 0195132815.

Weinblatt, Michael E. *The Arthritis Action Program: An Integrated Plan of Traditional and Complementary Therapies.* New York, NY: Fireside Books, 2001. ISBN 0684868024.

Magazine and Journal Articles about Arthritis and Rheumatology

Allaire, S.; Li, W.; LaValley, M. "Reduction of Job Loss in Persons with Rheumatic Diseases Receiving Vocational Rehabilitation." *Arthritis and Rheumatism,* vol. 48, no. 11, pp. 3212–3218, 2003.

Bolen, J.; Helmick, C.G.; Sacks, J.J.; Langmaid, G. "Prevalence of Self-Reported Arthritis or Chronic Joint Symptoms Among Adults—United States, 2001." *Morbidity and Mortality Weekly Report,* vol. 51, pp. 948–950, 2002.

Boutry, N.; Larde, A.; Lapegue, F.; Solau-Gervais, E; Flipo, R.M.; Cotton, A. "Magnetic Resonance Imaging Appearance of the Hands and Feet in Patients With Early Rheumatoid Arthritis." *Journal of Rheumatology,* vol. 30, no. 4, pp. 671–679, 2003.

Bren, L. "Joint Replacement: An Inside Look," *FDA Consumer,* vol. 38, no. 2, March 2004.

Buvanendran, Asokumar; Kroin, Jeffrey S.; Tuman, Kenneth J.; Lubenow, Timothy R.; Elmofty, Dalia; Moric, Mario; Rosenberg, Aaron G. "Effects of Perioperative Administration of a Selective Cyclooxygenase 2 Inhibitor on Pain Management and Recovery of Function after Knee Replacement: A Randomized Controlled Trial." *Journal of the American Medical Association,* vol. 290, pp. 2411–2418, 2003.

Demissie, S.; Cupples, L.; Myers, R.; Aliabadi, P.; Levy, D.; Felson, D. "Genome Scan for Quantity of Hand Osteoarthritis." *Arthritis and Rheumatism,* vol. 46, no. 4, pp. 946–952, 2002.

Dunlop, D.D.; Song, J.; Manheim, L.M.; Chang, R.W. "Racial Disparities in Joint Replacement Use among Older Adults." *Medical Care,* vol. 41, no. 2, pp. 288–298, February 2003.

Felson, D.T.; McLaughlin, S.; Goggins, J.; LaValley, M.P.; Gale, M.E.; Totterman, S.; Li, W.; Hill, C.; Gale, D. "Bone Marrow Edema and Its Relation to Progression of Knee Osteoarthritis. *Annals of Internal Medicine,* vol. 139, no. 5, part 1, pp. 330–336. September 2, 2003.

Fortin, Paul R.; Penrod, John R.; Clarke, Ann E.; St-Pierre, Yvan; Joseph, Lawrence; Belisle, Patrick; Liang, Matthew H.; Ferland, Diane; Phillips, Charlotte B.; Mahomed, Nizar; Tanzer, Michael; Sledge, Clement; Fossel, Anne H.; Katz, Jeffrey N. "Timing of Total Joint Replacement Affects Clinical Outcomes Among Patients with Osteoarthritis of the Hip or Knee." *Arthritis and Rheumatism,* vol. 46, no. 12, pp. 3327–3330, 2002.

Grant, E.P.; Pickard, M.D.; Briskin, M.J.; Gutierrez-Ramos, J.C. "Gene Expression Profiles: Creating New Perspectives in Arthritis Research." *Arthritis and Rheumatism,* vol. 46, no. 4, pp. 874–884, 2002.

Heisel, C.; Silva, M.; Schmalzried, T.P. "Bearing Surface Options for Total Hip Replacement in Young Patients." *Journal of Bone and Joint Surgery,* vol. 85A, no. 7, pp. 1366–1379, July 2003.

Helms, C., et al. "A Putative RUNX1 Binding Site Variant between SLC9A3R1 and NAT9 Is Associated with Susceptibility to Psoriasis." *Nature Genetics,* vol. 35, pp. 349–356, 2003.

Hoffman, G.S.; Cid, M.C.; Hellmann, D.B.; et al. "A Multicenter, Randomized, Double-Blind, Placebo-Controlled Trial of Adjuvant Methotrexate Treatment for Giant Cell Arteritis." *Arthritis and Rheumatism,* vol. 46, no. 5, pp. 1309–1318, 2002.

Jasmin, L.; Rabkin, S.D.; Granato, A.; Boudah, A.; Ohara, P.T. "Analgesia and Hyperalgesia from GABA-Mediated Modulation of the Cerebral Cortex." *Nature,* vol. 424, no. 6946, pp. 316–320, 2003.

Klein, R.; et al. "Regulation of Bone Mass in Mice by the Lipoxygenase Gene Alox15." *Science,* vol. 303, no. 5655, pp. 229–232, 2004.

Kousteni, S.; Han, L.; Chen, J.R.; Almeida, M.; Plotkin, L.I.; Bellido, T.; Manolagas, S.C. "Kinase-Mediated Regulation of Common Transcription Factors Accounts for the Bone-Protective Effects of Sex Steroids." *Journal of Clinical Investigation,* vol. 111, no. 11, pp. 1651–64, June 2003.

Krishnan, E.; Fries, J. "Reduction in Long-Term Functional Disability in Rheumatoid Arthritis from 1977 to 1998: A Longitudinal Study of 3,035 Patients." *American Journal of Medicine,* vol. 115, no. 5, pp. 371–376, 2003.

Leung, B.P.; Sattar, N.; Crilly, A.; Prach, M.; McCarey, D.W.; Payne, H.; Madhok, R.; Campbell, C.; Gracie, J.A.; Liew, F.Y.; McInnes, I.B. "A Novel Anti-Inflammatory Role for Simvastatin in Inflammatory Arthritis." *Journal of Immunology,* vol. 170, no. 3, pp. 1524–1530, February 1, 2003.

McCarey, D.W.; Sattar, N.; Hampson, R.; Madhok, R.; Capell, H.A.; McInnes, I.B. "A Randomised, Placebo Controlled Trial Comparing the Anti-inflammatory and Vascular Risk Modulatory Effects of Atorvastatin in Rheumatoid Arthritis (RA)." *Arthritis and Rheumatism,* vol. 48, no. 9, Supplement: S666, September 2003.

Meadows, M. "Managing Chronic Pain," *FDA Consumer,* vol. 38, no. 2, March 2004.

Minor, M.A. "Exercise and Arthritis: We Know a Little Bit about a Lot of Things." *Arthritis and Rheumatism,* vol. 49, no. 1, pp. 1–2, February 15, 2003.

National Academy of Sciences. *Proceedings of the National Academy of Sciences, USA,* vol. 100, no. 5, pp. 2610–2615, March 4, 2003.

O'Dell, J.R.; Leff, R.; Paulsen, G.; et al. "Treatment of Rheumatoid Arthritis with Methotrexate and Hydroxychloroquine, Methotrexate and Sulfasalazine, or a Combination of the Three Medications: Results of a Two-Year, Randomized, Double-Blind, Placebo-Controlled Trial." *Arthritis and Rheumatism,* vol. 46, no. 5, pp. 1164–1170, 2002.

Ogilvie, E.M. "The -174 Allele of the Interleukin-6 Gene Confers Susceptibility to Systemic Arthritis in Children." *Arthritis and Rheumatism,* vol. 48, no. 11, pp. 3202–3206, 2003.

Rantapaa-Dahlqvist, S.; De Jong, B.A.; Berglin, E.; Hallmans, G.; Wadell, G.; Stenlund, H., Sundin, U., Van Venrooij, W.J. "Antibodies against Cyclic Citrullinated Peptide and IgA Rheumatoid Factor Predict the Development of Rheumatoid Arthritis." *Arthritis and Rheumatism,* vol. 48, no. 10, pp. 2741–2749, October 2003.

Raynauld, J.P.; Kauffmann, C.; Beaudoin, G.; Berthiaume, M.J.; de Guise, J.A.; Bloch, D.A.; Camacho, F.; Godbout, B.; Altman, R.D.; Hochberg, M.; Meyer, J.M.; Cline, G.; Pelletier, J.P.; Martel-Pelletier, J. "Reliability of a Quantification Imaging System Using Magnetic Resonance Images to Measure Cartilage Thickness and Volume in Human Normal and Osteoarthritic Knees." *Osteoarthritis and Cartilage,* vol. 11, no. 5, pp. 351–360, May 2003.

Roman, M.J.; et al. "Prevalence and Correlates of Accelerated Atherosclerosis in Systemic Lupus Erythematosus." *New England Journal of Medicine,* vol. 349, pp. 2397–2404, 2003.

Roubenoff, R. "Exercise and Inflammatory Disease." *Arthritis Care and Research,* vol. 49, no. 2, pp. 263–266, 2003.

Salvarani, C.; Silingardi, M.; Ghirarduzzi, A.; et al. "Is Duplex Ultrasonography Useful for the Diagnosis of Giant-Cell Arteritis?" *Annals of Internal Medicine,* vol. 137, no. 4, pp. 232–238, 2002.

Skinner, J.; Weinstein, J.N.; Sporer, S.M.; Wennberg, J.E. "Racial, Ethnic, and Geographic Disparities in Rates of Knee Arthroplasty among Medicare Patients." *New England Journal of Medicine,* vol. 349, no. 14, pp. 1350–1359, October 2, 2003.

Soderlin, M.K.; Kautiainen, H.; Puolakkainen, M.; et al. "Infections Preceding Early Arthritis in Southern Sweden: A Prospective Population-Based Study." *Journal of Rheumatology,* vol. 30, no. 3, pp. 459–464, 2003.

Solomon, D.H.; Karlson, E.W.; Rimm, E.B.; Cannuscio, C.C.; Mandl, L.A.; Manson, J.E.; Stampfer, M.J.; Curhan, G.C. "Cardiovascular Morbidity and Mortality in Women Diagnosed with Rheumatoid Arthritis." *Circulation,* vol. 107, no. 9, pp. 1303–1307, March 11, 2003.

Taniguchi, N.; Kawahara, K.; Yone, K.; et al. "High Mobility Group Box Chromosomal Protein 1 Plays a Role in the Pathogenesis of Rheumatoid Arthritis as a Novel Cytokine." *Arthritis and Rheumatism,* vol. 48, no. 4, pp. 971–981, 2003.

Thornburg, C.; Ward, M. "Hospitalizations for Coronary Heart Disease among Patients with Systemic Lupus Erythematosus." *Arthritis and Rheumatism,* vol. 48, no. 9, pp. 2519–2523, 2003.

Van Doornum, S.; McColl, G.; Wicks, I.P. "Accelerated Atherosclerosis: An Extraarticular Feature of Rheumatoid Arthritis?" *Arthritis and Rheumatism,* vol. 46, no. 4, pp. 862–873, 2002.

Websites That Provide Arthritis and Rheumatology Information

American Academy of Orthopaedic Surgeons (AAOS)
http://www.aaos.org

American College of Rheumatology
http://www.rheumatology.org

American Physical Therapy Association
http://www.apta.org

American Society for Bone and Mineral Research
http://www.asbmr.org

Annals of Internal Medicine
http://www.annals.org/

Arthritis Foundation
http://www.arthritis.org

Arthritis Research Campaign
http://www.arc.org.uk

Arthritis Society
http://www.arthritis.ca

Arthritis Source
http://www.orthop.washington.edu/arthritis

Australian Rheumatology Association
http://www.rheumatology.org.au/index.asp

CenterWatch
http://www.centerwatch.com/patient/trials.html

Clinical Immunology Society
http://www.clinimmsoc.org

ClinicalTrials.gov
http://www.clinicaltrials.gov

Hospital for Special Surgery—Rheumatology Division
http://www.rheumatology.hss.edu

International League of Associations for Rheumatology
http://www.ilar.org

Johns Hopkins Arthritis Center
http://www.hopkins-arthritis.org

JointandBone.org
http://www.jointandbone.org

MedlinePLUS Health Information from the National Library of Medicine
http://www.medlineplus.org

National Institute of Arthritis and Musculoskeletal and Skin Diseases
http://www.niams.nih.gov

Rheuma21st
http://www.rheuma21st.com

RheumatologyWeb
http://www.rheumatologyweb.com

Journals That Publish Rheumatology Research

Annals of the Rheumatic Diseases
http://ard.bmjjournals.com

Archives of Internal Medicine
http://pubs.ama-assn.org

Arthritis & Rheumatism
http://www3.interscience.wiley.com/cgi-bin/jhome/76509746

Arthritis Care & Research
http://www3.interscience.wiley.com/cgi-bin/jhome/77005015

Arthritis Research and Therapy
http://arthritis-research.com

Arthritis Today
http://www.arthritis.org/resources/arthritistoday

Arthroscopy
http://www2.us.elsevierhealth.com

Best Practice and Research Clinical Rheumatology
http://www.harcourt-international.com/journals/berh

Clinical and Experimental Rheumatology
http://www.clinexprheumatol.org

Clinical Rheumatology
http://www.springerlink.com

Current Opinion in Rheumatology
http://www.co-rheumatology.com

Journal of the American Medical Association
http://pubs.ama-assn.org

Journal of Bone and Mineral Research
http://www.jbmr-online.org

Journal of Clinical Rheumatology
http://www.jbmr-online.org

Journal of Joint and Bone Surgery
http://www.ejbjs.org

Journal of Pain and Syndrome Management
http://www.elsevier.com

Journal of Rheumatology
http://www.jrheum.com

Lupus
http://www.arnoldpublishers.com/journals/pages/lupus/09612033.htm

Modern Rheumatology
http://www.springerlink.com

Morbidity and Mortality Weekly Report
http://www.cdc.gov/mmwr

New England Journal of Medicine
http://content.nejm.org

Rheumatology
http://www.springerlink.com

Year Book of Rheumatology, Arthritis, and Musculoskeletal Disease
http://www.us.elsevierhealth.com

Index

Index

Page numbers followed by 'n' indicate a footnote. Page numbers in *italics* indicate a table or illustration.

A

Health Reference Series
COMPLETE CATALOG

Adolescent Health Sourcebook

Basic Consumer Health Information about Common Medical, Mental, and Emotional Concerns in Adolescents, Including Facts about Acne, Body Piercing, Mononucleosis, Nutrition, Eating Disorders, Stress, Depression, Behavior Problems, Peer Pressure, Violence, Gangs, Drug Use, Puberty, Sexuality, Pregnancy, Learning Disabilities, and More

Along with a Glossary of Terms and Other Resources for Further Help and Information

Edited by Chad T. Kimball. 658 pages. 2002. 0-7808-0248-9. $78.

"It is written in clear, nontechnical language aimed at general readers. . . . Recommended for public libraries, community colleges, and other agencies serving health care consumers."
— *American Reference Books Annual, 2003*

"Recommended for school and public libraries. Parents and professionals dealing with teens will appreciate the easy-to-follow format and the clearly written text. This could become a 'must have' for every high school teacher." — *E-Streams, Jan '03*

"A good starting point for information related to common medical, mental, and emotional concerns of adolescents." — *School Library Journal, Nov '02*

"This book provides accurate information in an easy to access format. It addresses topics that parents and caregivers might not be aware of and provides practical, useable information." — *Doody's Health Sciences Book Review Journal, Sep-Oct '02*

"Recommended reference source."
— *Booklist, American Library Association, Sep '02*

▪

AIDS Sourcebook, 3rd Edition

Basic Consumer Health Information about Acquired Immune Deficiency Syndrome (AIDS) and Human Immunodeficiency Virus (HIV) Infection, Including Facts about Transmission, Prevention, Diagnosis, Treatment, Opportunistic Infections, and Other Complications, with a Section for Women and Children, Including Details about Associated Gynecological Concerns, Pregnancy, and Pediatric Care

Along with Updated Statistical Information, Reports on Current Research Initiatives, a Glossary, and Directories of Internet, Hotline, and Other Resources

Edited by Dawn D. Matthews. 664 pages. 2003. 0-7808-0631-X. $78.

ALSO AVAILABLE: *AIDS Sourcebook, 1st Edition.* Edited by Karen Bellenir and Peter D. Dresser. 831 pages. 1995. 0-7808-0031-1. $78.

AIDS Sourcebook, 2nd Edition. Edited by Karen Bellenir. 751 pages. 1999. 0-7808-0225-X. $78.

"The 3rd edition of the *AIDS Sourcebook*, part of Omnigraphics' *Health Reference Series*, is a welcome update. . . . This resource is highly recommended for academic and public libraries."
— *American Reference Books Annual, 2004*

"Excellent sourcebook. This continues to be a highly recommended book. There is no other book that provides as much information as this book provides."
— *AIDS Book Review Journal, Dec-Jan 2000*

"Recommended reference source."
— *Booklist, American Library Association, Dec '99*

"A solid text for college-level health libraries."
— *The Bookwatch, Aug '99*

Cited in *Reference Sources for Small and Medium-Sized Libraries, American Library Association, 1999*

▪

Alcoholism Sourcebook

Basic Consumer Health Information about the Physical and Mental Consequences of Alcohol Abuse, Including Liver Disease, Pancreatitis, Wernicke-Korsakoff Syndrome (Alcoholic Dementia), Fetal Alcohol Syndrome, Heart Disease, Kidney Disorders, Gastrointestinal Problems, and Immune System Compromise and Featuring Facts about Addiction, Detoxification, Alcohol Withdrawal, Recovery, and the Maintenance of Sobriety

Along with a Glossary and Directories of Resources for Further Help and Information

Edited by Karen Bellenir. 613 pages. 2000. 0-7808-0325-6. $78.

"This title is one of the few reference works on alcoholism for general readers. For some readers this will be a welcome complement to the many self-help books on the market. Recommended for collections serving general readers and consumer health collections."
— *E-Streams, Mar '01*

"This book is an excellent choice for public and academic libraries."
— *American Reference Books Annual, 2001*

"Recommended reference source."
— *Booklist, American Library Association, Dec '00*

"Presents a wealth of information on alcohol use and abuse and its effects on the body and mind, treatment, and prevention." — *SciTech Book News, Dec '00*

"Important new health guide which packs in the latest consumer information about the problems of alcoholism." — *Reviewer's Bookwatch, Nov '00*

SEE ALSO *Drug Abuse Sourcebook, Substance Abuse Sourcebook*

Allergies Sourcebook, 2nd Edition

Basic Consumer Health Information about Allergic Disorders, Triggers, Reactions, and Related Symptoms, Including Anaphylaxis, Rhinitis, Sinusitis, Asthma, Dermatitis, Conjunctivitis, and Multiple Chemical Sensitivity

Along with Tips on Diagnosis, Prevention, and Treatment, Statistical Data, a Glossary, and a Directory of Sources for Further Help and Information

Edited by Annemarie S. Muth. 598 pages. 2002. 0-7808-0376-0. $78.

ALSO AVAILABLE: Allergies Sourcebook, 1st Edition. Edited by Allan R. Cook. 611 pages. 1997. 0-7808-0036-2. $78.

"This book brings a great deal of useful material together. . . . This is an excellent addition to public and consumer health library collections."
— *American Reference Books Annual, 2003*

"This second edition would be useful to laypersons with little or advanced knowledge of the subject matter. This book would also serve as a resource for nursing and other health care professions students. It would be useful in public, academic, and hospital libraries with consumer health collections." — *E-Streams, Jul '02*

Alternative Medicine Sourcebook, 2nd Edition

Basic Consumer Health Information about Alternative and Complementary Medical Practices, Including Acupuncture, Chiropractic, Herbal Medicine, Homeopathy, Naturopathic Medicine, Mind-Body Interventions, Ayurveda, and Other Non-Western Medical Traditions

Along with Facts about such Specific Therapies as Massage Therapy, Aromatherapy, Qigong, Hypnosis, Prayer, Dance, and Art Therapies, a Glossary, and Resources for Further Information

Edited by Dawn D. Matthews. 618 pages. 2002. 0-7808-0605-0. $78.

ALSO AVAILABLE: Alternative Medicine Sourcebook, 1st Edition. Edited by Allan R. Cook. 737 pages. 1999. 0-7808-0200-4. $78.

"Recommended for public, high school, and academic libraries that have consumer health collections. Hospital libraries that also serve the public will find this to be a useful resource." — *E-Streams, Feb '03*

"Recommended reference source."
— *Booklist, American Library Association, Jan '03*

"An important alternate health reference."
— *MBR Bookwatch, Oct '02*

"A great addition to the reference collection of every type of library." — *American Reference Books Annual, 2000*

Alzheimer's Disease Sourcebook, 3rd Edition

Basic Consumer Health Information about Alzheimer's Disease, Other Dementias, and Related Disorders, Including Multi-Infarct Dementia, AIDS Dementia Complex, Dementia with Lewy Bodies, Huntington's Disease, Wernicke-Korsakoff Syndrome (Alcohol-Reated Dementia), Delirium, and Confusional States

Along with Information for People Newly Diagnosed with Alzheimer's Disease and Caregivers, Reports Detailing Current Research Efforts in Prevention, Diagnosis, and Treatment, Facts about Long-Term Care Issues, and Listings of Sources for Additional Information

Edited by Karen Bellenir. 645 pages. 2003. 0-7808-0666-2. $78.

ALSO AVAILABLE: Alzheimer's, Stroke & 29 Other Neurological Disorders Sourcebook, 1st Edition. Edited by Frank E. Bair. 579 pages. 1993. 1-55888-748-2. $78.

ALSO AVAILABLE: Alzheimer's Disease Sourcebook, 2nd Edition. Edited by Karen Bellenir. 524 pages. 1999. 0-7808-0223-3. $78.

"This very informative and valuable tool will be a great addition to any library serving consumers, students and health care workers."
— *American Reference Books Annual, 2004*

"This is a valuable resource for people affected by dementias such as Alzheimer's. It is easy to navigate and includes important information and resources."
— *Doody's Review Service, Feb. 2004*

"Recommended reference source."
— *Booklist, American Library Association, Oct '99*

SEE ALSO Brain Disorders Sourcebook

Arthritis Sourcebook, 2nd Edition

Basic Consumer Health Information about Osteoarthritis, Rheumatoid Arthritis, Other Rheumatic Disorders, Infectious Forms of Arthritis, and Diseases with Symptoms Linked to Arthritis, Featuring Facts about Diagnosis, Pain Management, and Surgical Therapies

Along with Coping Strategies, Research Updates, a Glossary, and Resources for Additional Help and Information

Edited by Amy L. Sutton. 593 pages. 2004. 0-7808-0667-0. $78.

ALSO AVAILABLE: Arthritis Sourcebook, 1st Edition. Edited by Allan R. Cook. 550 pages. 1998. 0-7808-0201-2. $78.

". . . accessible to the layperson."
— *Reference and Research Book News, Feb '99*

Asthma Sourcebook

Basic Consumer Health Information about Asthma, Including Symptoms, Traditional and Nontraditional Remedies, Treatment Advances, Quality-of-Life Aids, Medical Research Updates, and the Role of Allergies, Exercise, Age, the Environment, and Genetics in the Development of Asthma

Along with Statistical Data, a Glossary, and Directories of Support Groups, and Other Resources for Further Information

Edited by Annemarie S. Muth. 628 pages. 2000. 0-7808-0381-7. $78.

"A worthwhile reference acquisition for public libraries and academic medical libraries whose readers desire a quick introduction to the wide range of asthma information." — *Choice, Association of College & Research Libraries, Jun '01*

"Recommended reference source."
— *Booklist, American Library Association, Feb '01*

"Highly recommended." — *The Bookwatch, Jan '01*

"There is much good information for patients and their families who deal with asthma daily."
— *American Medical Writers Association Journal, Winter '01*

"This informative text is recommended for consumer health collections in public, secondary school, and community college libraries and the libraries of universities with a large undergraduate population."
— *American Reference Books Annual, 2001*

Attention Deficit Disorder Sourcebook

Basic Consumer Health Information about Attention Deficit/Hyperactivity Disorder in Children and Adults, Including Facts about Causes, Symptoms, Diagnostic Criteria, and Treatment Options Such as Medications, Behavior Therapy, Coaching, and Homeopathy

Along with Reports on Current Research Initiatives, Legal Issues, and Government Regulations, and Featuring a Glossary of Related Terms, Internet Resources, and a List of Additional Reading Material

Edited by Dawn D. Matthews. 470 pages. 2002. 0-7808-0624-7. $78.

"Recommended reference source."
— *Booklist, American Library Association, Jan '03*

"This book is recommended for all school libraries and the reference or consumer health sections of public libraries." — *American Reference Books Annual, 2003*

Back & Neck Sourcebook, 2nd Edition

Basic Consumer Health Information about Spinal Pain, Spinal Cord Injuries, and Related Disorders, Such as Degenerative Disk Disease, Osteoarthritis, Scoliosis,

Sciatica, Spina Bifida, and Spinal Stenosis, and Featuring Facts about Maintaining Spinal Health, Self-Care, Pain Management, Rehabilitative Care, Chiropractic Care, Spinal Surgeries, and Complementary Therapies

Along with Suggestions for Preventing Back and Neck Pain, a Glossary of Related Terms, and a Directory of Resources

Edited by Amy L. Sutton. 600 pages. 2004. 0-7808-0738-3 $78.

ALSO AVAILABLE: Back & Neck Disorders Sourcebook, 1st Edition. Edited by Karen Bellenir. 548 pages. 1997. 0-7808-0202-0. $78.

"The strength of this work is its basic, easy-to-read format. Recommended."
— *Reference and User Services Quarterly, American Library Association, Winter '97*

Blood & Circulatory Disorders Sourcebook

Basic Information about Blood and Its Components, Anemias, Leukemias, Bleeding Disorders, and Circulatory Disorders, Including Aplastic Anemia, Thalassemia, Sickle Cell Disease, Hemochromatosis, Hemophilia, Von Willebrand Disease, and Vascular Diseases

Along with a Special Section on Blood Transfusions and Blood Supply Safety, a Glossary, and Source Listings for Further Help and Information

Edited by Karen Bellenir and Linda M. Shin. 554 pages. 1998. 0-7808-0203-9. $78.

"Recommended reference source."
— *Booklist, American Library Association, Feb '99*

"An important reference sourcebook written in simple language for everyday, non-technical users."
— *Reviewer's Bookwatch, Jan '99*

Brain Disorders Sourcebook

Basic Consumer Health Information about Strokes, Epilepsy, Amyotrophic Lateral Sclerosis (ALS/Lou Gehrig's Disease), Parkinson's Disease, Brain Tumors, Cerebral Palsy, Headache, Tourette Syndrome, and More

Along with Statistical Data, Treatment and Rehabilitation Options, Coping Strategies, Reports on Current Research Initiatives, a Glossary, and Resource Listings for Additional Help and Information

Edited by Karen Bellenir. 481 pages. 1999. 0-7808-0229-2. $78.

"Belongs on the shelves of any library with a consumer health collection." — *E-Streams, Mar '00*

"Recommended reference source."
— *Booklist, American Library Association, Oct '99*

SEE ALSO Alzheimer's Disease Sourcebook

Breast Cancer Sourcebook, 2nd Edition

Basic Consumer Health Information about Breast Cancer, Including Facts about Risk Factors, Prevention, Screening and Diagnostic Methods, Treatment Options, Complementary and Alternative Therapies, Post-Treatment Concerns, Clinical Trials, Special Risk Populations, and New Developments in Breast Cancer Research

Along with Breast Cancer Statistics, a Glossary of Related Terms, and a Directory of Resources for Additional Help and Information

Edited by Sandra J. Judd. 600 pages. 2004. 0-7808-0668-9. $78.

ALSO AVAILABLE: Breast Cancer Sourcebook, 1st Edition. Edited by Edward J. Prucha and Karen Bellenir. 580 pages. 2001. 0-7808-0244-6. $78.

"It would be a useful reference book in a library or on loan to women in a support group."
— *Cancer Forum, Mar '03*

"Recommended reference source."
— *Booklist, American Library Association, Jan '02*

"This reference source is highly recommended. It is quite informative, comprehensive and detailed in nature, and yet it offers practical advice in easy-to-read language. It could be thought of as the 'bible' of breast cancer for the consumer." — *E-Streams, Jan '02*

"The broad range of topics covered in lay language make the *Breast Cancer Sourcebook* an excellent addition to public and consumer health library collections."
— *American Reference Books Annual 2002*

"From the pros and cons of different screening methods and results to treatment options, *Breast Cancer Sourcebook* provides the latest information on the subject."
— *Library Bookwatch, Dec '01*

"This thoroughgoing, very readable reference covers all aspects of breast health and cancer. . . . Readers will find much to consider here. Recommended for all public and patient health collections."
— *Library Journal, Sep '01*

SEE ALSO Cancer Sourcebook for Women, Women's Health Concerns Sourcebook

■

Breastfeeding Sourcebook

Basic Consumer Health Information about the Benefits of Breastmilk, Preparing to Breastfeed, Breastfeeding as a Baby Grows, Nutrition, and More, Including Information on Special Situations and Concerns Such as Mastitis, Illness, Medications, Allergies, Multiple Births, Prematurity, Special Needs, and Adoption

Along with a Glossary and Resources for Additional Help and Information

Edited by Jenni Lynn Colson. 388 pages. 2002. 0-7808-0332-9. $78.

SEE ALSO Pregnancy & Birth Sourcebook

"Particularly useful is the information about professional lactation services and chapters on breastfeeding when returning to work. . . . *Breastfeeding Sourcebook* will be useful for public libraries, consumer health libraries, and technical schools offering nurse assistant training, especially in areas where Internet access is problematic."
— *American Reference Books Annual, 2003*

■

Burns Sourcebook

Basic Consumer Health Information about Various Types of Burns and Scalds, Including Flame, Heat, Cold, Electrical, Chemical, and Sun Burns

Along with Information on Short-Term and Long-Term Treatments, Tissue Reconstruction, Plastic Surgery, Prevention Suggestions, and First Aid

Edited by Allan R. Cook. 604 pages. 1999. 0-7808-0204-7. $78.

"This is an exceptional addition to the series and is highly recommended for all consumer health collections, hospital libraries, and academic medical centers."
— *E-Streams, Mar '00*

"This key reference guide is an invaluable addition to all health care and public libraries in confronting this ongoing health issue."
— *American Reference Books Annual, 2000*

"Recommended reference source."
— *Booklist, American Library Association, Dec '99*

SEE ALSO Skin Disorders Sourcebook

■

Cancer Sourcebook, 4th Edition

Basic Consumer Health Information about Major Forms and Stages of Cancer, Featuring Facts about Head and Neck Cancers, Lung Cancers, Gastrointestinal Cancers, Genitourinary Cancers, Lymphomas, Blood Cell Cancers, Endocrine Cancers, Skin Cancers, Bone Cancers, Sarcomas, and Others, and Including Information about Cancer Treatments and Therapies, Identifying and Reducing Cancer Risks, and Strategies for Coping with Cancer and the Side Effects of Treatment

Along with a Cancer Glossary, Statistical and Demographic Data, and a Directory of Sources for Additional Help and Information

Edited by Karen Bellenir. 1,119 pages. 2003. 0-7808-0633-6. $78.

ALSO AVAILABLE: Cancer Sourcebook, 1st Edition. Edited by Frank E. Bair. 932 pages. 1990. 1-55888-888-8. $78.

New Cancer Sourcebook, 2nd Edition. Edited by Allan R. Cook. 1,313 pages. 1996. 0-7808-0041-9. $78.

Cancer Sourcebook, 3rd Edition. Edited by Edward J. Prucha. 1,069 pages. 2000. 0-7808-0227-6. $78.

"With cancer being the second leading cause of death for Americans, a prodigious work such as this one, which locates centrally so much cancer-related information, is clearly an asset to this nation's citizens and others." — *Journal of the National Medical Association, 2004*

"This title is recommended for health sciences and public libraries with consumer health collections."
— *E-Streams, Feb '01*

"... can be effectively used by cancer patients and their families who are looking for answers in a language they can understand. Public and hospital libraries should have it on their shelves."
— *American Reference Books Annual, 2001*

"Recommended reference source."
—*Booklist, American Library Association, Dec '00*

Cited in *Reference Sources for Small and Medium-Sized Libraries*, American Library Association, 1999

"The amount of factual and useful information is extensive. The writing is very clear, geared to general readers. Recommended for all levels."
— *Choice,* Association of College & Research Libraries, Jan '97

SEE ALSO *Breast Cancer Sourcebook, Cancer Sourcebook for Women, Pediatric Cancer Sourcebook, Prostate Cancer Sourcebook*

■

Cancer Sourcebook for Women, 2nd Edition

Basic Consumer Health Information about Gynecologic Cancers and Related Concerns, Including Cervical Cancer, Endometrial Cancer, Gestational Trophoblastic Tumor, Ovarian Cancer, Uterine Cancer, Vaginal Cancer, Vulvar Cancer, Breast Cancer, and Common Non-Cancerous Uterine Conditions, with Facts about Cancer Risk Factors, Screening and Prevention, Treatment Options, and Reports on Current Research Initiatives

Along with a Glossary of Cancer Terms and a Directory of Resources for Additional Help and Information

Edited by Karen Bellenir. 604 pages. 2002. 0-7808-0226-8. $78.

ALSO AVAILABLE: *Cancer Sourcebook for Women, 1st Edition.* Edited by Allan R. Cook and Peter D. Dresser. 524 pages. 1996. 0-7808-0076-1. $78.

"An excellent addition to collections in public, consumer health, and women's health libraries."
— *American Reference Books Annual, 2003*

"Overall, the information is excellent, and complex topics are clearly explained. As a reference book for the consumer it is a valuable resource to assist them to make informed decisions about cancer and its treatments."
— *Cancer Forum, Nov '02*

"Highly recommended for academic and medical reference collections."
— *Library Bookwatch, Sep '02*

"This is a highly recommended book for any public or consumer library, being reader friendly and containing accurate and helpful information."
— *E-Streams, Aug '02*

"Recommended reference source."
— *Booklist, American Library Association, Jul '02*

SEE ALSO *Breast Cancer Sourcebook, Women's Health Concerns Sourcebook*

Cardiovascular Diseases & Disorders Sourcebook, 1st Edition

SEE *Heart Diseases & Disorders Sourcebook, 2nd Edition*

■

Caregiving Sourcebook

Basic Consumer Health Information for Caregivers, Including a Profile of Caregivers, Caregiving Responsibilities and Concerns, Tips for Specific Conditions, Care Environments, and the Effects of Caregiving

Along with Facts about Legal Issues, Financial Information, and Future Planning, a Glossary, and a Listing of Additional Resources

Edited by Joyce Brennfleck Shannon. 600 pages. 2001. 0-7808-0331-0. $78.

"Essential for most collections."
— *Library Journal, Apr 1, 2002*

"An ideal addition to the reference collection of any public library. Health sciences information professionals may also want to acquire the *Caregiving Sourcebook* for their hospital or academic library for use as a ready reference tool by health care workers interested in aging and caregiving."
— *E-Streams, Jan '02*

"Recommended reference source."
— *Booklist, American Library Association, Oct '01*

■

Child Abuse Sourcebook

Basic Consumer Health Information about the Physical, Sexual, and Emotional Abuse of Children, with Additional Facts about Neglect, Munchausen Syndrome by Proxy (MSBP), Shaken Baby Syndrome, and Controversial Issues Related to Child Abuse, Such as Withholding Medical Care, Corporal Punishment, and Child Maltreatment in Youth Sports, and Featuring Facts about Child Protective Services, Foster Care, Adoption, Parenting Challenges, and Other Abuse Prevention Efforts

Along with a Glossary of Related Terms and Resources for Additional Help and Information

Edited by Dawn D. Matthews. 620 pages. 2004. 0-7808-0705-7. $78.

■

Childhood Diseases & Disorders Sourcebook

Basic Consumer Health Information about Medical Problems Often Encountered in Pre-Adolescent Children, Including Respiratory Tract Ailments, Ear Infections, Sore Throats, Disorders of the Skin and Scalp, Digestive and Genitourinary Diseases, Infectious Diseases, Inflammatory Disorders, Chronic Physical and Developmental Disorders, Allergies, and More

Along with Information about Diagnostic Tests, Common Childhood Surgeries, and Frequently Used Medications, with a Glossary of Important Terms and Resource Directory

Edited by Chad T. Kimball. 662 pages. 2003. 0-7808-0458-9. $78.

"This is an excellent book for new parents and should be included in all health care and public libraries."
— *American Reference Books Annual, 2004*

■

Colds, Flu & Other Common Ailments Sourcebook

Basic Consumer Health Information about Common Ailments and Injuries, Including Colds, Coughs, the Flu, Sinus Problems, Headaches, Fever, Nausea and Vomiting, Menstrual Cramps, Diarrhea, Constipation, Hemorrhoids, Back Pain, Dandruff, Dry and Itchy Skin, Cuts, Scrapes, Sprains, Bruises, and More

Along with Information about Prevention, Self-Care, Choosing a Doctor, Over-the-Counter Medications, Folk Remedies, and Alternative Therapies, and Including a Glossary of Important Terms and a Directory of Resources for Further Help and Information

Edited by Chad T. Kimball. 638 pages. 2001. 0-7808-0435-X. $78.

"A good starting point for research on common illnesses. It will be a useful addition to public and consumer health library collections."
— *American Reference Books Annual 2002*

"Will prove valuable to any library seeking to maintain a current, comprehensive reference collection of health resources. . . . Excellent reference."
— *The Bookwatch, Aug '01*

"Recommended reference source."
— *Booklist, American Library Association, July '01*

■

Communication Disorders Sourcebook

Basic Information about Deafness and Hearing Loss, Speech and Language Disorders, Voice Disorders, Balance and Vestibular Disorders, and Disorders of Smell, Taste, and Touch

Edited by Linda M. Ross. 533 pages. 1996. 0-7808-0077-X. $78.

"This is skillfully edited and is a welcome resource for the layperson. It should be found in every public and medical library." — *Booklist Health Sciences Supplement, American Library Association, Oct '97*

■

Congenital Disorders Sourcebook

Basic Information about Disorders Acquired during Gestation, Including Spina Bifida, Hydrocephalus, Cerebral Palsy, Heart Defects, Craniofacial Abnormalities, Fetal Alcohol Syndrome, and More

Along with Current Treatment Options and Statistical Data

Edited by Karen Bellenir. 607 pages. 1997. 0-7808-0205-5. $78.

"Recommended reference source."
— *Booklist, American Library Association, Oct '97*

SEE ALSO Pregnancy & Birth Sourcebook

■

Consumer Issues in Health Care Sourcebook

Basic Information about Health Care Fundamentals and Related Consumer Issues, Including Exams and Screening Tests, Physician Specialties, Choosing a Doctor, Using Prescription and Over-the-Counter Medications Safely, Avoiding Health Scams, Managing Common Health Risks in the Home, Care Options for Chronically or Terminally Ill Patients, and a List of Resources for Obtaining Help and Further Information

Edited by Karen Bellenir. 618 pages. 1998. 0-7808-0221-7. $78.

"Both public and academic libraries will want to have a copy in their collection for readers who are interested in self-education on health issues."
— *American Reference Books Annual, 2000*

"The editor has researched the literature from government agencies and others, saving readers the time and effort of having to do the research themselves. Recommended for public libraries."
— *Reference and User Services Quarterly, American Library Association, Spring '99*

"Recommended reference source."
— *Booklist, American Library Association, Dec '98*

■

Contagious Diseases Sourcebook

Basic Consumer Health Information about Infectious Diseases Spread by Person-to-Person Contact through Direct Touch, Airborne Transmission, Sexual Contact, or Contact with Blood or Other Body Fluids, Including Hepatitis, Herpes, Influenza, Lice, Measles, Mumps, Pinworm, Ringworm, Severe Acute Respiratory Syndrome (SARS), Streptococcal Infections, Tuberculosis, and Others

Along with Facts about Disease Transmission, Antimicrobial Resistance, and Vaccines, with a Glossary and Directories of Resources for More Information

Edited by Karen Bellenir. 625 pages. 2004. 0-7808-0736-7. $78.

■

Contagious & Non-Contagious Infectious Diseases Sourcebook

Basic Information about Contagious Diseases like Measles, Polio, Hepatitis B, and Infectious Mononucleosis, and Non-Contagious Infectious Diseases like Tetanus and Toxic Shock Syndrome, and Diseases Occurring as Secondary Infections Such as Shingles and Reye Syndrome

Along with Vaccination, Prevention, and Treatment Information, and a Section Describing Emerging Infectious Disease Threats

Edited by Karen Bellenir and Peter D. Dresser. 566 pages. 1996. 0-7808-0075-3. $78.

Death & Dying Sourcebook

Basic Consumer Health Information for the Layperson about End-of-Life Care and Related Ethical and Legal Issues, Including Chief Causes of Death, Autopsies, Pain Management for the Terminally Ill, Life Support Systems, Insurance, Euthanasia, Assisted Suicide, Hospice Programs, Living Wills, Funeral Planning, Counseling, Mourning, Organ Donation, and Physician Training

Along with Statistical Data, a Glossary, and Listings of Sources for Further Help and Information

Edited by Annemarie S. Muth. 641 pages. 1999. 0-7808-0230-6. $78.

"Public libraries, medical libraries, and academic libraries will all find this sourcebook a useful addition to their collections."
— American Reference Books Annual, 2001

"An extremely useful resource for those concerned with death and dying in the United States."
— Respiratory Care, Nov '00

"Recommended reference source."
— Booklist, American Library Association, Aug '00

"This book is a definite must for all those involved in end-of-life care." — Doody's Review Service, 2000

■

Dental Care & Oral Health Sourcebook, 2nd Edition

Basic Consumer Health Information about Dental Care, Including Oral Hygiene, Dental Visits, Pain Management, Cavities, Crowns, Bridges, Dental Implants, and Fillings, and Other Oral Health Concerns, Such as Gum Disease, Bad Breath, Dry Mouth, Genetic and Developmental Abnormalities, Oral Cancers, Orthodontics, and Temporomandibular Disorders

Along with Updates on Current Research in Oral Health, a Glossary, a Directory of Dental and Oral Health Organizations, and Resources for People with Dental and Oral Health Disorders

Edited by Amy L. Sutton. 609 pages. 2003. 0-7808-0634-4. $78.

ALSO AVAILABLE: Oral Health Sourcebook, 1st Edition. Edited by Allan R. Cook. 558 pages. 1997. 0-7808-0082-6. $78.

"This book could serve as a turning point in the battle to educate consumers in issues concerning oral health."
— American Reference Books Annual, 2004

"Unique source which will fill a gap in dental sources for patients and the lay public. A valuable reference tool even in a library with thousands of books on dentistry. Comprehensive, clear, inexpensive, and easy to read and use. It fills an enormous gap in the health care literature." — Reference and User Services Quarterly, American Library Association, Summer '98

"Recommended reference source."
— Booklist, American Library Association, Dec '97

Depression Sourcebook

Basic Consumer Health Information about Unipolar Depression, Bipolar Disorder, Postpartum Depression, Seasonal Affective Disorder, and Other Types of Depression in Children, Adolescents, Women, Men, the Elderly, and Other Selected Populations

Along with Facts about Causes, Risk Factors, Diagnostic Criteria, Treatment Options, Coping Strategies, Suicide Prevention, a Glossary, and a Directory of Sources for Additional Help and Information

Edited by Karen Belleni. 602 pages. 2002. 0-7808-0611-5. $78.

"Depression Sourcebook is of a very high standard. Its purpose, which is to serve as a reference source to the lay reader, is very well served."
— Journal of the National Medical Association, 2004

"Invaluable reference for public and school library collections alike." — Library Bookwatch, Apr '03

"Recommended for purchase."
— American Reference Books Annual, 2003

■

Diabetes Sourcebook, 3rd Edition

Basic Consumer Health Information about Type 1 Diabetes (Insulin-Dependent or Juvenile-Onset Diabetes), Type 2 Diabetes (Noninsulin-Dependent or Adult-Onset Diabetes), Gestational Diabetes, Impaired Glucose Tolerance (IGT), and Related Complications, Such as Amputation, Eye Disease, Gum Disease, Nerve Damage, and End-Stage Renal Disease, Including Facts about Insulin, Oral Diabetes Medications, Blood Sugar Testing, and the Role of Exercise and Nutrition in the Control of Diabetes

Along with a Glossary and Resources for Further Help and Information

Edited by Dawn D. Matthews. 622 pages. 2003. 0-7808-0629-8. $78.

ALSO AVAILABLE: Diabetes Sourcebook, 1st Edition. Edited by Karen Bellenir and Peter D. Dresser. 827 pages. 1994. 1-55888-751-2. $78.

Diabetes Sourcebook, 2nd Edition. Edited by Karen Bellenir. 688 pages. 1998. 0-7808-0224-1. $78.

"This edition is even more helpful than earlier versions. . . . It is a truly valuable tool for anyone seeking readable and authoritative information on diabetes."
— American Reference Books Annual, 2004

"An invaluable reference." — Library Journal, May '00

Selected as one of the 250 "Best Health Sciences Books of 1999." — Doody's Rating Service, Mar-Apr 2000

"Provides useful information for the general public."
— Healthlines, University of Michigan Health Management Research Center, Sep/Oct '99

". . . provides reliable mainstream medical information . . . belongs on the shelves of any library with a consumer health collection." — E-Streams, Sep '99

"Recommended reference source."
— Booklist, American Library Association, Feb '99

Diet & Nutrition Sourcebook, 2nd Edition

Basic Consumer Health Information about Dietary Guidelines, Recommended Daily Intake Values, Vitamins, Minerals, Fiber, Fat, Weight Control, Dietary Supplements, and Food Additives

Along with Special Sections on Nutrition Needs throughout Life and Nutrition for People with Such Specific Medical Concerns as Allergies, High Blood Cholesterol, Hypertension, Diabetes, Celiac Disease, Seizure Disorders, Phenylketonuria (PKU), Cancer, and Eating Disorders, and Including Reports on Current Nutrition Research and Source Listings for Additional Help and Information

Edited by Karen Bellenir. 650 pages. 1999. 0-7808-0228-4. $78.

ALSO AVAILABLE: *Diet & Nutrition Sourcebook, 1st Edition.* Edited by Dan R. Harris. 662 pages. 1996. 0-7808-0084-2. $78.

"This book is an excellent source of basic diet and nutrition information." — *Booklist Health Sciences Supplement, American Library Association, Dec '00*

"This reference document should be in any public library, but it would be a very good guide for beginning students in the health sciences. If the other books in this publisher's series are as good as this, they should all be in the health sciences collections."
—*American Reference Books Annual, 2000*

"This book is an excellent general nutrition reference for consumers who desire to take an active role in their health care for prevention. Consumers of all ages who select this book can feel confident they are receiving current and accurate information." — *Journal of Nutrition for the Elderly, Vol. 19, No. 4, '00*

"Recommended reference source."
—*Booklist, American Library Association, Dec '99*

SEE ALSO *Digestive Diseases & Disorders Sourcebook, Eating Disorders Sourcebook, Gastrointestinal Diseases & Disorders Sourcebook, Vegetarian Sourcebook*

Digestive Diseases & Disorders Sourcebook

Basic Consumer Health Information about Diseases and Disorders that Impact the Upper and Lower Digestive System, Including Celiac Disease, Constipation, Crohn's Disease, Cyclic Vomiting Syndrome, Diarrhea, Diverticulosis and Diverticulitis, Gallstones, Heartburn, Hemorrhoids, Hernias, Indigestion (Dyspepsia), Irritable Bowel Syndrome, Lactose Intolerance, Ulcers, and More

Along with Information about Medications and Other Treatments, Tips for Maintaining a Healthy Digestive Tract, a Glossary, and Directory of Digestive Diseases Organizations

Edited by Karen Bellenir. 335 pages. 2000. 0-7808-0327-2. $78.

"This title would be an excellent addition to all public or patient-research libraries."
—*American Reference Books Annual, 2001*

"This title is recommended for public, hospital, and health sciences libraries with consumer health collections." —*E-Streams, Jul-Aug '00*

"Recommended reference source."
—*Booklist, American Library Association, May '00*

SEE ALSO *Diet & Nutrition Sourcebook, Eating Disorders Sourcebook, Gastrointestinal Diseases & Disorders Sourcebook*

Disabilities Sourcebook

Basic Consumer Health Information about Physical and Psychiatric Disabilities, Including Descriptions of Major Causes of Disability, Assistive and Adaptive Aids, Workplace Issues, and Accessibility Concerns

Along with Information about the Americans with Disabilities Act, a Glossary, and Resources for Additional Help and Information

Edited by Dawn D. Matthews. 616 pages. 2000. 0-7808-0389-2. $78.

"It is a must for libraries with a consumer health section." — *American Reference Books Annual 2002*

"A much needed addition to the Omnigraphics *Health Reference Series*. A current reference work to provide people with disabilities, their families, caregivers or those who work with them, a broad range of information in one volume, has not been available until now. . . . It is recommended for all public and academic library reference collections." —*E-Streams, May '01*

"An excellent source book in easy-to-read format covering many current topics; highly recommended for all libraries." — *Choice, Association of College and Research Libraries, Jan '01*

"Recommended reference source."
—*Booklist, American Library Association, Jul '00*

Domestic Violence Sourcebook, 2nd Edition

Basic Consumer Health Information about the Causes and Consequences of Abusive Relationships, Including Physical Violence, Sexual Assault, Battery, Stalking, and Emotional Abuse, and Facts about the Effects of Violence on Women, Men, Young Adults, and the Elderly, with Reports about Domestic Violence in Selected Populations, and Featuring Facts about Medical Care, Victim Assistance and Protection, Prevention Strategies, Mental Health Services, and Legal Issues

Along with a Glossary of Related Terms and Resources for Additional Help and Information

Edited by Dawn D. Matthews. 628 pages. 2004. 0-7808-0669-7. $78.

ALSO AVAILABLE: *Domestic Violence & Child Abuse Sourcebook, 1st Edition.* Edited by Helene Henderson. 1,064 pages. 2001. 0-7808-0235-7. $78.

"Interested lay persons should find the book extremely beneficial. . . . A copy of *Domestic Violence and Child Abuse Sourcebook* should be in every public library in the United States."
— *Social Science & Medicine*, No. 56, 2003

"This is important information. The Web has many resources but this sourcebook fills an important societal need. I am not aware of any other resources of this type." — *Doody's Review Service, Sep '01*

"Recommended for all libraries, scholars, and practitioners." — *Choice,*
Association of College & Research Libraries, Jul '01

"Recommended reference source."
— *Booklist, American Library Association, Apr '01*

"Important pick for college-level health reference libraries." — *The Bookwatch, Mar '01*

"Because this problem is so widespread and because this book includes a lot of issues within one volume, this work is recommended for all public libraries."
— *American Reference Books Annual, 2001*

■

Drug Abuse Sourcebook, 2nd Edition

Basic Consumer Health Information about Illicit Substances of Abuse and the Misuse of Prescription and Over-the-Counter Medications, Including Depressants, Hallucinogens, Inhalants, Marijuana, Stimulants, and Anabolic Steroids

Along with Facts about Related Health Risks, Treatment Programs, Prevention Programs, a Glossary of Abuse and Addiction Terms, a Glossary of Drug-Related Street Terms, and a Directory Resources for More Information

Edited by Catherine Ginther. 600 pages. 2004. 0-7808-0740-5. $78.

ALSO AVAILABLE: Drug Abuse Sourcebook, 1st Edition. Edited by Karen Bellenir. 629 pages. 2000. 0-7808-0242 X. $78.

"Containing a wealth of information . . . . This resource belongs in libraries that serve a lower-division undergraduate or community college clientele as well as the general public." — *Choice, Association of*
College and Research Libraries, Jun '01

"Recommended reference source."
— *Booklist, American Library Association, Feb '01*

"Highly recommended." — *The Bookwatch, Jan '01*

"Even though there is a plethora of books on drug abuse, this volume is recommended for school, public, and college libraries."
—*American Reference Books Annual, 2001*

SEE ALSO Alcoholism Sourcebook, Substance Abuse Sourcebook

Ear, Nose & Throat Disorders Sourcebook

Basic Information about Disorders of the Ears, Nose, Sinus Cavities, Pharynx, and Larynx, Including Ear Infections, Tinnitus, Vestibular Disorders, Allergic and Non-Allergic Rhinitis, Sore Throats, Tonsillitis, and Cancers That Affect the Ears, Nose, Sinuses, and Throat

Along with Reports on Current Research Initiatives, a Glossary of Related Medical Terms, and a Directory of Sources for Further Help and Information

Edited by Karen Bellenir and Linda M. Shin. 576 pages. 1998. 0-7808-0206-3. $78.

"Overall, this sourcebook is helpful for the consumer seeking information on ENT issues. It is recommended for public libraries."
—*American Reference Books Annual, 1999*

"Recommended reference source."
—*Booklist, American Library Association, Dec '98*

■

Eating Disorders Sourcebook

Basic Consumer Health Information about Eating Disorders, Including Information about Anorexia Nervosa, Bulimia Nervosa, Binge Eating, Body Dysmorphic Disorder, Pica, Laxative Abuse, and Night Eating Syndrome

Along with Information about Causes, Adverse Effects, and Treatment and Prevention Issues, and Featuring a Section on Concerns Specific to Children and Adolescents, a Glossary, and Resources for Further Help and Information

Edited by Dawn D. Matthews. 322 pages. 2001. 0-7808-0335-3. $78.

"Recommended for health science libraries that are open to the public, as well as hospital libraries. This book is a good resource for the consumer who is concerned about eating disorders." — *E-Streams, Mar '02*

"This volume is another convenient collection of excerpted articles. Recommended for school and public library patrons; lower-division undergraduates; and two-year technical program students." — *Choice,*
Association of College & Research Libraries, Jan '02

"Recommended reference source." — *Booklist,*
American Library Association, Oct '01

SEE ALSO Diet & Nutrition Sourcebook, Digestive Diseases & Disorders Sourcebook, Gastrointestinal Diseases & Disorders Sourcebook

■

Emergency Medical Services Sourcebook

Basic Consumer Health Information about Preventing, Preparing for, and Managing Emergency Situations, When and Who to Call for Help, What to Expect in the Emergency Room, the Emergency Medical Team, Patient Issues, and Current Topics in Emergency Medicine

Along with Statistical Data, a Glossary, and Sources of Additional Help and Information

577

Edited by Jenni Lynn Colson. 494 pages. 2002. 0-7808-0420-1. $78.

"Handy and convenient for home, public, school, and college libraries. Recommended."
— *Choice, Association of College and Research Libraries, Apr '03*

"This reference can provide the consumer with answers to most questions about emergency care in the United States, or it will direct them to a resource where the answer can be found."
— *American Reference Books Annual, 2003*

"Recommended reference source."
— *Booklist, American Library Association, Feb '03*

■

Endocrine & Metabolic Disorders Sourcebook

Basic Information for the Layperson about Pancreatic and Insulin-Related Disorders Such as Pancreatitis, Diabetes, and Hypoglycemia; Adrenal Gland Disorders Such as Cushing's Syndrome, Addison's Disease, and Congenital Adrenal Hyperplasia; Pituitary Gland Disorders Such as Growth Hormone Deficiency, Acromegaly, and Pituitary Tumors; Thyroid Disorders Such as Hypothyroidism, Graves' Disease, Hashimoto's Disease, and Goiter; Hyperparathyroidism; and Other Diseases and Syndromes of Hormone Imbalance or Metabolic Dysfunction

Along with Reports on Current Research Initiatives

Edited by Linda M. Shin. 574 pages. 1998. 0-7808-0207-1. $78.

"Omnigraphics has produced another needed resource for health information consumers."
— *American Reference Books Annual, 2000*

"Recommended reference source."
— *Booklist, American Library Association, Dec '98*

■

Environmental Health Sourcebook, 2nd Edition

Basic Consumer Health Information about the Environment and Its Effect on Human Health, Including the Effects of Air Pollution, Water Pollution, Hazardous Chemicals, Food Hazards, Radiation Hazards, Biological Agents, Household Hazards, Such as Radon, Asbestos, Carbon Monoxide, and Mold, and Information about Associated Diseases and Disorders, Including Cancer, Allergies, Respiratory Problems, and Skin Disorders

Along with Information about Environmental Concerns for Specific Populations, a Glossary of Related Terms, and Resources for Further Help and Information

Edited by Dawn D. Matthews. 673 pages. 2003. 0-7808-0632-8. $78.

ALSO AVAILABLE: *Environmentally Induced Disorders Sourcebook, 1st Edition.* Edited by Allan R. Cook. 620 pages. 1997. 0-7808-0083-4. $78.

"This recently updated edition continues the level of quality and the reputation of the numerous other volumes in Omnigraphics' *Health Reference Series.*"
— *American Reference Books Annual, 2004*

"Recommended reference source."
— *Booklist, American Library Association, Sep '98*

"This book will be a useful addition to anyone's library." — *Choice Health Sciences Supplement, Association of College and Research Libraries, May '98*

". . . a good survey of numerous environmentally induced physical disorders . . . a useful addition to anyone's library."
— *Doody's Health Sciences Book Reviews, Jan '98*

". . . provide[s] introductory information from the best authorities around. Since this volume covers topics that potentially affect everyone, it will surely be one of the most frequently consulted volumes in the *Health Reference Series.*" — *Rettig on Reference, Nov '97*

■

Environmentally Induced Disorders Sourcebook, 1st Edition

SEE *Environmental Health Sourcebook, 2nd Edition*

■

Ethnic Diseases Sourcebook

Basic Consumer Health Information for Ethnic and Racial Minority Groups in the United States, Including General Health Indicators and Behaviors, Ethnic Diseases, Genetic Testing, the Impact of Chronic Diseases, Women's Health, Mental Health Issues, and Preventive Health Care Services

Along with a Glossary and a Listing of Additional Resources

Edited by Joyce Brennfleck Shannon. 664 pages. 2001. 0-7808-0336-1. $78.

"Recommended for health sciences libraries where public health programs are a priority."
— *E-Streams, Jan '02*

"Not many books have been written on this topic to date, and the *Ethnic Diseases Sourcebook* is a strong addition to the list. It will be an important introductory resource for health consumers, students, health care personnel, and social scientists. It is recommended for public, academic, and large hospital libraries."
— *American Reference Books Annual 2002*

"Recommended reference source."
— *Booklist, American Library Association, Oct '01*

"Will prove valuable to any library seeking to maintain a current, comprehensive reference collection of health resources. . . . An excellent source of health information about genetic disorders which affect particular ethnic and racial minorities in the U.S."
— *The Bookwatch, Aug '01*

Eye Care Sourcebook, 2nd Edition

Basic Consumer Health Information about Eye Care and Eye Disorders, Including Facts about the Diagnosis, Prevention, and Treatment of Common Refractive Problems Such as Myopia, Hyperopia, Astigmatism, and Presbyopia, and Eye Diseases, Including Glaucoma, Cataract, Age-Related Macular Degeneration, and Diabetic Retinopathy

Along with a Section on Vision Correction and Refractive Surgeries, Including LASIK and LASEK, a Glossary, and Directories of Resources for Additional Help and Information

Edited by Amy L. Sutton. 543 pages. 2003. 0-7808-0635-2. $78.

ALSO AVAILABLE: Ophthalmic Disorders Sourcebook, 1st Edition. Edited by Linda M. Ross. 631 pages. 1996. 0-7808-0081-8. $78.

". . . a solid reference tool for eye care and a valuable addition to a collection."
— *American Reference Books Annual, 2004*

∎

Family Planning Sourcebook

Basic Consumer Health Information about Planning for Pregnancy and Contraception, Including Traditional Methods, Barrier Methods, Hormonal Methods, Permanent Methods, Future Methods, Emergency Contraception, and Birth Control Choices for Women at Each Stage of Life

Along with Statistics, a Glossary, and Sources of Additional Information

Edited by Amy Marcaccio Keyzer. 520 pages. 2001. 0-7808-0379-5. $78.

"Recommended for public, health, and undergraduate libraries as part of the circulating collection."
— *E-Streams, Mar '02*

"Information is presented in an unbiased, readable manner, and the sourcebook will certainly be a necessary addition to those public and high school libraries where Internet access is restricted or otherwise problematic." — *American Reference Books Annual 2002*

"Recommended reference source."
— *Booklist, American Library Association, Oct '01*

"Will prove valuable to any library seeking to maintain a current, comprehensive reference collection of health resources. . . . Excellent reference."
— *The Bookwatch, Aug '01*

SEE ALSO Pregnancy & Birth Sourcebook

∎

Fitness & Exercise Sourcebook, 2nd Edition

Basic Consumer Health Information about the Fundamentals of Fitness and Exercise, Including How to Begin and Maintain a Fitness Program, Fitness as a Lifestyle, the Link between Fitness and Diet, Advice for Specific Groups of People, Exercise as It Relates to

Specific Medical Conditions, and Recent Research in Fitness and Exercise

Along with a Glossary of Important Terms and Resources for Additional Help and Information

Edited by Kristen M. Gledhill. 646 pages. 2001. 0-7808-0334-5. $78.

ALSO AVAILABLE: Fitness & Exercise Sourcebook, 1st Edition. Edited by Dan R. Harris. 663 pages. 1996. 0-7808-0186-5. $78.

"This work is recommended for all general reference collections."
— *American Reference Books Annual 2002*

"Highly recommended for public, consumer, and school grades fourth through college."
— *E-Streams, Nov '01*

"Recommended reference source." — *Booklist, American Library Association, Oct '01*

"The information appears quite comprehensive and is considered reliable. . . . This second edition is a welcomed addition to the series."
— *Doody's Review Service, Sep '01*

"This reference is a valuable choice for those who desire a broad source of information on exercise, fitness, and chronic-disease prevention through a healthy lifestyle." — *American Medical Writers Association Journal, Fall '01*

"Will prove valuable to any library seeking to maintain a current, comprehensive reference collection of health resources. . . . Excellent reference."
— *The Bookwatch, Aug '01*

∎

Food & Animal Borne Diseases Sourcebook

Basic Information about Diseases That Can Be Spread to Humans through the Ingestion of Contaminated Food or Water or by Contact with Infected Animals and Insects, Such as Botulism, E. Coli, Hepatitis A, Trichinosis, Lyme Disease, and Rabies

Along with Information Regarding Prevention and Treatment Methods, and Including a Special Section for International Travelers Describing Diseases Such as Cholera, Malaria, Travelers' Diarrhea, and Yellow Fever, and Offering Recommendations for Avoiding Illness

Edited by Karen Bellenir and Peter D. Dresser. 535 pages. 1995. 0-7808-0033-8. $78.

"Targeting general readers and providing them with a single, comprehensive source of information on selected topics, this book continues, with the excellent caliber of its predecessors, to catalog topical information on health matters of general interest. Readable and thorough, this valuable resource is highly recommended for all libraries."
— *Academic Library Book Review, Summer '96*

"A comprehensive collection of authoritative information." — *Emergency Medical Services, Oct '95*

579

Food Safety Sourcebook

Basic Consumer Health Information about the Safe Handling of Meat, Poultry, Seafood, Eggs, Fruit Juices, and Other Food Items, and Facts about Pesticides, Drinking Water, Food Safety Overseas, and the Onset, Duration, and Symptoms of Foodborne Illnesses, Including Types of Pathogenic Bacteria, Parasitic Protozoa, Worms, Viruses, and Natural Toxins

Along with the Role of the Consumer, the Food Handler, and the Government in Food Safety; a Glossary, and Resources for Additional Help and Information

Edited by Dawn D. Matthews. 339 pages. 1999. 0-7808-0326-4. $78.

"This book is recommended for public libraries and universities with home economic and food science programs." — *E-Streams, Nov '00*

"Recommended reference source."
—*Booklist, American Library Association, May '00*

"This book takes the complex issues of food safety and foodborne pathogens and presents them in an easily understood manner. [It does] an excellent job of covering a large and often confusing topic."
—*American Reference Books Annual, 2000*

■

Forensic Medicine Sourcebook

Basic Consumer Information for the Layperson about Forensic Medicine, Including Crime Scene Investigation, Evidence Collection and Analysis, Expert Testimony, Computer-Aided Criminal Identification, Digital Imaging in the Courtroom, DNA Profiling, Accident Reconstruction, Autopsies, Ballistics, Drugs and Explosives Detection, Latent Fingerprints, Product Tampering, and Questioned Document Examination

Along with Statistical Data, a Glossary of Forensics Terminology, and Listings of Sources for Further Help and Information

Edited by Annemarie S. Muth. 574 pages. 1999. 0-7808-0232-2. $78.

"Given the expected widespread interest in its content and its easy to read style, this book is recommended for most public and all college and university libraries."
— *E-Streams, Feb '01*

"Recommended for public libraries."
—*Reference & User Services Quarterly, American Library Association, Spring 2000*

"Recommended reference source."
—*Booklist, American Library Association, Feb '00*

"A wealth of information, useful statistics, references are up-to-date and extremely complete. This wonderful collection of data will help students who are interested in a career in any type of forensic field. It is a great resource for attorneys who need information about types of expert witnesses needed in a particular case. It also offers useful information for fiction and nonfiction writers whose work involves a crime. A fascinating compilation. All levels." — *Choice, Association of College and Research Libraries, Jan 2000*

"There are several items that make this book attractive to consumers who are seeking certain forensic data. . . . This is a useful current source for those seeking general forensic medical answers."
—*American Reference Books Annual, 2000*

■

Gastrointestinal Diseases & Disorders Sourcebook

Basic Information about Gastroesophageal Reflux Disease (Heartburn), Ulcers, Diverticulosis, Irritable Bowel Syndrome, Crohn's Disease, Ulcerative Colitis, Diarrhea, Constipation, Lactose Intolerance, Hemorrhoids, Hepatitis, Cirrhosis, and Other Digestive Problems, Featuring Statistics, Descriptions of Symptoms, and Current Treatment Methods of Interest for Persons Living with Upper and Lower Gastrointestinal Maladies

Edited by Linda M. Ross. 413 pages. 1996. 0-7808-0078-8. $78.

". . . very readable form. The successful editorial work that brought this material together into a useful and understandable reference makes accessible to all readers information that can help them more effectively understand and obtain help for digestive tract problems."
—*Choice, Association of College & Research Libraries, Feb '97*

SEE ALSO *Diet & Nutrition Sourcebook, Digestive Diseases & Disorders, Eating Disorders Sourcebook*

■

Genetic Disorders Sourcebook, 3rd Edition

Basic Consumer Health Information about Hereditary Diseases and Disorders, Including Facts about the Human Genome, Genetic Inheritance Patterns, Disorders Associated with Specific Genes, such as Sickle Cell Disease, Hemophilia, and Cystic Fibrosis, Chromosome Disorders, such as Down Syndrome, Fragile X Syndrome, and Turner Syndrome, and Complex Diseases and Disorders Resulting from the Interaction of Environmental and Genetic Factors, such as Allergies, Cancer, and Obesity

Along with Facts about Genetic Testing, Suggestions for Parents of Children with Special Needs, Reports on Current Research Initiatives, a Glossary of Genetic Terminology, and Resources for Additional Help and Information

Edited by Karen Bellenir. 750 pages. 2004. 0-7808-0742-1. $78.

ALSO AVAILABLE: Genetic Disorders Sourcebook, 1st Edition. Edited by Karen Bellenir. 642 pages. 1996. 0-7808-0034-6. $78.

Genetic Disorders Sourcebook, 2nd Edition. Edited by Kathy Massimini. 768 pages. 2001. 0-7808-0241-1. $78.

"Recommended for public libraries and medical and hospital libraries with consumer health collections."
—*E-Streams, May '01*

■

Head Trauma Sourcebook

Basic Information for the Layperson about Open-Head and Closed-Head Injuries, Treatment Advances, Recovery, and Rehabilitation

Along with Reports on Current Research Initiatives

Edited by Karen Bellenir. 414 pages. 1997. 0-7808-0208-X. $78.

■

Headache Sourcebook

Basic Consumer Health Information about Migraine, Tension, Cluster, Rebound and Other Types of Headaches, with Facts about the Cause and Prevention of Headaches, the Effects of Stress and the Environment, Headaches during Pregnancy and Menopause, and Childhood Headaches

Along with a Glossary and Other Resources for Additional Help and Information

Edited by Dawn D. Matthews. 362 pages. 2002. 0-7808-0337-X. $78.

"Highly recommended for academic and medical reference collections." — *Library Bookwatch, Sep '02*

■

Health Insurance Sourcebook

Basic Information about Managed Care Organizations, Traditional Fee-for-Service Insurance, Insurance Portability and Pre-Existing Conditions Clauses, Medicare, Medicaid, Social Security, and Military Health Care

Along with Information about Insurance Fraud

Edited by Wendy Wilcox. 530 pages. 1997. 0-7808-0222-5. $78.

"Particularly useful because it brings much of this information together in one volume. This book will be a handy reference source in the health sciences library, hospital library, college and university library, and medium to large public library."
— *Medical Reference Services Quarterly, Fall '98*

Awarded "Books of the Year Award"
— *American Journal of Nursing, 1997*

"The layout of the book is particularly helpful as it provides easy access to reference material. A most useful addition to the vast amount of information about health insurance. The use of data from U.S. government agencies is most commendable. Useful in a library or learning center for healthcare professional students."
— *Doody's Health Sciences Book Reviews, Nov '97*

Health Reference Series Cumulative Index 1999

A Comprehensive Index to the Individual Volumes of the Health Reference Series, Including a Subject Index, Name Index, Organization Index, and Publication Index

Along with a Master List of Acronyms and Abbreviations

Edited by Edward J. Prucha, Anne Holmes, and Robert Rudnick. 990 pages. 2000. 0-7808-0382-5. $78.

"This volume will be most helpful in libraries that have a relatively complete collection of the Health Reference Series." — *American Reference Books Annual, 2001*

"Essential for collections that hold any of the numerous *Health Reference Series* titles."
— *Choice, Association of College and Research Libraries, Nov '00*

■

Healthy Aging Sourcebook

Basic Consumer Health Information about Maintaining Health through the Aging Process, Including Advice on Nutrition, Exercise, and Sleep, Help in Making Decisions about Midlife Issues and Retirement, and Guidance Concerning Practical and Informed Choices in Health Consumerism

Along with Data Concerning the Theories of Aging, Different Experiences in Aging by Minority Groups, and Facts about Aging Now and Aging in the Future; and Featuring a Glossary, a Guide to Consumer Help, Additional Suggested Reading, and Practical Resource Directory

Edited by Jenifer Swanson. 536 pages. 1999. 0-7808-0390-6. $78.

"Recommended reference source."
— *Booklist, American Library Association, Feb '00*

SEE ALSO *Physical & Mental Issues in Aging Sourcebook*

■

Healthy Children Sourcebook

Basic Consumer Health Information about the Physical and Mental Development of Children between the Ages of 3 and 12, Including Routine Health Care, Preventative Health Services, Safety and First Aid, Healthy Sleep, Dental Care, Nutrition, and Fitness, and Featuring Parenting Tips on Such Topics as Bedwetting, Choosing Day Care, Monitoring TV and Other Media, and Establishing a Foundation for Substance Abuse Prevention

Along with a Glossary of Commonly Used Pediatric Terms and Resources for Additional Help and Information.

Edited by Chad T. Kimball. 647 pages. 2003. 0-7808-0247-0. $78.

"It is hard to imagine that any other single resource exists that would provide such a comprehensive guide

of timely information on health promotion and disease prevention for children aged 3 to 12."
— *American Reference Books Annual, 2004*

"The strengths of this book are many. It is clearly written, presented and structured."
— *Journal of the National Medical Association, 2004*

■

Healthy Heart Sourcebook for Women

Basic Consumer Health Information about Cardiac Issues Specific to Women, Including Facts about Major Risk Factors and Prevention, Treatment and Control Strategies, and Important Dietary Issues

Along with a Special Section Regarding the Pros and Cons of Hormone Replacement Therapy and Its Impact on Heart Health, and Additional Help, Including Recipes, a Glossary, and a Directory of Resources

Edited by Dawn D. Matthews. 336 pages. 2000. 0-7808-0329-9. $78.

"A good reference source and recommended for all public, academic, medical, and hospital libraries."
— *Medical Reference Services Quarterly, Summer '01*

"Because of the lack of information specific to women on this topic, this book is recommended for public libraries and consumer libraries."
— *American Reference Books Annual, 2001*

"Contains very important information about coronary artery disease that all women should know. The information is current and presented in an easy-to-read format. The book will make a good addition to any library."
— *American Medical Writers Association Journal, Summer '00*

"Important, basic reference."
— *Reviewer's Bookwatch, Jul '00*

SEE ALSO *Heart Diseases & Disorders Sourcebook, Women's Health Concerns Sourcebook*

■

Heart Diseases & Disorders Sourcebook, 2nd Edition

Basic Consumer Health Information about Heart Attacks, Angina, Rhythm Disorders, Heart Failure, Valve Disease, Congenital Heart Disorders, and More, Including Descriptions of Surgical Procedures and Other Interventions, Medications, Cardiac Rehabilitation, Risk Identification, and Prevention Tips

Along with Statistical Data, Reports on Current Research Initiatives, a Glossary of Cardiovascular Terms, and Resource Directory

Edited by Karen Bellenir. 612 pages. 2000. 0-7808-0238-1. $78.

ALSO AVAILABLE: *Cardiovascular Diseases & Disorders Sourcebook, 1st Edition.* Edited by Karen Bellenir and Peter D. Dresser. 683 pages. 1995. 0-7808-0032-X. $78.

"This work stands out as an imminently accessible resource for the general public. It is recommended for the reference and circulating shelves of school, public, and academic libraries."
— *American Reference Books Annual, 2001*

"Recommended reference source."
— *Booklist, American Library Association, Dec '00*

"Provides comprehensive coverage of matters related to the heart. This title is recommended for health sciences and public libraries with consumer health collections."
— *E-Streams, Oct '00*

SEE ALSO *Healthy Heart Sourcebook for Women*

■

Household Safety Sourcebook

Basic Consumer Health Information about Household Safety, Including Information about Poisons, Chemicals, Fire, and Water Hazards in the Home

Along with Advice about the Safe Use of Home Maintenance Equipment, Choosing Toys and Nursery Furniture, Holiday and Recreation Safety, a Glossary, and Resources for Further Help and Information

Edited by Dawn D. Matthews. 606 pages. 2002. 0-7808-0338-8. $78.

"This work will be useful in public libraries with large consumer health and wellness departments."
— *American Reference Books Annual, 2003*

"As a sourcebook on household safety this book meets its mark. It is encyclopedic in scope and covers a wide range of safety issues that are commonly seen in the home."
— *E-Streams, Jul '02*

■

Hypertension Sourcebook

Basic Consumer Health Information about the Causes, Diagnosis, and Treatment of High Blood Pressure, with Facts about Consequences, Complications, and Co-Occurring Disorders, Such as Coronary Heart Disease, Diabetes, Stroke, Kidney Disease, and Hypertensive Retinopathy, and Issues in Blood Pressure Control, Including Dietary Choices, Stress Management, and Medications

Along with Reports on Current Research Initiatives and Clinical Trials, a Glossary, and Resources for Additional Help and Information

Edited by Dawn D. Matthews and Karen Bellenir. 600 pages. 2004. 0-7808-0674-3. $78.

■

Immune System Disorders Sourcebook

Basic Information about Lupus, Multiple Sclerosis, Guillain-Barré Syndrome, Chronic Granulomatous Disease, and More

Along with Statistical and Demographic Data and Reports on Current Research Initiatives

Edited by Allan R. Cook. 608 pages. 1997. 0-7808-0209-8. $78.

Infant & Toddler Health Sourcebook

Basic Consumer Health Information about the Physical and Mental Development of Newborns, Infants, and Toddlers, Including Neonatal Concerns, Nutrition Recommendations, Immunization Schedules, Common Pediatric Disorders, Assessments and Milestones, Safety Tips, and Advice for Parents and Other Caregivers

Along with a Glossary of Terms and Resource Listings for Additional Help

Edited by Jenifer Swanson. 585 pages. 2000. 0-7808-0246-2. $78.

"As a reference for the general public, this would be useful in any library." — *E-Streams, May '01*

"Recommended reference source."
— *Booklist, American Library Association, Feb '01*

"This is a good source for general use."
— *American Reference Books Annual, 2001*

■

Infectious Diseases Sourcebook

Basic Consumer Health Information about Non-Contagious Bacterial, Viral, Prion, Fungal, and Parasitic Diseases Spread by Food and Water, Insects and Animals, or Environmental Contact, Including Botulism, E. Coli, Encephalitis, Legionnaires' Disease, Lyme Disease, Malaria, Plague, Rabies, Salmonella, Tetanus, and Others, and Facts about Newly Emerging Diseases, Such as Hantavirus, Mad Cow Disease, Monkeypox, and West Nile Virus

Along with Information about Preventing Disease Transmission, the Threat of Bioterrorism, and Current Research Initiatives, with a Glossary and Directory of Resources for More Information

Edited by Karen Bellenir. 634 pages. 2004. 0-7808-0675-1. $78.

■

Injury & Trauma Sourcebook

Basic Consumer Health Information about the Impact of Injury, the Diagnosis and Treatment of Common and Traumatic Injuries, Emergency Care, and Specific Injuries Related to Home, Community, Workplace, Transportation, and Recreation

Along with Guidelines for Injury Prevention, a Glossary, and a Directory of Additional Resources

Edited by Joyce Brennfleck Shannon. 696 pages. 2002. 0-7808-0421-X. $78.

"This publication is the most comprehensive work of its kind about injury and trauma."
— *American Reference Books Annual, 2003*

"This sourcebook provides concise, easily readable, basic health information about injuries. . . . This book is well organized and an easy to use reference resource suitable for hospital, health sciences and public libraries with consumer health collections."
— *E-Streams, Nov '02*

"Practitioners should be aware of guides such as this in order to facilitate their use by patients and their families." — *Doody's Health Sciences Book Review Journal, Sep-Oct '02*

"Recommended reference source."
— *Booklist, American Library Association, Sep '02*

"Highly recommended for academic and medical reference collections." — *Library Bookwatch, Sep '02*

■

Kidney & Urinary Tract Diseases & Disorders Sourcebook

Basic Information about Kidney Stones, Urinary Incontinence, Bladder Disease, End Stage Renal Disease, Dialysis, and More

Along with Statistical and Demographic Data and Reports on Current Research Initiatives

Edited by Linda M. Ross. 602 pages. 1997. 0-7808-0079-6. $78.

■

Learning Disabilities Sourcebook, 2nd Edition

Basic Consumer Health Information about Learning Disabilities, Including Dyslexia, Developmental Speech and Language Disabilities, Non-Verbal Learning Disorders, Developmental Arithmetic Disorder, Developmental Writing Disorder, and Other Conditions That Impede Learning Such as Attention Deficit/ Hyperactivity Disorder, Brain Injury, Hearing Impairment, Klinefelter Syndrome, Dyspraxia, and Tourette Syndrome

Along with Facts about Educational Issues and Assistive Technology, Coping Strategies, a Glossary of Related Terms, and Resources for Further Help and Information

Edited by Dawn D. Matthews. 621 pages. 2003. 0-7808-0626-3. $78.

ALSO AVAILABLE: Learning Disabilities Sourcebook, 1st Edition. Edited by Linda M. Shin. 579 pages. 1998. 0-7808-0210-1. $78.

"The second edition of *Learning Disabilities Sourcebook* far surpasses the earlier edition in that it is more focused on information that will be useful as a consumer health resource."
— *American Reference Books Annual, 2004*

"Teachers as well as consumers will find this an essential guide to understanding various syndromes and their latest treatments. [An] invaluable reference for public and school library collections alike."
— *Library Bookwatch, Apr '03*

Named **"Outstanding Reference Book of 1999."**
— *New York Public Library, Feb 2000*

"An excellent candidate for inclusion in a public library reference section. It's a great source of information. Teachers will also find the book useful. Definitely worth reading."
— *Journal of Adolescent & Adult Literacy, Feb 2000*

"Readable . . . provides a solid base of information regarding successful techniques used with individuals who have learning disabilities, as well as practical suggestions for educators and family members. Clear language, concise descriptions, and pertinent information for contacting multiple resources add to the strength of this book as a useful tool." — *Choice, Association of College and Research Libraries, Feb '99*

"Recommended reference source."
— *Booklist, American Library Association, Sep '98*

"A useful resource for libraries and for those who don't have the time to identify and locate the individual publications." — *Disability Resources Monthly, Sep '98*

■

Leukemia Sourcebook

Basic Consumer Health Information about Adult and Childhood Leukemias, Including Acute Lymphocytic Leukemia (ALL), Chronic Lymphocytic Leukemia (CLL), Acute Myelogenous Leukemia (AML), Chronic Myelogenous Leukemia (CML), and Hairy Cell Leukemia, and Treatments Such as Chemotherapy, Radiation Therapy, Peripheral Blood Stem Cell and Marrow Transplantation, and Immunotherapy

Along with Tips for Life During and After Treatment, a Glossary, and Directories of Additional Resources

Edited by Joyce Brennfleck Shannon. 587 pages. 2003. 0-7808-0627-1. $78.

"Unlike other medical books for the layperson, . . . the language does not talk down to the reader. . . . This volume is highly recommended for all libraries."
— *American Reference Books Annual, 2004*

■

Liver Disorders Sourcebook

Basic Consumer Health Information about the Liver and How It Works; Liver Diseases, Including Cancer, Cirrhosis, Hepatitis, and Toxic and Drug Related Diseases; Tips for Maintaining a Healthy Liver; Laboratory Tests, Radiology Tests, and Facts about Liver Transplantation

Along with a Section on Support Groups, a Glossary, and Resource Listings

Edited by Joyce Brennfleck Shannon. 591 pages. 2000. 0-7808-0383-3. $78.

"A valuable resource."
— *American Reference Books Annual, 2001*

"This title is recommended for health sciences and public libraries with consumer health collections."
— *E-Streams, Oct '00*

"Recommended reference source."
— *Booklist, American Library Association, Jun '00*

■

Lung Disorders Sourcebook

Basic Consumer Health Information about Emphysema, Pneumonia, Tuberculosis, Asthma, Cystic Fibrosis, and Other Lung Disorders, Including Facts about

Diagnostic Procedures, Treatment Strategies, Disease Prevention Efforts, and Such Risk Factors as Smoking, Air Pollution, and Exposure to Asbestos, Radon, and Other Agents

Along with a Glossary and Resources for Additional Help and Information

Edited by Dawn D. Matthews. 678 pages. 2002. 0-7808-0339-6. $78.

"This title is a great addition for public and school libraries because it provides concise health information on the lungs."
— *American Reference Books Annual, 2003*

"Highly recommended for academic and medical reference collections." — *Library Bookwatch, Sep '02*

■

Medical Tests Sourcebook, 2nd Edition

Basic Consumer Health Information about Medical Tests, Including Age-Specific Health Tests, Important Health Screenings and Exams, Home-Use Tests, Blood and Specimen Tests, Electrical Tests, Scope Tests, Genetic Testing, and Imaging Tests, Such as X-Rays, Ultrasound, Computed Tomography, Magnetic Resonance Imaging, Angiography, and Nuclear Medicine

Along with a Glossary and Directory of Additional Resources

Edited by Joyce Brennfleck Shannon. 654 pages. 2004. 0-7808-0670-0. $78.

ALSO AVAILABLE: Medical Tests, 1st Edition. Edited by Joyce Brennfleck Shannon. 691 pages. 1999. 0-7808-0243-8. $78.

"Recommended for hospital and health sciences libraries with consumer health collections."
— *E-Streams, Mar '00*

"This is an overall excellent reference with a wealth of general knowledge that may aid those who are reluctant to get vital tests performed."
— *Today's Librarian, Jan 2000*

"A valuable reference guide."
— *American Reference Books Annual, 2000*

■

Men's Health Concerns Sourcebook, 2nd Edition

Basic Consumer Health Information about the Medical and Mental Concerns of Men, Including Theories about the Shorter Male Lifespan, the Leading Causes of Death and Disability, Physical Concerns of Special Significance to Men, Reproductive and Sexual Concerns, Sexually Transmitted Diseases, Men's Mental and Emotional Health, and Lifestyle Choices That Affect Wellness, Such as Nutrition, Fitness, and Substance Use

Along with a Glossary of Related Terms and a Directory of Organizational Resources in Men's Health

Edited by Robert Aquinas McNally. 644 pages. 2004. 0-7808-0671-9. $78.

Mental Health Disorders Sourcebook, 2nd Edition

Basic Consumer Health Information about Anxiety Disorders, Depression and Other Mood Disorders, Eating Disorders, Personality Disorders, Schizophrenia, and More, Including Disease Descriptions, Treatment Options, and Reports on Current Research Initiatives

Along with Statistical Data, Tips for Maintaining Mental Health, a Glossary, and Directory of Sources for Additional Help and Information

Edited by Karen Bellenir. 605 pages. 2000. 0-7808-0240-3. $78.

Mental Retardation Sourcebook

Basic Consumer Health Information about Mental Retardation and Its Causes, Including Down Syndrome, Fetal Alcohol Syndrome, Fragile X Syndrome, Genetic Conditions, Injury, and Environmental Sources

Along with Preventive Strategies, Parenting Issues, Educational Implications, Health Care Needs, Employment and Economic Matters, Legal Issues, a Glossary, and a Resource Listing for Additional Help and Information

Edited by Joyce Brennfleck Shannon. 642 pages. 2000. 0-7808-0377-9. $78.

Movement Disorders Sourcebook

Basic Consumer Health Information about Neurological Movement Disorders, Including Essential Tremor, Parkinson's Disease, Dystonia, Cerebral Palsy, Huntington's Disease, Myasthenia Gravis, Multiple Sclerosis, and Other Early-Onset and Adult-Onset Movement Disorders, Their Symptoms and Causes, Diagnostic Tests, and Treatments

Along with Mobility and Assistive Technology Information, a Glossary, and a Directory of Additional Resources

Edited by Joyce Brennfleck Shannon. 655 pages. 2003. 0-7808-0628-X. $78.

Muscular Dystrophy Sourcebook

Basic Consumer Health Information about Congenital, Childhood-Onset, and Adult-Onset Forms of Muscular Dystrophy, Such as Duchenne, Becker, Emery-Dreifuss, Distal, Limb-Girdle, Facioscapulohumeral (FSHD), Myotonic, and Ophthalmoplegic Muscular Dystrophies, Including Facts about Diagnostic Tests, Medical and Physical Therapies, Management of Co-Occurring Conditions, and Parenting Guidelines

Along with Practical Tips for Home Care, a Glossary, and Directories of Additional Resources

Edited by Joyce Brennfleck Shannon. 577 pages. 2004. 0-7808-0676-X. $78.

Obesity Sourcebook

Basic Consumer Health Information about Diseases and Other Problems Associated with Obesity, and Including Facts about Risk Factors, Prevention Issues, and Management Approaches

Along with Statistical and Demographic Data, Information about Special Populations, Research Updates, a Glossary, and Source Listings for Further Help and Information

Edited by Wilma Caldwell and Chad T. Kimball. 376 pages. 2001. 0-7808-0333-7. $78.

Ophthalmic Disorders Sourcebook, 1st Edition

SEE Eye Care Sourcebook, 2nd Edition

■

Oral Health Sourcebook

SEE Dental Care & Oral Health Sourcebook, 2nd Ed.

■

Osteoporosis Sourcebook

Basic Consumer Health Information about Primary and Secondary Osteoporosis and Juvenile Osteoporosis and Related Conditions, Including Fibrous Dysplasia, Gaucher Disease, Hyperthyroidism, Hypophosphatasia, Myeloma, Osteopetrosis, Osteogenesis Imperfecta, and Paget's Disease

Along with Information about Risk Factors, Treatments, Traditional and Non-Traditional Pain Management, a Glossary of Related Terms, and a Directory of Resources

Edited by Allan R. Cook. 584 pages. 2001. 0-7808-0239-X. $78.

"This would be a book to be kept in a staff or patient library. The targeted audience is the layperson, but the therapist who needs a quick bit of information on a particular topic will also find the book useful."
— Physical Therapy, Jan '02

"This resource is recommended as a great reference source for public, health, and academic libraries, and is another triumph for the editors of Omnigraphics."
— American Reference Books Annual 2002

"Recommended for all public libraries and general health collections, especially those supporting patient education or consumer health programs."
— E-Streams, Nov '01

"Will prove valuable to any library seeking to maintain a current, comprehensive reference collection of health resources. . . . From prevention to treatment and associated conditions, this provides an excellent survey."
— The Bookwatch, Aug '01

"Recommended reference source."
— Booklist, American Library Association, July '01

SEE ALSO Women's Health Concerns Sourcebook

■

Pain Sourcebook, 2nd Edition

Basic Consumer Health Information about Specific Forms of Acute and Chronic Pain, Including Muscle and Skeletal Pain, Nerve Pain, Cancer Pain, and Disorders Characterized by Pain, Such as Fibromyalgia, Shingles, Angina, Arthritis, and Headaches

Along with Information about Pain Medications and Management Techniques, Complementary and Alternative Pain Relief Options, Tips for People Living with Chronic Pain, a Glossary, and a Directory of Sources for Further Information

Edited by Karen Bellenir. 670 pages. 2002. 0-7808-0612-3. $78.

ALSO AVAILABLE: Pain Sourcebook, 1st Edition. Edited by Allan R. Cook. 667 pages. 1997. 0-7808-0213-6. $78.

"A source of valuable information. . . . This book offers help to nonmedical people who need information about pain and pain management. It is also an excellent reference for those who participate in patient education."
— Doody's Review Service, Sep '02

"The text is readable, easily understood, and well indexed. This excellent volume belongs in all patient education libraries, consumer health sections of public libraries, and many personal collections."
— American Reference Books Annual, 1999

"A beneficial reference." — Booklist Health Sciences Supplement, American Library Association, Oct '98

"The information is basic in terms of scholarship and is appropriate for general readers. Written in journalistic style . . . intended for non-professionals. Quite thorough in its coverage of different pain conditions and summarizes the latest clinical information regarding pain treatment." — Choice, Association of College and Research Libraries, Jun '98

"Recommended reference source."
— Booklist, American Library Association, Mar '98

■

Pediatric Cancer Sourcebook

Basic Consumer Health Information about Leukemias, Brain Tumors, Sarcomas, Lymphomas, and Other Cancers in Infants, Children, and Adolescents, Including Descriptions of Cancers, Treatments, and Coping Strategies

Along with Suggestions for Parents, Caregivers, and Concerned Relatives, a Glossary of Cancer Terms, and Resource Listings

Edited by Edward J. Prucha. 587 pages. 1999. 0-7808-0245-4. $78.

"An excellent source of information. Recommended for public, hospital, and health science libraries with consumer health collections." — E-Streams, Jun '00

"Recommended reference source."
— Booklist, American Library Association, Feb '00

"A valuable addition to all libraries specializing in health services and many public libraries."
— American Reference Books Annual, 2000

■

Physical & Mental Issues in Aging Sourcebook

Basic Consumer Health Information on Physical and Mental Disorders Associated with the Aging Process, Including Concerns about Cardiovascular Disease, Pulmonary Disease, Oral Health, Digestive Disorders, Musculoskeletal and Skin Disorders, Metabolic Changes, Sexual and Reproductive Issues, and Changes in Vision, Hearing, and Other Senses

Along with Data about Longevity and Causes of Death, Information on Acute and Chronic Pain, Descriptions of Mental Concerns, a Glossary of Terms, and Resource Listings for Additional Help

Edited by Jenifer Swanson. 660 pages. 1999. 0-7808-0233-0. $78.

"This is a treasure of health information for the layperson." — *Choice Health Sciences Supplement, Association of College & Research Libraries, May 2000*

"Recommended for public libraries."
—*American Reference Books Annual, 2000*

"Recommended reference source."
— *Booklist, American Library Association, Oct '99*

SEE ALSO *Healthy Aging Sourcebook*

Podiatry Sourcebook

Basic Consumer Health Information about Foot Conditions, Diseases, and Injuries, Including Bunions, Corns, Calluses, Athlete's Foot, Plantar Warts, Hammertoes and Clawtoes, Clubfoot, Heel Pain, Gout, and More

Along with Facts about Foot Care, Disease Prevention, Foot Safety, Choosing a Foot Care Specialist, a Glossary of Terms, and Resource Listings for Additional Information

Edited by M. Lisa Weatherford. 380 pages. 2001. 0-7808-0215-2. $78.

"Recommended reference source."
— *Booklist, American Library Association, Feb '02*

"There is a lot of information presented here on a topic that is usually only covered sparingly in most larger comprehensive medical encyclopedias."
— *American Reference Books Annual 2002*

Pregnancy & Birth Sourcebook, 2nd Edition

Basic Consumer Health Information about Conception and Pregnancy, Including Facts about Fertility, Infertility, Pregnancy Symptoms and Complications, Fetal Growth and Development, Labor, Delivery, and the Postpartum Period, as Well as Information about Maintaining Health and Wellness during Pregnancy and Caring for a Newborn

Along with Information about Public Health Assistance for Low-Income Pregnant Women, a Glossary, and Directories of Agencies and Organizations Providing Help and Support

Edited by Amy L. Sutton. 626 pages. 2004. 0-7808-0672-7. $78.

ALSO AVAILABLE: *Pregnancy & Birth Sourcebook, 1st Edition.* Edited by Heather E. Aldred. 737 pages. 1997. 0-7808-0216-0. $78.

"A well-organized handbook. Recommended."
— *Choice, Association of College and Research Libraries, Apr '98*

"Recommended reference source."
— *Booklist, American Library Association, Mar '98*

"Recommended for public libraries."
— *American Reference Books Annual, 1998*

SEE ALSO *Congenital Disorders Sourcebook, Family Planning Sourcebook*

Prostate Cancer Sourcebook

Basic Consumer Health Information about Prostate Cancer, Including Information about the Associated Risk Factors, Detection, Diagnosis, and Treatment of Prostate Cancer

Along with Information on Non-Malignant Prostate Conditions, and Featuring a Section Listing Support and Treatment Centers and a Glossary of Related Terms

Edited by Dawn D. Matthews. 358 pages. 2001. 0-7808-0324-8. $78.

"Recommended reference source."
— *Booklist, American Library Association, Jan '02*

"A valuable resource for health care consumers seeking information on the subject. . . . All text is written in a clear, easy-to-understand language that avoids technical jargon. Any library that collects consumer health resources would strengthen their collection with the addition of the *Prostate Cancer Sourcebook*."
— *American Reference Books Annual 2002*

Public Health Sourcebook

Basic Information about Government Health Agencies, Including National Health Statistics and Trends, Healthy People 2000 Program Goals and Objectives, the Centers for Disease Control and Prevention, the Food and Drug Administration, and the National Institutes of Health

Along with Full Contact Information for Each Agency

Edited by Wendy Wilcox. 698 pages. 1998. 0-7808-0220-9. $78.

"Recommended reference source."
— *Booklist, American Library Association, Sep '98*

"This consumer guide provides welcome assistance in navigating the maze of federal health agencies and their data on public health concerns."
— *SciTech Book News, Sep '98*

Reconstructive & Cosmetic Surgery Sourcebook

Basic Consumer Health Information on Cosmetic and Reconstructive Plastic Surgery, Including Statistical Information about Different Surgical Procedures, Things to Consider Prior to Surgery, Plastic Surgery Techniques and Tools, Emotional and Psychological Considerations, and Procedure-Specific Information

Along with a Glossary of Terms and a Listing of Resources for Additional Help and Information

Edited by M. Lisa Weatherford. 374 pages. 2001. 0-7808-0214-4. $78.

"An excellent reference that addresses cosmetic and medically necessary reconstructive surgeries. . . . The

style of the prose is calm and reassuring, discussing the many positive outcomes now available due to advances in surgical techniques."
— *American Reference Books Annual 2002*

"Recommended for health science libraries that are open to the public, as well as hospital libraries that are open to the patients. This book is a good resource for the consumer interested in plastic surgery."
— *E-Streams, Dec '01*

"Recommended reference source."
— *Booklist, American Library Association, July '01*

■

Rehabilitation Sourcebook

Basic Consumer Health Information about Rehabilitation for People Recovering from Heart Surgery, Spinal Cord Injury, Stroke, Orthopedic Impairments, Amputation, Pulmonary Impairments, Traumatic Injury, and More, Including Physical Therapy, Occupational Therapy, Speech/ Language Therapy, Massage Therapy, Dance Therapy, Art Therapy, and Recreational Therapy

Along with Information on Assistive and Adaptive Devices, a Glossary, and Resources for Additional Help and Information

Edited by Dawn D. Matthews. 531 pages. 1999. 0-7808-0236-5. $78.

"This is an excellent resource for public library reference and health collections."
— *American Reference Books Annual, 2001*

"Recommended reference source."
— *Booklist, American Library Association, May '00*

■

Respiratory Diseases & Disorders Sourcebook

Basic Information about Respiratory Diseases and Disorders, Including Asthma, Cystic Fibrosis, Pneumonia, the Common Cold, Influenza, and Others, Featuring Facts about the Respiratory System, Statistical and Demographic Data, Treatments, Self-Help Management Suggestions, and Current Research Initiatives

Edited by Allan R. Cook and Peter D. Dresser. 771 pages. 1995. 0-7808-0037-0. $78.

"Designed for the layperson and for patients and their families coping with respiratory illness. . . . an extensive array of information on diagnosis, treatment, management, and prevention of respiratory illnesses for the general reader." — *Choice, Association of College and Research Libraries, Jun '96*

"A highly recommended text for all collections. It is a comforting reminder of the power of knowledge that good books carry between their covers."
— *Academic Library Book Review, Spring '96*

"A comprehensive collection of authoritative information presented in a nontechnical, humanitarian style for patients, families, and caregivers." — *Association of Operating Room Nurses, Sep/Oct '95*

SEE ALSO Lung Disorders Sourcebook

Sexually Transmitted Diseases Sourcebook, 2nd Edition

Basic Consumer Health Information about Sexually Transmitted Diseases, Including Information on the Diagnosis and Treatment of Chlamydia, Gonorrhea, Hepatitis, Herpes, HIV, Mononucleosis, Syphilis, and Others

Along with Information on Prevention, Such as Condom Use, Vaccines, and STD Education; And Featuring a Section on Issues Related to Youth and Adolescents, a Glossary, and Resources for Additional Help and Information

Edited by Dawn D. Matthews. 538 pages. 2001. 0-7808-0249-7. $78.

ALSO AVAILABLE: Sexually Transmitted Diseases Sourcebook, 1st Edition. Edited by Linda M. Ross. 550 pages. 1997. 0-7808-0217-9. $78.

"Recommended for consumer health collections in public libraries, and secondary school and community college libraries."
— *American Reference Books Annual 2002*

"Every school and public library should have a copy of this comprehensive and user-friendly reference book."
— *Choice, Association of College & Research Libraries, Sep '01*

"This is a highly recommended book. This is an especially important book for all school and public libraries." — *AIDS Book Review Journal, Jul-Aug '01*

"Recommended reference source."
— *Booklist, American Library Association, Apr '01*

"Recommended pick both for specialty health library collections and any general consumer health reference collection." — *The Bookwatch, Apr '01*

■

Skin Disorders Sourcebook

Basic Information about Common Skin and Scalp Conditions Caused by Aging, Allergies, Immune Reactions, Sun Exposure, Infectious Organisms, Parasites, Cosmetics, and Skin Traumas, Including Abrasions, Cuts, and Pressure Sores

Along with Information on Prevention and Treatment

Edited by Allan R. Cook. 647 pages. 1997. 0-7808-0080-X. $78.

". . . comprehensive, easily read reference book."
— *Doody's Health Sciences Book Reviews, Oct '97*

SEE ALSO Burns Sourcebook

■

Sleep Disorders Sourcebook

Basic Consumer Health Information about Sleep and Its Disorders, Including Insomnia, Sleepwalking, Sleep Apnea, Restless Leg Syndrome, and Narcolepsy

Along with Data about Shiftwork and Its Effects, Information on the Societal Costs of Sleep Deprivation, Descriptions of Treatment Options, a Glossary of Terms, and Resource Listings for Additional Help

Edited by Jenifer Swanson. 439 pages. 1998. 0-7808-0234-9. $78.

"This text will complement any home or medical library. It is user-friendly and ideal for the adult reader."
— *American Reference Books Annual, 2000*

"A useful resource that provides accurate, relevant, and accessible information on sleep to the general public. Health care providers who deal with sleep disorders patients may also find it helpful in being prepared to answer some of the questions patients ask."
— *Respiratory Care, Jul '99*

"Recommended reference source."
— *Booklist, American Library Association, Feb '99*

■

Smoking Concerns Sourcebook

Basic Consumer Health Information about Nicotine Addiction and Smoking Cessation, Featuring Facts about the Health Effects of Tobacco Use, Including Lung and Other Cancers, Heart Disease, Stroke, and Respiratory Disorders, Such as Emphysema and Chronic Bronchitis

Along with Information about Smoking Prevention Programs, Suggestions for Achieving and Maintaining a Smoke-Free Lifestyle, Statistics about Tobacco Use, Reports on Current Research Initiatives, a Glossary of Related Terms, and Directories of Resources for Additional Help and Information

Edited by Karen Bellenir. 625 pages. 2004. 0-7808-0323-X. $78.

■

Sports Injuries Sourcebook, 2nd Edition

Basic Consumer Health Information about the Diagnosis, Treatment, and Rehabilitation of Common Sports-Related Injuries in Children and Adults

Along with Suggestions for Conditioning and Training, Information and Prevention Tips for Injuries Frequently Associated with Specific Sports and Special Populations, a Glossary, and a Directory of Additional Resources

Edited by Joyce Brennfleck Shannon. 614 pages. 2002. 0-7808-0604-2. $78.

ALSO AVAILABLE: Sports Injuries Sourcebook, 1st Edition. Edited by Heather E. Aldred. 624 pages. 1999. 0-7808-0218-7. $78.

"This is an excellent reference for consumers and it is recommended for public, community college, and undergraduate libraries."
— *American Reference Books Annual, 2003*

"Recommended reference source."
— *Booklist, American Library Association, Feb '03*

Stress-Related Disorders Sourcebook

Basic Consumer Health Information about Stress and Stress-Related Disorders, Including Stress Origins and Signals, Environmental Stress at Work and Home, Mental and Emotional Stress Associated with Depression, Post-Traumatic Stress Disorder, Panic Disorder, Suicide, and the Physical Effects of Stress on the Cardiovascular, Immune, and Nervous Systems

Along with Stress Management Techniques, a Glossary, and a Listing of Additional Resources

Edited by Joyce Brennfleck Shannon. 610 pages. 2002. 0-7808-0560-7. $78.

"Well written for a general readership, the *Stress-Related Disorders Sourcebook* is a useful addition to the health reference literature."
— *American Reference Books Annual, 2003*

"I am impressed by the amount of information. It offers a thorough overview of the causes and consequences of stress for the layperson. . . . A well-done and thorough reference guide for professionals and nonprofessionals alike."
— *Doody's Review Service, Dec '02*

■

Stroke Sourcebook

Basic Consumer Health Information about Stroke, Including Ischemic, Hemorrhagic, Transient Ischemic Attack (TIA), and Pediatric Stroke, Stroke Triggers and Risks, Diagnostic Tests, Treatments, and Rehabilitation Information

Along with Stroke Prevention Guidelines, Legal and Financial Information, a Glossary, and a Directory of Additional Resources

Edited by Joyce Brennfleck Shannon. 606 pages. 2003. 0-7808-0630-1. $78.

"This volume is highly recommended and should be in every medical, hospital, and public library."
— *American Reference Books Annual, 2004*

■

Substance Abuse Sourcebook

Basic Health-Related Information about the Abuse of Legal and Illegal Substances Such as Alcohol, Tobacco, Prescription Drugs, Marijuana, Cocaine, and Heroin; and Including Facts about Substance Abuse Prevention Strategies, Intervention Methods, Treatment and Recovery Programs, and a Section Addressing the Special Problems Related to Substance Abuse during Pregnancy

Edited by Karen Bellenir. 573 pages. 1996. 0-7808-0038-9. $78.

"A valuable addition to any health reference section. Highly recommended."
— *The Book Report, Mar/Apr '97*

". . . a comprehensive collection of substance abuse information that's both highly readable and compact. Families and caregivers of substance abusers will find

the information enlightening and helpful, while teachers, social workers and journalists should benefit from the concise format. Recommended."
— *Drug Abuse Update, Winter '96/'97*

SEE ALSO *Alcoholism Sourcebook, Drug Abuse Sourcebook*

■

Surgery Sourcebook

Basic Consumer Health Information about Inpatient and Outpatient Surgeries, Including Cardiac, Vascular, Orthopedic, Ocular, Reconstructive, Cosmetic, Gynecologic, and Ear, Nose, and Throat Procedures and More

Along with Information about Operating Room Policies and Instruments, Laser Surgery Techniques, Hospital Errors, Statistical Data, a Glossary, and Listings of Sources for Further Help and Information

Edited by Annemarie S. Muth and Karen Bellenir. 596 pages. 2002. 0-7808-0380-9. $78.

"Large public libraries and medical libraries would benefit from this material in their reference collections."
— *American Reference Books Annual, 2004*

"Invaluable reference for public and school library collections alike." — *Library Bookwatch, Apr '03*

■

Transplantation Sourcebook

Basic Consumer Health Information about Organ and Tissue Transplantation, Including Physical and Financial Preparations, Procedures and Issues Relating to Specific Solid Organ and Tissue Transplants, Rehabilitation, Pediatric Transplant Information, the Future of Transplantation, and Organ and Tissue Donation

Along with a Glossary and Listings of Additional Resources

Edited by Joyce Brennfleck Shannon. 628 pages. 2002. 0-7808-0322-1. $78.

"Along with these advances [in transplantation technology] have come a number of daunting questions for potential transplant patients, their families, and their health care providers. This reference text is the best single tool to address many of these questions. . . . It will be a much-needed addition to the reference collections in health care, academic, and large public libraries."
— *American Reference Books Annual, 2003*

"Recommended for libraries with an interest in offering consumer health information." — *E-Streams, Jul '02*

"This is a unique and valuable resource for patients facing transplantation and their families."
— *Doody's Review Service, Jun '02*

■

Traveler's Health Sourcebook

Basic Consumer Health Information for Travelers, Including Physical and Medical Preparations, Transportation Health and Safety, Essential Information about Food and Water, Sun Exposure, Insect and Snake Bites, Camping and Wilderness Medicine, and Travel with Physical or Medical Disabilities

Along with International Travel Tips, Vaccination Recommendations, Geographical Health Issues, Disease Risks, a Glossary, and a Listing of Additional Resources

Edited by Joyce Brennfleck Shannon. 613 pages. 2000. 0-7808-0384-1. $78.

"Recommended reference source."
— *Booklist, American Library Association, Feb '01*

"This book is recommended for any public library, any travel collection, and especially any collection for the physically disabled."
— *American Reference Books Annual, 2001*

■

Vegetarian Sourcebook

Basic Consumer Health Information about Vegetarian Diets, Lifestyle, and Philosophy, Including Definitions of Vegetarianism and Veganism, Tips about Adopting Vegetarianism, Creating a Vegetarian Pantry, and Meeting Nutritional Needs of Vegetarians, with Facts Regarding Vegetarianism's Effect on Pregnant and Lactating Women, Children, Athletes, and Senior Citizens

Along with a Glossary of Commonly Used Vegetarian Terms and Resources for Additional Help and Information

Edited by Chad T. Kimball. 360 pages. 2002. 0-7808-0439-2. $78.

"Organizes into one concise volume the answers to the most common questions concerning vegetarian diets and lifestyles. This title is recommended for public and secondary school libraries." — *E-Streams, Apr '03*

"Invaluable reference for public and school library collections alike." — *Library Bookwatch, Apr '03*

"The articles in this volume are easy to read and come from authoritative sources. The book does not necessarily support the vegetarian diet but instead provides the pros and cons of this important decision. The *Vegetarian Sourcebook* is recommended for public libraries and consumer health libraries."
— *American Reference Books Annual, 2003*

■

Women's Health Concerns Sourcebook, 2nd Edition

Basic Consumer Health Information about the Medical and Mental Concerns of Women, Including Maintaining Health and Wellness, Gynecological Concerns, Breast Health, Sexuality and Reproductive Issues, Menopause, Cancer in Women, the Leading Causes of Death and Disability among Women, Physical Concerns of Special Significance to Women, and Women's Mental and Emotional Health

Along with a Glossary of Related Terms and Directories of Resources for Additional Help and Information

Edited by Amy L. Sutton. 748 pages. 2004. 0-7808-0673-5. $78.

ALSO AVAILABLE: *Women's Health Concerns Sourcebook, 1st Edition.* Edited by Heather E. Aldred. 567 pages. 1997. 0-7808-0219-5. $78.

"Handy compilation. There is an impressive range of diseases, devices, disorders, procedures, and other physical and emotional issues covered . . . well organized, illustrated, and indexed." — Choice, Association of College and Research Libraries, Jan '98

SEE ALSO Breast Cancer Sourcebook, Cancer Sourcebook for Women, Healthy Heart Sourcebook for Women, Osteoporosis Sourcebook

Workplace Health & Safety Sourcebook

Basic Consumer Health Information about Workplace Health and Safety, Including the Effect of Workplace Hazards on the Lungs, Skin, Heart, Ears, Eyes, Brain, Reproductive Organs, Musculoskeletal System, and Other Organs and Body Parts

Along with Information about Occupational Cancer, Personal Protective Equipment, Toxic and Hazardous Chemicals, Child Labor, Stress, and Workplace Violence

Edited by Chad T. Kimball. 626 pages. 2000. 0-7808-0231-4. $78.

"As a reference for the general public, this would be useful in any library." E Streams, Jun '01

"Provides helpful information for primary care physicians and other caregivers interested in occupational medicine. . . . General readers; professionals." — Choice, Association of College & Research Libraries, May '01

"Recommended reference source." — Booklist, American Library Association, Feb '01

"Highly recommended." — The Bookwatch, Jan '01

Worldwide Health Sourcebook

Basic Information about Global Health Issues, Including Malnutrition, Reproductive Health, Disease Dispersion and Prevention, Emerging Diseases, Risky Health Behaviors, and the Leading Causes of Death

Along with Global Health Concerns for Children, Women, and the Elderly, Mental Health Issues, Research and Technology Advancements, and Economic, Environmental, and Political Health Implications, a Glossary, and a Resource Listing for Additional Help and Information

Edited by Joyce Brennfleck Shannon. 614 pages. 2001. 0-7808-0330-2. $78.

"Named an Outstanding Academic Title." —Choice, Association of College & Research Libraries, Jan '02

"Yet another handy but also unique compilation in the extensive Health Reference Series, this is a useful work because many of the international publications reprinted or excerpted are not readily available. Highly recommended." —Choice, Association of College & Research Libraries, Nov '01

"Recommended reference source." —Booklist, American Library Association, Oct '01

Teen Health Series

Helping Young Adults Understand, Manage, and Avoid Serious Illness

Cancer Information for Teens

Health Tips about Cancer Awareness, Prevention, Diagnosis, and Treatment

Including Facts about Frequently Occurring Cancers, Cancer Risk Factors, and Coping Strategies for Teens Fighting Cancer or Dealing with Cancer in Friends or Family Members

Edited by Wilma R. Caldwell. 428 pages. 2004. 0-7808-0678-6. $58.

Diet Information for Teens

Health Tips about Diet and Nutrition

Including Facts about Nutrients, Dietary Guidelines, Breakfasts, School Lunches, Snacks, Party Food, Weight Control, Eating Disorders, and More

Edited by Karen Bellenir. 399 pages. 2001. 0-7808-0441-4. $58.

"Full of helpful insights and facts throughout the book. . . . An excellent resource to be placed in public libraries or even in personal collections."
—*American Reference Books Annual 2002*

"Recommended for middle and high school libraries and media centers as well as academic libraries that educate future teachers of teenagers. It is also a suitable addition to health science libraries that serve patrons who are interested in teen health promotion and education." —*E-Streams, Oct '01*

"This comprehensive book would be beneficial to collections that need information about nutrition, dietary guidelines, meal planning, and weight control. . . . This reference is so easy to use that its purchase is recommended." —*The Book Report, Sep-Oct '01*

"This book is written in an easy to understand format describing issues that many teens face every day, and then provides thoughtful explanations so that teens can make informed decisions. This is an interesting book that provides important facts and information for today's teens." —*Doody's Health Sciences Book Review Journal, Jul-Aug '01*

"A comprehensive compendium of diet and nutrition. The information is presented in a straightforward, plain-spoken manner. This title will be useful to those working on reports on a variety of topics, as well as to general readers concerned about their dietary health." —*School Library Journal, Jun '01*

Drug Information for Teens

Health Tips about the Physical and Mental Effects of Substance Abuse

Including Facts about Alcohol, Anabolic Steroids, Club Drugs, Cocaine, Depressants, Hallucinogens, Herbal Products, Inhalants, Marijuana, Narcotics, Stimulants, Tobacco, and More

Edited by Karen Bellenir. 452 pages. 2002. 0-7808-0444-9. $58.

"A clearly written resource for general readers and researchers alike." —*School Library Journal*

"The chapters are quick to make a connection to their teenage reading audience. The prose is straightforward and the book lends itself to spot reading. It should be useful both for practical information and for research, and it is suitable for public and school libraries." —*American Reference Books Annual, 2003*

"Recommended reference source." —*Booklist, American Library Association, Feb '03*

"This is an excellent resource for teens and their parents. Education about drugs and substances is key to discouraging teen drug abuse and this book provides this much needed information in a way that is interesting and factual." —*Doody's Review Service, Dec '02*

Fitness Information for Teens

Health Tips about Exercise, Physical Well-Being, and Health Maintenance

Including Facts about Aerobic and Anaerobic Conditioning, Stretching, Body Shape and Body Image, Sports Training, Nutrition, and Activities for Non-Athletes

Edited by Karen Bellenir. 425 pages. 2004. 0-7808-0679-4. $58.

Mental Health Information for Teens

Health Tips about Mental Health and Mental Illness

Including Facts about Anxiety, Depression, Suicide, Eating Disorders, Obsessive-Compulsive Disorders, Panic Attacks, Phobias, Schizophrenia, and More

Edited by Karen Bellenir. 406 pages. 2001. 0-7808-0442-2. $58.

"In both language and approach, this user-friendly entry in the *Teen Health Series* is on target for teens needing information on mental health concerns." —*Booklist, American Library Association, Jan '02*

"Readers will find the material accessible and informative, with the shaded notes, facts, and embedded glossary insets adding appropriately to the already interesting and succinct presentation."
—*School Library Journal, Jan '02*

"This title is highly recommended for any library that serves adolescents and parents/caregivers of adolescents."
—*E-Streams, Jan '02*

"Recommended for high school libraries and young adult collections in public libraries. Both health professionals and teenagers will find this book useful."
—*American Reference Books Annual 2002*

"This is a nice book written to enlighten the society, primarily teenagers, about common teen mental health issues. It is highly recommended to teachers and parents as well as adolescents."
—*Doody's Review Service, Dec '01*

■

Sexual Health Information for Teens
Health Tips about Sexual Development, Human Reproduction, and Sexually Transmitted Diseases

Including Facts about Puberty, Reproductive Health, Chlamydia, Human Papillomavirus, Pelvic Inflammatory Disease, Herpes, AIDS, Contraception, Pregnancy, and More

Edited by Deborah A. Stanley. 391 pages. 2003. 0-7808-0445-7. $58.

"This work should be included in all high school libraries and many larger public libraries. . . . highly recommended."
—*American Reference Books Annual 2004*

"Sexual Health approaches its subject with appropriate seriousness and offers easily accessible advice and information."
—*School Library Journal, Feb. 2004*

Skin Health Information For Teens
Health Tips about Dermatological Concerns and Skin Cancer Risks

Including Facts about Acne, Warts, Hives, and Other Conditions and Lifestyle Choices, Such as Tanning, Tattooing, and Piercing, That Affect the Skin, Nails, Scalp, and Hair

Edited by Robert Aquinas McNally. 430 pages. 2003. 0-7808-0446-5. $58.

"This volume, as with others in the series, will be a useful addition to school and public library collections."
—*American Reference Books Annual 2004*

"This volume serves as a one-stop source and should be a necessity for any health collection."
—*Library Media Connection*

■

Sports Injuries Information For Teens
Health Tips about Sports Injuries and Injury Protection

Including Facts about Specific Injuries, Emergency Treatment, Rehabilitation, Sports Safety, Competition Stress, Fitness, Sports Nutrition, Steroid Risks, and More

Edited by Joyce Brennfleck Shannon. 425 pages. 2003. 0-7808-0447-3. $58.

"This work will be useful in the young adult collections of public libraries as well as high school libraries."
—*American Reference Books Annual 2004*

Health Re<del>ference Series</del>

Adolescent Health Sourcebook

AIDS Sourcebook, 3rd Edition

Alcoholism Sourcebook

Allergies Sourcebook, 2nd Edition

Alternative Medicine Sourcebook,
2nd Edition

Alzheimer's Disease Sourcebook,
3rd Edition

Arthritis Sourcebook

Asthma Sourcebook

Attention Deficit Disorder Sourcebook

Back & Neck Disorders Sourcebook

Blood & Circulatory Disorders
Sourcebook

Brain Disorders Sourcebook

Breast Cancer Sourcebook

Breastfeeding Sourcebook

Burns Sourcebook

Cancer Sourcebook, 4th Edition

Cancer Sourcebook for Women,
2nd Edition

Caregiving Sourcebook

Child Abuse Sourcebook

Childhood Diseases & Disorders
Sourcebook

Colds, Flu & Other Common Ailments
Sourcebook

Communication Disorders
Sourcebook

Congenital Disorders Sourcebook

Consumer Issues in Health Care
Sourcebook

Contagious & Non-Contagious
Infectious Diseases Sourcebook

Death & Dying Sourcebook

Dental Care & Oral Health Sourcebook,
2nd Edition

Depression Sourcebook

2nd Edition

Digestive Diseases & Disorder
Sourcebook

Disabilities Sourcebook

Domestic Violence Sourcebook,
2nd Edition

Drug Abuse Sourcebook

Ear, Nose & Throat Disorders
Sourcebook

Eating Disorders Sourcebook

Emergency Medical Services
Sourcebook

Endocrine & Metabolic Disorders
Sourcebook

Environmentally Health Sourcebook,
2nd Edition

Ethnic Diseases Sourcebook

Eye Care Sourcebook, 2nd Edition

Family Planning Sourcebook

Fitness & Exercise Sourcebook,
2nd Edition

Food & Animal Borne Diseases
Sourcebook

Food Safety Sourcebook

Forensic Medicine Sourcebook

Gastrointestinal Diseases & Disorders
Sourcebook

Genetic Disorders Sourcebook,
2nd Edition

Head Trauma Sourcebook

Headache Sourcebook

Health Insurance Sourcebook

Health Reference Series Cumulative
Index 1999

Healthy Aging Sourcebook

Healthy Children Sourcebook